PROCEDURES
for the Primary Care Provider

PROCEDURES

for the Primary Care Provider

THIRD EDITION

Marilyn Winterton Edmunds, PhD, ANP/GNP, FAANP
Adjunct Faculty
Johns Hopkins University School of Nursing
Baltimore, Maryland
President, Nurse Practitioner Connections, Inc.
Ellicott City, Maryland

FOREWORDS BY

James F. Cawley, MPH, PA-C, DHL (Hon)
Professor of Physician Assistant Studies
School of Medicine and Health Sciences
Professor of Prevention and Community Health
Milken Institute School of Public Health
The George Washington University
Washington, DC

Janet S. Selway, DNSc, ANP-BC, CPNP-PC, FAANP
Director
Adult-Gerontology Nurse Practitioner Program
Assistant Professor
School of Nursing
The Catholic University of America
Washington, DC

ELSEVIER

ELSEVIER

3251 Riverport Lane
St. Louis, Missouri 63043

PROCEDURES FOR THE PRIMARY CARE PROVIDER,
THIRD EDITION

ISBN: 978-0-323-34003-8

Notices

Knowledge and best practice in this field are constantly changing. As new research and experience broaden our understanding, changes in research methods, professional practices, or medical treatment may become necessary.

Practitioners and researchers must always rely on their own experience and knowledge in evaluating and using any information, methods, compounds, or experiments described herein. In using such information or methods they should be mindful of their own safety and the safety of others, including parties for whom they have a professional responsibility.

With respect to any drug or pharmaceutical products identified, readers are advised to check the most current information provided (i) on procedures featured or (ii) by the manufacturer of each product to be administered, to verify the recommended dose or formula, the method and duration of administration, and contraindications. It is the responsibility of practitioners, relying on their own experience and knowledge of their patients, to make diagnoses, to determine dosages and the best treatment for each individual patient, and to take all appropriate safety precautions.

To the fullest extent of the law, neither the Publisher nor the authors, contributors, or editors, assume any liability for any injury and/or damage to persons or property as a matter of products liability, negligence or otherwise, or from any use or operation of any methods, products, instructions, or ideas contained in the material herein.

Library of Congress Cataloging-in-Publication Data

Procedures for primary care practitioners
Procedures for the primary care provider / [edited by] Marilyn Winterton Edmunds ; forewords by James F. Cawley, Janet S. Selway. — Third edition.
p. ; cm.
Preceded by Procedures for primary care practitioners / [edited by] Marilyn Winterton Edmunds, Maren Stewart Mayhew. 2nd ed. c2003.
Includes bibliographical references.
ISBN 978-0-323-34003-8 (alk. paper)
I. Edmunds, Marilyn W., editor. II. Title.
[DNLM: 1. Primary Nursing—methods—Handbooks. 2. Ambulatory Care—methods—Handbooks. 3. Nurse Practitioners—Handbooks. 4. Physician Assistants—Handbooks. 5. Primary Health Care—methods—Handbooks. WY 49]
R729
362.1—dc23

2015022064

Executive Content Strategist: Lee Henderson
Content Development Manager: Laurie Gower
Senior Content Development Specialist: Karen C. Turner
Publishing Services Manager: Jeffrey Patterson
Book Production Specialist: Carol O'Connell
Design Direction: Renée Duenow

Printed in India

Last digit is the print number: 9 8 7

Contributors

Tom Bartol, NP, APRN
Nurse Practitioner
Richmond Area Health Center
HealthReach Community Health Centers
Richmond, Maine

Kent D. Blad, DNP, FNP-c, ACNP-BC, FCCM, FAANP
Associate Dean, Teaching Professor
College of Nursing
Brigham Young University
Provo, Utah

Christy L. Crowther-Radulewicz, MS, CRNP
Nurse Practitioner
Orthopedic Surgery
Anne Arundel Orthopedic Surgeons
Annapolis, Maryland

Jan DiSantostefano, MS, FNP, WHNP
Nurse Practitioner
SAS Institute
Cary, North Carolina

Pegah C. Dixon Conk, MSN, APRN, WHNP-BC
Women's Health Nurse Practitioner
Intermountain Healthcare
Salt Lake City, Utah

Sabrina D. Jarvis, DNP, FNP-BC, ACNP-BC, FAANP
Associate Teaching Professor
College of Nursing
Brigham Young University
Provo, Utah

Joanne Rolls, MPAS, PA-C
Instructor (Clinical), Physician Assistant
Department of Family and Preventative Medicine
University of Utah School of Medicine
Salt Lake City, Utah

Jared Spackman, MPAS, PA-C
Association Program Director
Physician Assistant Program
University of Utah
Salt Lake City, Utah

Reviewers

Sameeya Ahmed-Winston, CPNP, CPHON, BMTCN
Pediatric Nurse Practitioner
Children's National Medical Center
Washington, DC

Katrina Allen-Thomas, RN, CCRN, MSN
Nursing Instructor
Faulkner State Community College
Bay Minette, Alabama

Jenny Bosley, RN, MS, CEN
Clinical Nurse Specialist
Department of Performance Improvement
Thomas Jefferson University Hospital
Philadelphia, Pennsylvania

Laura Crisanti, MSN, CCRN, CPNP-PC/AC
Pediatric Nurse Practitioner
Ann & Robert H. Lurie Children's Hospital of Chicago
Chicago, Illinois

Diane Daddario, MSN, ANP-C, ACNS-BC, RN-BC, CMSRN
Adjunct Faculty
Pennsylvania State University
University Park, Pennsylvania

Elizabeth L. Darling, MPAS, PA-C
Physician Assistant
Salt Lake City, Utah

Anna Dierenfeld, MSN, CPNP-PC
PICU Nurse Practitioner
Ann & Robert H. Lurie Children's Hospital of Chicago
Chicago, Illinois

Krista Estes, DNP, FNP-C
Assistant Professor
University of Colorado College of Nursing
Aurora, Colorado

Margie Francisco, EdD, MSN, RN
Nursing Professor
Illinois Valley Community College
Oglesby, Illinois

Kari Greenwood, RN (NP), BN, MN
Instructor
Faculty of Nursing
University of Regina
Regina, Saskatchewan

Jill Harpst-Rodgers, DNP, FNP-BC, MSN
Assistant Professor of Graduate Nursing
Carlow University
Pittsburgh, Pennsylvania

Mary Blaszko Helming, PhD, APRN, FNP-BC, AHN-BC
Professor of Nursing
School of Nursing
Quinnipiac University
Hamden, Connecticut

Kathleen S. Jordan, DNP, MS, FNP-BC, ENP-BC, SANE-P
Clinical Assistant Professor
UNC Charlotte, School of Nursing
Nurse Practitioner
Mid-Atlantic Emergency Medicine Associates
Charlotte, North Carolina

Tammie Kear, PhD, RN, CNS, CNN
Assistant Professor of Nursing
College of Nursing
Villanova University
Villanova, Pennsylvania

Andrea M. Kline-Tilford, MS, CPNP-AC/PC, FCCM
Pediatric Nurse Practitioner
Department of Cardiovascular Surgery
Children's Hospital of Michigan
Detroit, Michigan

Kari Ksar, RN, MS, CPNP
Pediatric Nurse Practitioner
Pediatric Gastroenterology, Hepatology and Nutrition
Lucile Packard Children's Hospital at Stanford
Palo Alto, California

Anna L. Petersen, MPAS, PA-C
Adjunct Faculty, Physician Assistant
Physician Assistant Program
University of Utah
Salt Lake City, Utah

Michael Sanchez, DNP, ARNP, FNP-B, AAHIVS
Nurse Practitioner
Camillus Health Concern
Miami, Florida

Diane Vail Skojec, DNP, MS, ANP-BC
Cardiac Surgery Nurse Practitioner
Johns Hopkins Hospital
Clinical Instructor
Johns Hopkins University School of Nursing
Baltimore, Maryland

Marcia Welsh, D Law, MSN, CNM
Associate Professor
West Chester University
West Chester, Pennsylvania

Susan Wilkinson, PhD, RN, CNS
Professor
Department of Nursing
Angelo State University
San Angelo, Texas

Foreword

In modern medicine in the United States, the capability to perform various types of medical procedures is a defining characteristic of health care providers. Procedures are often the major reason for an office-based medical encounter and this is particularly the case in primary care.

It was not so long ago when physicians were the only health care professionals authorized by law and training to perform specific diagnostic and therapeutic procedures. Today, with the spectacular growth and widespread acceptance of nurse practitioners and physician assistants, these health professionals have joined physicians in sharing a majority of tasks, duties, and procedures in clinical practice. The ability of nurse practitioners and physician assistants to master common, and often not-so-common, clinical procedures is related to the degree that these professionals ultimately become expert clinicians in their specific fields. Nurse practitioners and physician assistants have proven their capability to practice primary care medicine and to perform specific procedures at a level of quality and safety equivalent to physicians. In many instances, nurse practitioners have become autonomous providers of primary care for many rural and medically underserved communities. Proficiency in the performance of procedures also contributes to improvements in the delivery of quality health services to patients and makes these providers more marketable in the increasingly competitive workforce. Clearly, it is important for new graduates of both nurse practitioner and physician assistant programs to master both the theory of practice and the practical application of various clinical diagnostic and therapeutic procedures, and it is to this goal that this new edition is dedicated.

Because the performance of various clinical procedures is now part and parcel of the roles of nurse practitioners and physician assistants, particularly those in primary care practice, it is important for these providers to have a current and accurate source of information regarding the indications, limitations, and proper techniques for the performance of procedures. It is a reality that, for some nurse practitioner and physician assistant educational programs, there are increasing problems in terms of providing these types of experiences for students, yet at the same time, there is a growing need for the graduates to have these skills. It is this dilemma that led to the publication of the first edition of *Procedures for Primary Care Practitioners* and remains the intended goal for this updated and revised third edition.

A notable aspect of this book is that its intended audience is composed of students, new graduates, and established clinicians in both the nurse practitioner and physician assistant professions. Both professions typically focus their education and practice toward primary care, yet the number of books intended for both are precious few. Dr. Marilyn Edmunds, the author and editor of this book, is a leading educator, clinician, and researcher in the nurse practitioner profession. She is among the few national experts who possesses the depth and breadth of clinical educational and research experience and who has credibility in primary care practitioner fields to take on and successfully compile such a work. Edmunds has skillfully assembled a stellar cast of clinical experts drawn from both professions who have written clear and informative chapters that span the full range of important primary care clinical procedures. This new edition of *Procedures for Primary Care Practitioners* is a practical guide to more than 70 common procedures required in primary care clinical practice. Sections in this text include dermatology; ear, nose, and throat; respiratory; cardiovascular; gastrointestinal; orthopedic; genitourinary; women's health; men's health; and radiographic interpretation. Each section includes review of anatomy and physiology, pathophysiology, indications, precautions, assessment, patient preparation, equipment list, procedure, interpretation of results, patient education, follow-up, and current procedure technology billing information.

The author has delivered a new and updated version of a most valuable clinical reference that has proven its worth to thousands of clinicians, and is to be commended for continuing this most worthy text. This volume, in its new edition, provides both nurse practitioners and physician assistants with an authoritative reference for learning clinical procedures. This book meets the need for primary care providers to have a reference of timely and practical information for students and graduates to learn, perform, and ultimately master a variety of procedures necessary for clinicians to be fully effective in today's health care environment.

James F. Cawley, MPH, PA-C, DHL (Hon)
Professor of Physician Assistant Studies
School of Medicine and Health Sciences
Professor of Prevention and Community Health
Milken Institute School of Public Health
The George Washington University
Washington, DC

Foreword

Androcles and the lion is an ancient folktale that illustrates the value of a well-performed procedure. All versions of the fable describe Androcles as a humble man who stumbles into a cave where he discovers an unfortunate lion moaning in agony with a thorn embedded in a swollen paw. Knowing that he was in a rural health care professional shortage area, Androcles took immediate action. He adeptly pulled out the thorn and removed a large amount of pus, providing the poor lion immediate relief. Clearly Androcles was no stranger to the concept of patient-centered care. Despite the lack of clinical practice guidelines, proper equipment, or even rudimentary hand-washing facilities, Androcles achieved a successful patient outcome. The lion reported reduced pain and improved functional status, and there were no postoperative complications. The lion was especially happy that he did not have to wait for a specialist referral. Androcles' patient satisfaction scores soared. Even though there were no CPT codes in ancient times, Androcles, after many years, did receive adequate (although not monetary) compensation. As fate would have it, one day Androcles was forced into a gladiators' pit, only to find himself facing the same lion. Upon recognizing Androcles as an old friend, the lion's ferocity was quickly replaced with gratitude. Legend has it that Androcles and his lion entertained the emperor by engaging in a joyful reunion dance rather than bloody combat, sparing both of their lives.

Sparing oneself from a ferocious patient is, with hope, not the underlying motivation for the performance of procedures by the vast majority of primary care providers. There are many compelling reasons to consider that confer advantage. For example, quick relief, time and monetary savings, and increased patient satisfaction are highly important. Diagnostic procedures, such as obtaining a skin biopsy or aspirating joint fluid for analysis, often provide the advantage of quick results and improved diagnostic accuracy. Inadequate compensation for time spent, particularly for a provider who is overwhelmed in a busy practice, may be a disadvantage.

The Latin motto of my original basic nursing program was *age quod agis*—"Do well what you are doing." A hastily performed procedure by a provider who lacks a patient-centered perspective and knowledge and skill will certainly be a disadvantage for both the patient and provider. The patient's chances for a poor outcome or an unnecessary procedure will increase, as will the provider's medico-legal risk. A procedure that is performed in a thoughtful and accurate manner and with patient-centered actions and communication will mitigate this risk.

The term *procedure* is defined as "the mental and motor activities required to execute a manual task involving patient care."* When learning procedures, it is important to

* Wetmore S, Rivet C, Tepper J, et al: Defining core procedural skills for Canadian family medicine training, *Can Fam Physician* 51:1364-1365, 2005.

consider both domains. The primary care provider must understand the indications and the technologic performance aspects of the procedure. Taking the time to learn how to do the procedure correctly with the input and guidance of a capable preceptor or experienced provider is as important as learning the steps, indications, and appropriate tools. Proper patient follow up and taking measures to prevent complications are key to good outcomes and reduced medico-legal risk. The author and contributors of *Procedures for the Primary Care Provider,* 3rd edition, have created an outstanding work that covers a wealth of learning needs for all types of primary care providers. By enhancing the primary care provider's ability to perform procedures that are safe, technologically correct, and patient-centered, patients are well-served. The lion would agree.

Janet S. Selway, DNSc, ANP-BC, CPNP-PC, FAANP
Director
Adult-Gerontology Nurse Practitioner Program
Assistant Professor
School of Nursing
The Catholic University of America
Washington, DC

Preface

In the course of teaching nurse practitioners during the past 30 years, I have watched with interest the change in what primary care practitioners actually do when they assume clinical practice. Invariably, the reality of clinical practice is broader than what is taught in university programs. Even knowing that, academic curricula are frequently encumbered with bureaucracy and tradition and are often slow to change.

Primary care procedures are essential content that is difficult to teach in any formal program. There is wide diversity in the clinical sites used for student education, and there is substantial difficulty in providing clinical experiences for the broad numbers of procedures clinicians must master; however, many programs know that graduates will learn and master many procedures on the job and as dictated by the specific practice in which they work.

The first edition of this book was based on data from a research study of all nurse practitioners in Maryland comparing what procedures they were doing in their practices and what they had been taught to do in their educational programs. Because of the incongruence between these two sets of information, the book was developed to more adequately prepare students and new graduates for what they would face upon entering practice.

Over time, as the book became a standard in nurse practitioner programs, it became clear that physician assistants and medical students were also using the text. The commonalities that these providers share are ambulatory care practice and the need for basic information on procedures.

As this new edition is released, I want to emphasize again that this book is designed for the advanced practitioner. It presumes that the clinician already has substantial experience and education on which his or her practice is founded either in previous nursing, orderly, or medical assistant practice. As such, this book, with few exceptions, does not cover basic procedures, and we refer practitioners back to basic texts for those types of procedures.

This new edition is, again, built upon the procedures that clinicians are providing in their current practices and do not always correlate with what is taught in educational programs. Since publishing the first edition, many procedures, such as stress testing, have moved from primary care offices to specialty practice. This has required tailoring the current procedures included to the larger changes in primary care practice over time.

The procedures described in this text should serve as the core procedures all primary care clinicians should master. Some advanced procedures, particularly those requiring specific formal training or those completed in more specialty-oriented practices, are included in this text. These procedures are identified with the icon ■ to indicate that they are advanced techniques that may require special training.

A note about the references in this book: The procedure literature to date has been dominated by procedure articles and books developed for physicians. Many of the very best articles on some procedures were written many years ago and these articles still are the most precise in helping the novice clinician. Like almost every other procedure book on the market, we have retained some of these older references if they are still accessible; therefore older references do not mean that the book is outdated, but that these are still the best materials. Many times procedures really have not changed over time. Many of the newer references are to videos where we could find them available without charge to the viewer.

Although beginning medical students will find this text to be useful, it is not a book, in general, that is designed for the experienced or specialty physician. It is recognized that physicians' scope of practice often requires them to perform many acute care procedures in addition to the procedures listed in this book. There are a number of texts that clearly describe the additional in-patient procedures performed by physicians. This text remains focused on meeting the needs of those who are committed to working in primary care settings and are limited by law, opportunity, skill, or desire from performing many other procedures.

Although state practice acts may vary in which procedures nurse practitioners (NP) and physician assistants (PA) are legally allowed to perform, this text necessarily reflects the decisions of the editors about what practitioners are commonly allowed to perform. It does not, therefore, include what we believe most practitioners should not be doing in their primary care practices, although they may perform some of them in emergency departments or in specialty practices where they are employed. Not all practitioners will do all the procedures listed in this book, and there are some differences between what NPs and PAs do in their practices. The reader will note that there are some procedures that are noticeably absent. Specialized procedures that require specific training and certification, such as colposcopy and flexible sigmoidoscopy, have been omitted. We encourage practitioners to attend the educational courses designed to provide the didactic background and clinical supervision to prepare a practitioner in these procedures rather than to try to learn something out of a book. In addition, there are liability issues surrounding some procedures, including vasectomy, that preclude inclusion in a book of common procedures. This edition does include circumcision, which some PAs are now performing in primary care settings.

It is exciting to see the growth in the roles of primary care providers. With the implementation of the Affordable Care Act and the growing autonomy of clinicians in many states, we anticipate that there will be many more opportunities for changes in procedure patterns of all primary care providers. We desire all students, graduates, and experienced primary care practitioners to stay abreast of technologic changes, new information, guidelines, and legal issues that influence their ability to competently perform procedures as they care for today's patients.

Marilyn Winterton Edmunds, PhD, ANP/GNP, FAANP

Acknowledgments

I gratefully acknowledge the contributions of my patients and my students, who were really my *teachers*, and whose final examinations I ultimately had to pass as I worked in the "real world." I am particularly grateful to Maren Mayhew who assisted in the writing of the first two editions of this book.

For all of us who worked on this book, I also want to thank the staff at Elsevier, including Lee Henderson, Laurie Gower, Karen Turner, Jeff Patterson, Carol O'Connell, and Renée Duenow. In addition, we want to recognize the illustrators at Graphic World of St. Louis, Missouri, for their outstanding work.

I acknowledge the contributions of my former students and faculty colleagues who started me on this odyssey through their questions about these procedures. Their questions and ideas provided me with the impetus to revise and compile those procedures commonly performed by primary care nurse practitioners and physician assistants and to standardize the educational preparation of health care providers performing these procedures.

I would like to extend a special thank you to my husband and children for all their support and encouragement in this important revision. It sometimes takes a community to write a textbook also!

Contents

PROCEDURES
for the Primary Care Provider

1

Issues Related to Primary Care Procedures

Marilyn Winterton Edmunds

Reasons for Performing Clinical Procedures

Ambulatory care procedures are continuing to become an increasingly important skill for primary care practitioners (PCPs) to master. The ability to perform procedures has become essential in some clinical sites, especially in rural areas where specialists may not be available. Even when specialists are available, the advent of managed care may require the primary care professional to perform procedures that were once commonly referred to others, and some procedures that PCPs perform have now moved into more specialized settings. It is always a challenge for educators to know which procedures to emphasize in educational programs and even more difficult to predict which procedures students will actually have a chance to perform before they graduate.

The nonphysician primary care providers, particularly those who are now legally able to set up more independent practices, have financial incentives to learn to perform procedures. Their skills give them the ability to generate revenue that is commonly reimbursed at a high rate, making them more attractive to employers in the increasingly competitive employment environment or to surviving in their own practices. For practitioners who have been practicing for a number of years, the acquisition of new skills in the performance of procedures may allow them to begin to develop greater expertise or a specialty practice that rewards, challenges, and satisfies them. The ability to provide on-site total services for a patient is attractive to patients, providers, and insurers.

The Legal Environment

In hospitals, procedures are performed by practitioners who have met specific educational and practice requirements and are credentialed to perform those procedures. The standards of the Joint Committee on Accreditation of Healthcare Organizations (JCAHO) require a hospital credentialing committee to identify not only who can perform certain procedures but also what procedures cannot be performed.

Who is allowed to perform technical procedures in an office or ambulatory care clinic is less clearly controlled. State law, institutional policy, and the education and expertise of the practitioner are all factors that determine which procedures may be performed in a given setting. Common medical practice over the years has identified a core of office procedures that are usually performed in primary care settings and suggests those that require hospital inpatient, outpatient, or emergency department attention. However, the procedures that can be performed in an ambulatory care practice and the professionals who are allowed to perform them are commonly defined by state law, which may be very specific or very vague. These state definitions of the procedures practitioners are authorized to perform are often different for physicians, physician assistants, and nurse practitioners.

Even casual observation suggests that there is a set of procedures that are common in primary care practices, which may be categorized as *core office procedures.* These procedures make up the bulk of this book. Other office procedures may be performed in certain specialty practices or require specialized training and skill mastery before they can be performed. These procedures might be categorized as *advanced procedures.* Their very categorization implies that a more advanced or skilled practitioner should perform the procedures and that a beginner should not attempt them without taking additional specialized courses or training and without having adequate supervision and assistance until he or she has performed the procedures a number of times. There are several procedures in this book that fall into that category. The procedures identified as advanced are provided here to remind the novice clinician or the practitioner who does not have the opportunity to perform a particular procedure on a regular basis of the basic components of the procedure. The information provided is not a substitute for the more advanced courses that are required before the procedure is attempted.

There also are a variety of procedures that should not be performed in the primary care setting or should not be performed by persons who are not specialists. These are the procedures that require *referral.* Although a given primary care practitioner may acquire the skill to perform some of these procedures, as a general course, they are not attempted in the general setting by the general practitioner. This is especially true for nonphysician providers, for whom the legal authority to perform some procedures may be in a gray area. Therefore procedures such as colposcopy, cervical biopsy, vasectomy, and bone marrow aspiration are not included in this text, although some individuals may be performing them in primary care settings. The authority for some practitioners to perform some procedures will ultimately be more clearly defined through case law as litigation forces greater clarity of law over time.

Educational Preparation to Perform Procedures

Although many employers may see the services provided by physician assistants (PAs) and nurse practitioners (NPs) as interchangeable, they differ in many settings, particularly in regard to the procedures these professionals typically perform. PAs are hired because they are seen as very technically competent to perform a variety of procedures. NPs may or may not perform certain procedures in their practices or perform them as frequently as PAs, other than those related to women's health, because the primary role of NPs is often focused on educating and counseling the patient. These differences are reflected in hiring patterns based on the types of services the practice requires.

A recent study by Scheibmeir and colleagues in the *Journal for Nurse Practitioners* (2015) concerning the teaching of advanced diagnostic skills in 150 national NP and PA programs showed both similarities and differences between the two types of programs.

For example, many students enter NP programs after years of working as an RN and both seeing and performing a wide variety of procedures, whereas many students enter into PA programs without this medical background. Most NP programs require a significant amount of clinical experience before entering, but the type of experience can vary greatly, which may extend the amount of time required in certain curricular instruction.

Many core procedures are mastered by students as they progress through their basic educational programs. Some core content is usually taught in the health care curriculum, and students are expected to seize every opportunity to practice what they have learned in the clinical setting. Thus a good deal of what a student learns is dependent on fate, being determined by who walks in the door with a problem that requires a procedure when he or she happens to be on duty.

Faculty members stress the need for students to gain experience in clinical techniques, but they are powerless to guarantee that every student will have the opportunity to perform every procedure. Students therefore have to scout on their own for opportunities to perform procedures, and regardless of whether they are physicians, NPs, or PAs, many graduate without having performed or mastered the basic techniques for some procedures. On-the-job training is a reality for many new graduates; they are initially ill-prepared to carry out necessary procedures on patients who come to their office. How the necessary skills and expertise are developed is often left up to the practitioner. Their professional ethics should require them to obtain sufficient supervised experience before they attempt procedures on their own; however, this is often difficult in the busy primary care setting.

As graduates gain expertise and knowledge, and as technology changes over time, practitioners will have to learn to perform procedures to which they were not exposed during their educational programs or their initial years of practice. Continuing education for professionals is mandatory to stay abreast of new techniques. Many students and new graduates also rely on using smartphones and tablets to access online videos of procedures to remind them what they should do during a specific procedure.

A practitioner who performs a new procedure is often vulnerable to making mistakes or perhaps even to legal scrutiny or challenge of his or her work. One of the first things a practitioner must provide to an attorney in a lawsuit is the details of his or her basic professional education and training and the additional courses he or she has taken. One way of providing some proactive legal protection for new practitioners is to complete a certification checklist to document competency and training in the performance of each new procedure. An example of this checklist is given in Appendix A. The form is filled out as each new procedure is studied, practiced under supervision, and performed. These records are kept in a file or copies are sent to a state medical or nursing board or hospital accreditation committee, depending on the requirements within each state. Use of a format such as the one provided allows the practitioner to document growth in knowledge and skill far past his or her basic educational program.

Patient-Provider Relationships

Education of the patient both before and after the procedure is not just a legal requirement; it is good medicine. A cooperative relationship means that both the practitioner and the patient are working together for the best outcome. The "art" of providing health care is dominant here. The practitioner must explain enough about the risks and benefits of a procedure for the patient to provide true informed consent.

After the procedure, the patient may not be able to think clearly enough to understand the instructions he or she is given. Written instructions about what the patient should expect and when and how he or she should call the practitioner for help should always be provided.

Documentation of the preprocedural teaching and explanation and of the post-procedural instructions should always be included in the chart. The use of preprinted patient instructions for the follow-up of each type of procedure allows for standardized messages to always be conveyed to the patient.

Reimbursement

Procedures often provide a steady stream of revenue for a primary care practice. However, this is contingent on use of the proper codes to obtain reimbursement. Any practitioner who learns how to perform a procedure should also learn the appropriate billing codes and how to use them. Current procedural terminology (CPT) codes are listed in this book for most procedures, but which code should be used and what a given insurance company will reimburse are not standard.

Current Procedural Terminology: CPT Standard Edition by the American Medical Association (2015) is the source for the procedure code numbers. The codes are used as a uniform language to report medical services and procedures. They are also used as standard codes when billing for a procedure.

The American Medical Association does not decide what is a billable procedure. The Center for Medicare and Medicaid Service (CMS) decides what is considered a "billable procedure" for Medicare. Most insurance companies use Medicare as a guideline for what they consider a billable procedure and to determine how much they will reimburse. (See the CMS guidelines at www.cms.gov/Medicare/Coding/MedHCPCSGenInfo/index.html for up-to-date information.)

The billing codes are five-digit numbers, and there are modifiers that can be added to the code to more completely describe the service that was provided. For example, −50 is used for a bilateral procedure. The procedure code book is similar to the *International Classification of Diseases, Tenth Revision* (ICD-10) code book for diagnoses numbers.

Some procedures may not have CPT codes, and how standard office evaluation and management (E & M) codes are used to bill for a procedure performed during an office visit is often unclear. If a patient comes in for an office visit and has a new problem that requires a procedure, usual practice dictates that the practitioner bills for the procedure and does not bill for the office visit. (For example, if a patient comes in to have his or her blood pressure checked and, in the course of the examination, the practitioner discovers that the patient must have cerumen removed from his or her ears, the practitioner bills only for removal of the cerumen.) However, if the reimbursement for an office visit is higher than that for the procedure, some offices direct the practitioner to bill for the office visit. Other offices refuse to allow the practitioner to perform the procedure on that day and require the patient to return for another visit for the procedure. Thus practitioners must learn the policies of their offices.

Although Medicare policies should be standard throughout the United States, Medicare carriers vary from state to state on the codes for which they will reimburse.

Providers discover that they perform many procedures for which Medicare will not reimburse them, even though some have procedure codes. For some of these time-consuming and seemingly nonreimbursable procedures, it is better to fully document the E & M services and to code appropriately with the usual billing codes for an office visit. The E & M billing code should reflect the difficulty of the medical decision-making process and the time spent with the patient, including the reason the procedure was necessary. Prolonged E & M service is noted with the modifier −21. (It is beyond the scope of this book to fully discuss E & M billing codes; these codes are available at www.cms.gov/Outreach-and-Education/Medicare-Learning-Network-MLN/MLNProducts/Downloads/eval_mgmt_serv_guide-ICN006764.pdf.)

Billing guidelines are constantly changing. Medicare may put out new regulations, which changes codes and what is reimbursable and for how much. There also is wide variation in how the different state Medicare carriers interpret CMS regulations regarding for what and who is to be reimbursed. Increasingly CMS is covering the services provided by PAs and NPs. The utilization of electronic health records (EHR) and electronic billing will also standardize coding. Currently, most EMR systems automatically add a CPT code after a procedure is documented.

There are legal and financial consequences for the provider in submission of the claim. Ultimately, it is the health care provider who is responsible for accurate billing for the procedures performed, not the billing or office personnel. Reimbursement regulations require the health care provider to know the regulations involved in obtaining reimbursement and to follow them. Lack of knowledge of the regulations does not excuse the practitioner from legal liability. It is mandatory that each practitioner closely monitor the billing for all procedures he or she performs and ensure accuracy to avoid possible charges of fraud and abuse. Most PA program faculty and a growing number of NP program faculty are spending considerable time with students learning and practicing appropriate coding. Providers in most primary care practices are responsible for listing the correct billing code on patient encounter forms and also following up to confirm what code was used in the billing. Every provider should have a record of the services he or she has provided during the year, what was billing, and what was received. This helps ensure the provider has accurate financial information about revenue generation and his or her contributions to a practice.

Procedures Requiring Life-Span Modifications

There is a common format in performing a procedure, but some modifications are essential for pediatric patients. These changes commonly call for alternatives in the medications or dosages that are used, the positioning or restraint of patients, or protection for the site after the procedure is performed.

Many of these same factors apply for older or confused patients. It is especially important to keep track of the amount of anesthetic agent used in a procedure to avoid toxic reactions.

Few modifications are usually required for a pregnant woman or lactating mother. However, it is prudent for the practitioner to ask any woman of childbearing age about the possibility of pregnancy or whether she is breastfeeding so that any needed changes can be made in the anesthetic agent or antibiotic that is used.

Pediatric Considerations

One truism of health care is that children are not merely little adults. They present a special challenge in the performance of both diagnostic and therapeutic procedures. Depending on the age of a child, his or her behavior during any given procedure can range from frightened to ornery to docile to asleep. Even the youngest child deserves to have any questions answered and, if possible, any fears allayed.

A comforted and cooperative child is the key to success with any procedure. Parents should be used to the greatest extent possible. Many procedures can be safely performed with a young child seated in the mother's lap. In some situations, parents may be able to restrain a child safely and eliminate the need for frightening restraints, such as papoose boards. However, the decision must be an individual one. If the parent is unduly frightened or worried about holding the child, it is always wise to err on the side of safety and to use the appropriate restraint. In extreme situations where a child is exceptionally frightened and is unable to be easily restrained, the child may need to be referred to an emergency department for sedation before the procedure. Otherwise, there is increased risk of injury, such as a needlestick puncture, to the child, parent, clinician, and staff.

With the use of age-appropriate language, a procedure should always be explained to the child in advance. Young children who do not understand language can be familiarized with equipment through handling. It may be possible to perform a mock procedure on the child.

Procedures that involve a developing system, such as the eye, deserve special note. The goal in the care of a child is not preservation of an existing sensory system but optimal development. Special care must always be taken to ensure that damage to an organ will not affect development. Any procedure that involves the eye must be preceded by and followed by a visual acuity examination. Injuries that involve growth plates warrant meticulous evaluation and close follow-up. Always remember that development is symmetric in the young child. Vision, hearing, muscle mass, and strength should be compared on a side-by-side basis, and differences should trigger a more thorough evaluation and, often, a referral to a subspecialist.

A final note should be made about pain management. Any practicing pediatric health professional is familiar with situations in which children are presumed to not experience pain and as a result are not provided with appropriate analgesia. Many a child has been sent home after casting of a fracture with acetaminophen as the only pain medication. In the adult population, it is well recognized that anxiety compounds pain. A child's tears may certainly begin from fear and anxiety, but many continue because of pain. It is essential to evaluate pain and to treat it appropriately. The practitioner should give parents permission to contact him or her if they believe that their child is experiencing an unacceptable amount of pain. The practitioner should reevaluate children who are in pain when it is no longer expected and should ask the child questions about the pain rather than relying on parents as a sole source of information. Children deserve the same level of pain relief as adults.

Older Adult Considerations

The older adult population is extremely diverse. Each older person is a unique individual and must be evaluated specifically for appropriateness of the procedure. An elective procedure should not be withheld simply because the patient is an older adult.

Overall goals of care for that particular patient must be used to guide decisions about eligibility for a procedure.

Older adults are at increased risk for complications from a procedure; in general, they are slower to heal and are at an increased risk for infection.

The presence of a dementia, such as Alzheimer's disease, poses special problems in the completion of procedures. These patients tend to have a very short attention span and may be unable to cooperate with the procedure. Their reaction to a small amount of pain or discomfort may make the procedure impossible. Attempts to restrain them usually make them more agitated. Premedication with a benzodiazepine, such as lorazepam, may help gain their cooperation.

Dermatology is an area for special consideration in older adults. They experience many skin changes as a part of the normal changes associated with aging, accelerated by exposure to the sun. Lesions suspicious for cancer should be referred to a dermatologist for biopsy. The skin of older persons is susceptible to damage, slow to heal, and vulnerable to infection.

Older adults are more likely to have cardiac problems and are the population in whom cardiac procedures are most often performed. One important normal change associated with aging is increased ectopic beats. Any arrhythmia should be properly evaluated. In the use of a Holter monitor, it is important to correlate ectopy with symptoms. (Interpretation of such cardiac procedures as electrocardiography and use of the Holter monitor will be found in current specialty texts.)

General Considerations to Address in Every Procedure

DESCRIPTION

Each procedure has a brief description of the procedure and when it is used. This description also discusses whether the procedure is performed on an emergency or an elective basis. Many procedures should be part of the core knowledge and skills of a primary care provider. Other procedures are confined to more specialty practice settings and represent advanced skills that a practitioner may gain over time through specialized courses and supervised clinical experience. These advanced procedures are summarized here as a reminder of the key points of that content and cannot substitute for the more comprehensive courses. The more advanced procedures are identified in this section.

ANATOMY AND PHYSIOLOGY, PATHOPHYSIOLOGY

The practitioner should understand the basic anatomy and physiology and the pathologic processes involved to evaluate whether a procedure should be performed. This book includes only a quick review of the most important points. The practitioner should refer to a standard anatomy and physiology textbook if the present description does not provide sufficient information to make the practitioner feel comfortable with moving ahead with the procedure.

INDICATIONS

Both general indications and specific indications for a procedure may be identified in this section. The practitioner should not move ahead with a procedure if the patient does not have a clear indication for it.

CONTRAINDICATIONS

Considerations or conditions that would prohibit the procedure from being performed are listed in this section. A procedure should never be performed if the patient has a contraindication. If the procedure is absolutely necessary despite a contraindication, the patient should be referred to a specialist. Performing a contraindicated procedure places the patient at risk for complications and the practitioner at risk for litigation.

PRECAUTIONS

This section identifies "red flags" or considerations that cause the practitioner to proceed with caution. Each precaution must be evaluated relative to the individual patient to determine whether the procedure is appropriate for that patient. The practitioner must be clear about when a problem should be referred to another provider. Practitioners should not attempt procedures independently that are beyond their level of skill or training; professionals are held legally responsible for whatever they accept responsibility for doing.

ASSESSMENT

A targeted history and physical examination ensure the appropriateness of the procedure and help limit the development of unexpected problems. Included in the evaluation is the ability of the patient to cooperate with the examination. Practitioners should make certain that the patient is able to cooperate with the procedure not only by remaining quiet and not moving, but also by following through with postprocedure requirements.

PATIENT PREPARATION

It is mandatory to explain the procedure to every patient, without exception, and to obtain verbal consent.

With certain procedures, it is necessary to have the patient, or a legal guardian, sign a consent form for the procedure. The section of each procedure protocol indicates whether a signed consent is necessary; however, there are significant variations among institution requirements for whether a signed consent is necessary. Hospitals have policies requiring patients to not only sign a written consent, but to do so after they have had time to think about the procedure and ask questions about the procedure. It is the responsibility of the practitioner to confirm at least two patient identifiers to make sure the consent is from the correct patient. Outpatient clinics and private offices usually do not have these requirements. When a patient comes in for one discrete procedure, he or she gives verbal consent and there is no confusion among the providers about the identity of the patient. Before any procedure is started, the patient must be reassured, and everything possible must be done to help him or her remain calm. The practitioner should be honest about the amount of discomfort that is expected. The patient should be told approximately how long the procedure will take, what he or she should expect to see and feel, and what he or she is expected to do during the procedure.

TREATMENT ALTERNATIVES

Sometimes choices can be made about the type of procedure that will resolve a problem. This section helps the practitioner in discussing available alternatives with the patient so that the best procedure can be selected for the individual patient. The choice is based on what is best for the particular patient and on the preferences of the provider and patient. The patient should be included in the decision-making process whenever possible.

EQUIPMENT

It is essential to have all the recommended equipment and to have it prepared or laid out before beginning the procedure. If materials are assembled in the order in which they are used, the practitioner is prompted about the next step to take.

Procedure

1. Every procedure begins with the practitioner washing his or her hands. It is good practice to do this in the presence of the patient; this sends the proper message to the patient about the practitioner's general standard of practice.
2. All resources that are needed should be assembled before the procedure is started. This includes arranging the equipment; gowning, gloving, and masking of personnel as required; and ensuring the presence of any assistive personnel required for the procedure.
3. Important components of any procedure involve following universal precautions and cleaning and replacing equipment after the procedure. Disposal of sharps or infectious material should follow standard agency protocol.
4. At the beginning of the procedure, practitioners should position the patient so that the site of the procedure is accessible and easily visualized. The patient should be made as comfortable as possible so that he or she can remain quiet throughout the procedure. It is also very important for practitioners to find a comfortable position; stress from standing or bending will unnecessarily tire the practitioner and make it difficult to remain focused on what he or she is doing.
5. The final component of the procedure should be documentation of what has been done, the findings, and the patient's response. Documentation should be noted for any instructions that were given to the patient and that the patient has been told to call back if he or she has any problems or concerns.

PATIENT EDUCATION POSTPROCEDURE

- Explain any findings to the patient.
- Provide instructions for any follow-up care requirements and any particular problems that the patient might experience. Research indicates that patients often remember only three things, and they tend to remember them in the order presented. Keep it simple. Use written instructions. Develop instruction sheets to be copied, modified, and given to patients; adapt these sheets to the particular needs of each patient.
- Always tell the patient to call or return if the problem remains, returns, or does not follow the expected postprocedural course.

COMPLICATIONS

Practitioners should always be alert for the development of complications, such as infection or hemorrhage. Practitioners should not hesitate to refer the patient if the postprocedural course does not proceed as usual.

PRACTITIONER FOLLOW-UP

- Tell the patient if and when he or she is to return for follow-up.
- Make sure the problem is resolved and documented in the chart. If the procedure is very safe with very little risk of complications, you may simply ask the patient to call if he or she has any problems. For more complicated procedures, either have the patient call you to confirm resolution or schedule a follow-up visit.

REFERENCES AND RELATED RESOURCES

American Medical Association: *Current procedural terminology: CPT*, Professional edition, Chicago, 2015, AMA.

Scheibmeir M, Stevens C, Fund MB, Carrico K, Crenshaw J: Advanced diagnostic content in nurse practitioner and physician assistant programs, *J Nurse Pract* 11:633–639, 2015.

2

Dermatologic Procedures

Tom Bartol, Kent D. Blad, Marilyn Winterton Edmunds, and Sabrina Jarvis

DESCRIPTION

There are several general components of care that are involved in many dermatologic procedures.

- Skin preparation
- Anesthesia
- Wound care
- Wound hemostasis

This chapter discusses the general principles of skin preparation, hemostasis, and wound care before and after a procedure. Any variations from these guidelines are detailed in sections on specific procedures. Anesthesia is covered in "Anesthesia: Topical, Local, and Digital Nerve Block."

ANATOMY AND PHYSIOLOGY

An understanding of the basic anatomy and physiology of the skin is required as foundational knowledge for all dermatologic procedures. The skin provides the first line of defense and protection for the body from bacterial invasion, mechanical trauma, and injury caused by temperature extremes while also preventing water loss and regulating temperature. In addition, the skin serves as a sensory organ. Skin thickness varies depending on body site. Areas of thicker skin, such as the soles of the feet, require a larger needle for skin closure, whereas areas with thin skin, such as the face, are more effectively closed with a smaller needle.

The skin consists of two layers: the epidermis and the dermis (Figure 2-1). Under the skin are the subcutaneous layer and then the deep fascia. The *epidermis* is the outermost layer of the skin, and it is composed of squamous epithelial cells. It contains no nerve endings or blood vessels. The epidermis consists of a basal layer, the *stratum germinativum,* where new cells are formed during wound healing. The *stratum corneum* is the keratinized layer that is more superficial; it is composed of maturing cells.

The *dermis* is much thicker than the epidermis and lies immediately beneath the epidermis. Although it is a separate layer, it cannot be distinguished from the epidermis with the naked eye. The dermis is primarily composed of connective tissue and consists of fibroblasts. These fibroblasts produce collagen, which is the primary structural component of the skin. Macrophages, mast cells, and lymphocytes are also found in the dermis. The dermis contains nerve endings, hair follicles, sweat glands, sebaceous glands, and blood vessels.

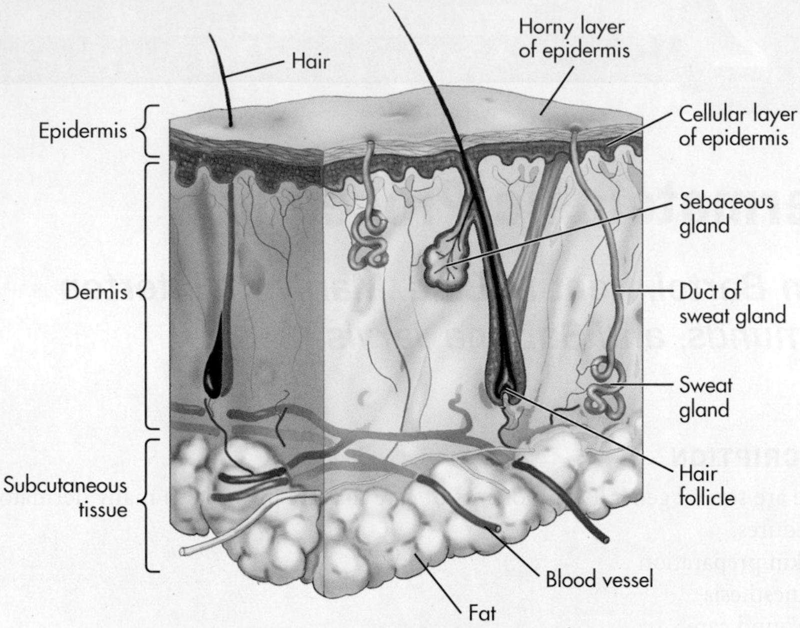

FIGURE 2-1 Three-dimensional schematic of the skin.

Beneath the dermis is the subcutaneous layer, or *superficial fascia.* This layer of subcutaneous fat provides protection and insulation. If devitalized, this layer can easily host infection. Sutures should be avoided in this layer, and devitalized areas should be débrided before wound closure. The sensory nerves are located in this layer.

Deep to the subcutaneous layer is the *deep fascia.* It is a thick, fibrous layer that supports the outer layer and protects and supports the soft tissue and muscles deep to it. The deep fascia, along with the underlying muscles in a body area, causes skin tension lines. These lines are often apparent as wrinkles in the skin created by contraction of muscles. In some areas, they are less obvious (Figures 2-2 and 2-3).

SKIN PREPARATION

Proper skin preparation is essential in most dermatologic procedures to reduce the risk of infection. Whether closing a laceration or creating an opening in the skin, such as an incision or biopsy, the skin must be cleansed appropriately. Several preparations are available for skin cleansing (Table 2-1).

The antibacterial agent povidone-iodine surgical scrub or solution or chlorhexidine may be used to scrub the periphery of the wound but should not be used inside an open wound. Then, using a disposable irrigation setup or a large bore intravenous catheter with the needle removed, most wounds should be irrigated with short bursts of normal saline. For extremely dirty wounds with particulate matter embedded or for large wounds, a large syringe and a liter or more of normal saline solution may be required to cleanse the wound. Limited amounts of *hydrogen peroxide* may be used in very dirty wounds to help loosen and dislodge debris and other contaminants from the tissue. Avoid using large amounts of hydrogen peroxide because the solution itself may cause hemolysis of cells. Poloxamer 188 or Shur-Clens is used as an alternative wound cleanser, particularly on the face, although it has no antibacterial component itself.

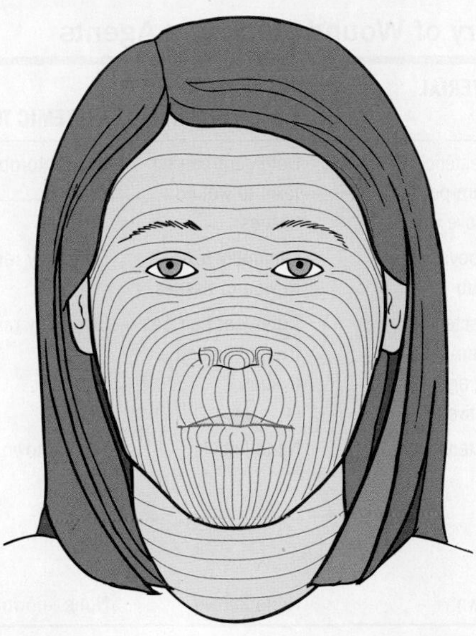

FIGURE 2-2 Skin tension lines of the face. Incisions or lacerations parallel to these lines are less likely to cause widened scars than are those made perpendicular to these lines.

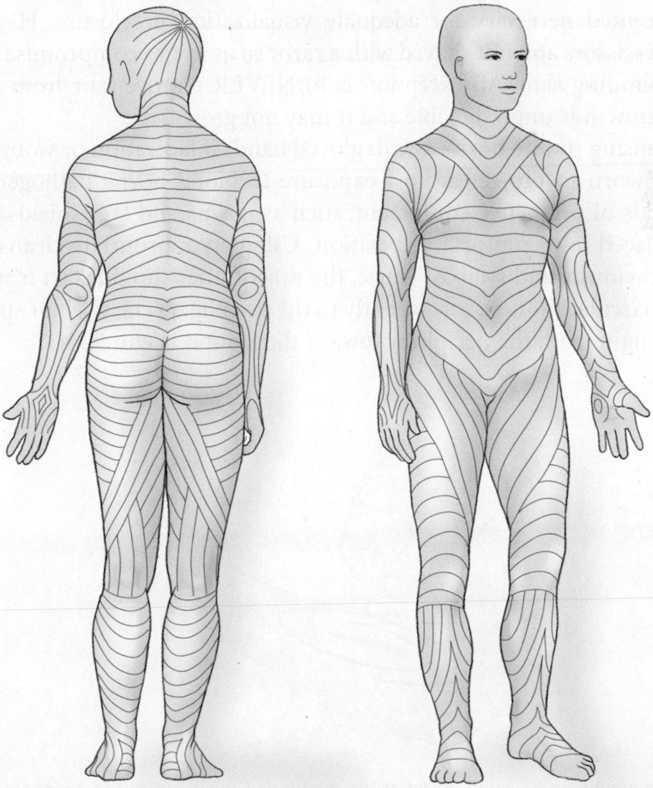

FIGURE 2-3 Skin tension lines of the body surface.

TABLE 2-1 Summary of Wound-Cleansing Agents

SKIN CLEANSER	ANTIBACTERIAL ACTIVITY	TISSUE TOXICITY	SYSTEMIC TOXICITY	POTENTIAL USES
Povidone-iodine surgical scrub	Strongly bactericidal against gram-positive and gram-negative viruses	Detergent can be toxic to wound tissues	Painful to open wounds	Hand cleanser
Povidone-iodine solution	Same as povidone-iodine scrub	Minimally toxic to wound tissues	Extremely rare	Wound-periphery cleanser
Chlorhexidine	Strongly bactericidal against gram-positives, less strong against gram-negatives	Detergent can be toxic to wound tissues	Extremely rare	Hand cleanser
Poloxamer 188	No antibacterial activity	None known	None known	Wound cleanser (useful on face) Alternative wound periphery cleanser
Saline	None known	None known	None known	Wound irrigant

From Trott AT: *Wounds and lacerations: emergency care and closure,* ed 4, Philadelphia, 2012, Saunders.

If the wound or incision is on a part of the body with hair, the hair may be removed if deemed necessary for adequate visualization or closure. Hair should be clipped with scissors and not shaved with a razor so as not to compromise the integrity of the surrounding skin. An exception is to NEVER remove hair from the eyebrow because its growth is unpredictable and it may not grow back.

Skin cleansing should be done with gloved hands if laceration or wound is present. Goggles are worn to protect against exposure to blood-borne pathogens as should other methods of protective equipment, such as gowns and face shields. The patient should be placed in a comfortable position. Using an appropriate cleansing agent as described previously and swab or gauze, the practitioner should start from the center and, using a circular motion, scrub gently to the periphery. The swab or sponge should never be brought from the periphery toward the wound (Figure 2-4).

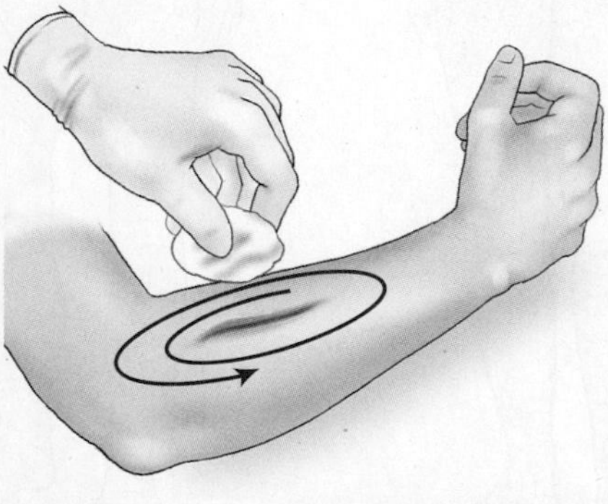

FIGURE 2-4 In scrubbing a wound, begin at the center and move out to the periphery in increasingly larger circles.

Wound Care

Marilyn Winterton Edmunds

DESCRIPTION

A moist wound bed promotes healing. Aseptic technique is used to minimize bacterial contamination.

Wound care includes tetanus prophylaxis (if indicated), dressing application (if needed), and instructions to the patient regarding wound care, signs and symptoms of infection, and follow-up. It is helpful to have written instructions to give to the patient, which are reinforced at the end of the procedure.

Recommendations for tetanus prophylaxis are given in Table 2-2. One dose of tetanus toxoid with diphtheria toxoid (Tdap or Td) is now recommended for anyone, regardless of the last time he or she had a tetanus immunization. There are special guidelines for some individuals older than 65 years, women who are pregnant, and individuals who have not received the vaccine in the past. See the Centers for Disease Control and Prevention (CDC) for the latest updates. Patients should be given instructions about their wound care. Signs of wound infection should be discussed with all patients. The first sign of infection is usually increased pain at the site of the wound. This may be followed by purulent drainage and redness that extends beyond the wound margins (>5 mm), along with swelling, tenderness, regional lymphadenitis, and possibly fever. Patients should be told to contact the clinician if these symptoms develop, and then the patient should be seen for follow-up.

If a dressing is applied, the patient should be instructed to keep it in place for 24 to 48 hours, and then to change it as needed. The dressing must be kept clean and dry, and if it is soiled or wet, it must be changed. Patients who have sutures can usually begin bathing once a day after 12 to 24 hours, patting the wound dry with a towel after bathing. The application of an antibiotic ointment helps keep the wound moist, which will promote more rapid healing and prevent infection. Daily soaks may be needed for some wounds, but these should not be done with hydrogen peroxide because it is toxic to the healing tissue. Do not soak wounds that have been closed with sutures or glue.

TABLE 2-2 Summary Guide to Tetanus Prophylaxis in Routine Wound Management, 1991

HISTORY OF ADSORBED TETANUS TOXOID (DOSES)	CLEAN, MINOR WOUNDS		ALL OTHER WOUNDS*	
	Td	TIG (250 U)	Td	TIG (250 U)
Unknown or <3	Yes	Yes	Yes	Yes
≥ 3‡	Yes	Yes	Yes	Yes

From ACIP: Diphtheria, tetanus, and pertussis recommendations for vaccine use and other preventative measures, MMWR Morb Morta Wkly Rep October 27, 2010, recommended use of Tdap regardless of interval since the last tetanus- or diphtheria-containing vaccine. Subsequent reports have also recommended use of Tdap in women who are pregnant, in certain adults ages 65 and older, and use of Tdap in under vaccinated children ages 7 through 10 years. See http://www.cdc.gov/vaccines/vpd-vac/combo-vaccines/DTaP-Td-DT/Tdap.htm for all reports. Last accessed December 21, 2014.

*Such as, but not limited to, wounds contaminated with dirt, feces, soil, and saliva; puncture wounds, avulsions, and wounds resulting from missiles, crushing burns, and frostbite.

Td, Tetanus toxoid with diphtheria toxoid; *TIG,* tetanus immunoglobulin.

After an injury, elevation of the affected area may reduce swelling and thus promote healing as well.

Wounds with a high risk of infection or in critical areas, such as the hands, may need to be reevaluated within 48 hours. If there is a high risk of infection, such as wounds caused by an animal or a human bite, a crushing injury, those involving joint spaces or ear cartilage, or severely contaminated wounds, antibiotic prophylaxis should be considered.

INDICATIONS

Office treatment is indicated for minor wounds such as skin tears, first- and minor second-degree burns, and uncomplicated lacerations. (Refer to "Suturing Simple Lacerations, Procedure" to evaluate the need for sutures.)

CONTRAINDICATIONS/PRECAUTIONS

Wounds that require special caution occur in the following situations:

- An older patient who has poor psychosocial support or concomitant disease.
- A noncooperative child who is younger than 2 years.
- Existing conditions that predispose a patient to infection, such as diabetes, corticosteroid therapy, or immunodeficiency.
- The patient who has a chemical, electrical, explosion, inhalation, or abuse-related injury; he or she should be referred to an emergency department because of the higher level of care that is required.
- As a precaution, the practitioner should assess for iodine and sulfa medication allergies before beginning the procedure.

EQUIPMENT

- Gloves
- 4 × 4 gauze pads
- Antiseptic ointment
- Tongue blade (burns)
- Choice of dressing
  - Semipermeable film (Op-Site Flexigrid; Smith & Nephew, Germantown, Wis)
  - Hydrocolloid sterile dressing (DuoDERM CGF; ConvaTec Connection, Princeton, NJ)
  - Nonadherent gauze dressing (Telfa; Tyco Healthcare, Kendall Company, Mansfield, Mass)
  - Kling (various sizes; Johnson & Johnson, Piscataway, NJ)
- Tape
- Tetanus toxoid (as indicated)

Standard Cleansing and Wrapping Procedure

1. Clean the wound using sterile normal saline or soap and water. Pat dry with sterile gauze. Apply antibacterial ointment.
2. Apply nonadherent dressing (Telfa).
3. Wrap with gauze dressing (Kling) in layers, forming a soft, bulky dressing if required, and secure with tape or coban.

4. Administer 0.5 ml of tetanus toxoid (Tdap or Td) IM in the deltoid muscle if the patient has not received a booster in the past 5 years.
5. Consider an analgesic agent or antibiotic as indicated.
6. For semipermeable and hydrocolloid dressings, dry the skin around the wound with a sterile 4 × 4 gauze pad. Apply the dressing according to the package directions. No cover dressing is necessary.

PATIENT EDUCATION POSTPROCEDURE

- Instruct the patient who has Telfa dressing to perform daily wound care: clean with sterile normal saline or soap and water, apply antibiotic cream, and redress. Tell the patient to return for follow-up in 3 to 5 days.
- Instruct the patient who has semipermeable films and hydrocolloids to leave the dressing on for 3 to 5 days and then return to the provider.
- Advise patients to notify the practitioner if signs of infection occur (e.g., erythema, purulent drainage, odor, increase in pain, elevated temperature).

PRACTITIONER FOLLOW-UP/COMPLICATIONS

- The patient should be seen in 3 to 5 days.
- To assess for signs of infection, practitioners look for redness, swelling, blisters, drainage, and fever.

▶ RED FLAG

The patient should be referred to a surgeon or ER physician if the wound is not healing.

REFERENCES AND RELATED RESOURCES

Dehn RW, Asprey DP: *Essential clinical procedures*, ed 3, New York, 2013, Saunders.
Papadakis MA, McPhee SJ: *CURRENT medical diagnosis and treatment 2014*, ed 53, New York, 2014, McGraw-Hill.

Topical Application of Hemostatic Agents

Marilyn Winterton Edmunds

DESCRIPTION

A variety of agents may be applied to superficial wounds to decrease bleeding via rapid vasoconstriction of small areas of tissue or when rapid hemostasis is essential. There are also several agents specifically designed for use in traumatic injuries, primarily in the military setting, that are not appropriate for the general primary care population and are not discussed here.

ANATOMY AND PHYSIOLOGY

Hemostasis of capillaries and small blood vessels following procedures or minor surgery may be achieved through the use of direct pressure, electrocautery, laser, or chemical agents. Each of these techniques has advantages and disadvantages. Vasoconstrictors, vaso-occlusive agents, or denaturing agents are the more traditional forms of hemostasis. These agents physically cause some tissue damage and produce an eschar. Some of the newer agents that act through chemicals that affect the clotting mechanism are effective, but may be cost-prohibitive.

INDICATIONS

- Hemostasis is used primarily to control bleeding in the removal of skin lesions, shave biopsies, removal of nail bed, or in minor surgery.
    - Hemostasis may be used for lacerations and cuts or open wounds that will be left open or closed secondarily.
- Hemostasis may also be used to cauterize lesions caused by impetigo.
    - Hemostasis may be used following granulation of tissue cauterization.

CONTRAINDICATIONS

- Hemostasis should not be used in surgery or injuries that involve the distal digits or on skin appendages because it may produce ischemia.
    - Topical agents are absolutely contraindicated when trying to control profusely bleeding vessels.
- Hemostatic agents should not be used in patients who have had hypopigmentation or hyperpigmentation skin reactions.
    - Some individuals may have an allergy to the hemostatic agent.
    - A deep or very large wound that will require primary surgical closure with sutures, staples, or skin glue would require manual pressure rather than a hemostatic agent.
    - Electrosurgery (not electrocautery) should not be performed on patients who have cardiac pacemakers.

PRECAUTIONS

- Hemostasis should be used with caution in patients who have a history of poor healing.

ASSESSMENT

- Assess for history of sensitivity to the chemical agent being used or any contraindications to the use of epinephrine.
- Assess for previous lacerations or surgical scars that have exaggerated hypopigmentation or hyperpigmentation of the skin caused by chemical agents.

PATIENT PREPARATION

This procedure is commonly a part of other procedures to remove lesions or to rectify small dermatologic problems. Informed written consent is not usually obtained for this procedure alone, but rather as part of the other procedure that is being performed.

The procedure should be explained to the patient. The patient should be informed of the risks of additional bleeding, infection, scarring, and nerve damage. If using any products that might permanently or temporarily stain the skin (such as silver nitrate), discuss this risk with the patient. Answer any questions the patient may have.

TREATMENT ALTERNATIVE

- Electrocautery

TABLE 2-3 Common Topical Hemostatic Agents

AGENT	CHARACTERISTICS	USES	LIMITATIONS
Aluminum chloride 30% (Drysol)	Fast hemolysis; reduced irritation of skin; rare incidence of pigment changes or staining	Apply as liquid directly to skin or on cotton applicator	
Epinephrine	Extremely potent vasoconstriction	Apply topically with cotton applicators (may also be injected intradermally or subcutaneously)	Must be used in only small amounts or tissue necrosis and sloughing may develop; cannot be used on digits or with skin appendages
Ferric subsulfate (Monsel's Solution)	Produces rapid hemolysis	Especially useful with seborrheic keratoses or basal cell carcinoma	Frequently causes pigment changes and staining of the skin
Silver nitrate sticks	Fast hemolysis; relatively inexpensive	Silver nitrate is impregnated in the cotton-tipped applicators	Most likely to cause pigment changes and staining of the skin; silver nitrate sticks must be kept dry or they deteriorate

2

EQUIPMENT

- Nonsterile gloves
- Sterile fenestrated drape
- Sterile cotton-tipped applicators
- Sterile 4 × 4 gauze pads
- Topical hemostatic agent (Table 2-3). Agents may be vaso-occlusive denaturing agents, agents producing a physical meshwork, physiologic hemostasis agents, or combination products.
- Mechanical methods may include direct pressure with finger, pressure dressings, ice or chemical cold packs, Shaw scalpel, electrocautery, electrosurgery, or laser. These mechanical methods are addressed as relevant in other procedures where control of hemostasis is an integral part of the procedural process.

Procedure using chemical hemostatic agents

1. Position the patient comfortably with the area involved well illuminated with light.
2. Clean the area if this has not already been done.
3. Drape area with sterile fenestrated drapes.
4. Apply vaso-occlusive denaturing agents.
   i. Silver nitrate: Available as 20% or 50% solutions and as a solid on a wooden applicator. Either remove two silver nitrate sticks from the sealed container for use or dip a cotton-tipped applicator into the hemostatic solution. Then squeeze the cotton applicator against the side of the container top to ensure that extra solution runs back into the bottle so it will not drip or run when applied to the skin.
      - Wearing gloves and using two fingers, stretch the skin tightly over the area where hemostasis is required.

- Wipe off any excess blood from the skin with sterile gauze and immediately apply the chemically filled, cotton-tipped applicator or wooden stick applicator to the area for at least 15 seconds. The solid silver nitrate on the stick is activated when the tip is placed in a moist wound.
- Discard the applicator and then release tension on the skin.
- As silver salts may stain the tissue black, some tattooing may remain for several months. Care should be exercised to touch only the wound area and no surrounding tissues. Because of this risk, silver nitrate is now most commonly restricted to nonvisible areas.

ii. Ferric subsulfate solution (20%; Monsel's Solution)

- Follow steps above. After cleaning, drying, and stretching the skin as above, the dark brown, thick solution is applied with very light pressure with a cotton-tipped swab. Any excess black, coagulated solution can be wiped away after the bleeding is stopped. Because there is the potential for permanent or semipermanent "tattooing," many clinicians decline to use this chemical on the face or in very fair-complexioned individuals.

iii. Aluminum chloride 30% (Lumicaine, Drysol)

- Using the process above, apply aluminum chloride topically with a swab using light pressure to a wound. This does not cause tattooing.

iv. QR powder (Potassium salts and hydrophilic polymers)

- These products are available over the counter where active bleeding is involved. The product comes in individual dose packets filled with a thin powder, which can be applied to the wound with pressure applied for 15 to 60 seconds or until bleeding stops. Repeat if bleeding reoccurs. The resulting eschar should be left in place until it sloughs off. It can be used in wounds left to heal by secondary intention. It is often effective in nose bleeds. It should not be used on sutured wounds.

5. The procedure may need to be repeated more than once until successful hemostasis is achieved.
6. If the base of a lesion is being cauterized with this chemical method, make certain that the chemical is applied to the whole base of the lesion.
7. Treatment site is usually left open to the air.

Procedure using physical meshwork agents

1. Position the patient comfortably with the area involved well illuminated with light.
2. Clean the area if this has not already been done.
3. Drape area with sterile fenestrated drapes.
4. Apply chemical directly to the wound area:

i. Absorbable gelatin sponge (Gelfoam)

- Gelatin sponges may be applied as a dry powder or moistened with saline or thrombin. Apply to the wound bed with light pressure and only to the area of bleeding. Avoid use near the tendons. Excessive granuloma formation and fibrosis may be a side effect especially around the tendons.

ii. Cyanoacrylates (Dermabond, IsoDent)

- These products are tissue glues and can seal wound edges, thus bleeding is stopped.

- Follow manufactures' directions carefully. Apply thin amounts to wound edges and manually compress until glue has fixed.

iii. Microfibrillar collagen (Avitene)

- This product is only used in office settings by the experienced clinician. The collagen adheres to wet gloves and any wet surface. It must be applied with dry instruments. It comes as a web or as a granular form, which is applied directly to the wound and held in place. Platelets aggregate on their surface. It is often used at biopsy sites. It cannot be used at skin closure sites because the wound edge healing is impeded.

iv. Oxidized cellulose (Surgicel)

- This product is composed of absorbable cellulose fibers, which are cut and held with firm pressure on the wound bed. It provides a meshwork where blood coagulation is facilitated. It may be left inside some wounds (not under skin grafts) or removed. Removal may provoke rebleeding.

5. Surgical wound closure and bandaging is used after most of these treatments.
   - Treat wound site as a surgical site.

Procedure using hemostatic agents

1. Position the patient comfortably with the area involved well illuminated with light.
2. Clean the area if this has not already been done.
3. Drape area with sterile fenestrated drapes.
4. Apply chemical to the bleeding site:

i. Epinephrine

- Epinephrine is readily available in local anesthetics (as adrenaline chloride solution or lidocaine with epinephrine). Apply topically to local areas, such as the nose, or inject into a bleeding site. Reduction of bleeding allows use of other topical agents or electrocoagulation if necessary.
- Action lasts about 2 hours.

RED FLAG

Avoid injection into end-arterial areas because of the risk of blood flow reduction, which may cause ischemia. This would be particularly problematic in the nose, finger, toes, or penis. Patients should be referred to a specialist if this procedure is considered essential. Watch for cardiac arrhythmias and neurologic adverse effects in patients.

ii. Fibrin sealant

- Fibrin sealant or fibrin glue is a unique product that employs mixing two human clotting factors together and applying them through a special spraying device just before application. The clot will form in about 30 seconds. Although it is highly effective, the risk of using human blood products, the awkward application process, and the cost make it uncommon to use.

iii. Thrombin (Thrombostat)

- Irrigate wound to remove excess blood and sponge dry. Then spray the freeze-dried powder mixed with isotonic saline on the wound bed, or apply the powder directly to the wound. Solution must be used within 6 hours and is used in superficial surgery or plastic surgery if diluted. It is expensive and thus not routinely used in office procedures.

5. Some of these treatment sites may be left open to air. In other cases, the resulting hemostasis precedes other surgery and a surgical dressing will be applied.

PATIENT EDUCATION POSTPROCEDURE

- Keep the treatment area clean and moist, but do not let the treatment area become soggy.
- Use a thick coat of antibiotic ointment on these sites to aid healing.
- Usually change any dressings two to three times a day and wash area gently with soap and water before applying clean dressing. Do not use hydrogen peroxide for cleaning.
- The skin will appear red and inflamed for up to 48 hours from the chemical irritation or may appear discolored if ferric subsulfate solution or silver nitrate is used.
- Pain is usually mild. Patient may take acetaminophen (Tylenol) every 4 hours as needed to decrease pain.
- Patient should return to the practitioner's office for evaluation immediately if bleeding or any signs of infection (swelling, warmth of tissues, drainage, foul-smelling odor, fever, chills, sweating, or purulent drainage) develop.

COMPLICATIONS

Rebound bleeding, infection, and local inflammatory reactions may develop. These are the most frequent complications. Also watch for nerve damage secondary to the wound itself or from the chemicals, swelling and/or excessive tissue damage, hypopigmentation or hyperpigmentation reactions of the skin, localized inflammation, scarring, or tattooing of the skin.

PRACTITIONER FOLLOW-UP

This is usually a self-limiting problem. No follow-up is required unless there is some suspicion about the etiology of the lesion being removed.

REFERENCES AND RELATED RESOURCES

Palm MD, Altman JS: Topical hemostatic agents: A review, *Dermatol Surg* 34:431–445, 2008.
Pfenninger JL, Fowler GC: *Procedures for primary care*, ed 3, Philadelphia, 2011, Mosby.
Take 5: Surgical Pearls: QR powder to control bleeding, *Pract Dermatol* 5:64, 2008.
Wang DS, Chu LF, Olson SE, et al: Comparative evaluation of noninvasive compression adjuncts for hemostasis in percutaneous arterial venous and arteriovenous dialysis access procedures, *J Vas Interv Radiol* 19:72–79, 2008.

Anesthesia: Topical, Local, and Digital Nerve Block

Marilyn Winterton Edmunds

Anesthesia is indicated for many of the procedures discussed in this book. Three methods—topical, local, and regional nerve block—are common in primary care settings.

DESCRIPTION

Topical anesthesia is a pain-free form of anesthesia in which a chemical or chemical mixture is applied directly to the skin. It is useful for very simple lacerations and is especially helpful in the pediatric patient, as well as in the adult patient who has a very low pain threshold or needle phobia. *Local anesthetic agents* are injected into the plane between the dermis and the subcutaneous layer at the site where anesthesia is desired. *Digital nerve blocks* involve the injection of an anesthetic agent at the base of a digit to anesthetize the entire digit and are useful for nail removal, paronychia drainage, and laceration repair of the fingers and toes. *Local* or *regional (nerve block)* anesthesia is used for many dermatologic procedures. Anesthesia facilitates patient comfort, which helps the clinician to perform the procedure. Choice of anesthesia type depends on the procedure, location, extent of the wound, length of time of the procedure, and the patient's age and emotional status.

ANATOMY AND PHYSIOLOGY

Topical anesthetics offer fairly easy and fairly rapid relief or prevention of pain in a localized area. This makes them appropriate for use in many dermatologic procedures or in treatment of minor skin injuries. Topical anesthetics are classified as those applied on intact skin, nonintact skin, and mucous membranes. Local anesthetics are used to prevent the generation and conduction of nerve impulses of pain at the molecular level. The local anesthetic agents infiltrate the tissues and diffuse across the neural sheaths, thereby inhibiting the transmission of impulses. Pain receptors have no myelin sheath and are of very small diameter, and thus can be easily blocked. Pressure receptors are larger and have a myelin sheath, and they are often not blocked with local anesthesia; the patient may have a sensation of pressure, but not of pain. It is important to inform the patient that he or she may feel pressure despite the anesthesia and that this is normal, but that he or she should not feel pain.

A digital nerve block involves infiltrating a local anesthetizing solution at the base of the four nerves to each finger or toe: the two palmar digital nerves and the two dorsal digital nerves (Figures 2-5 and 2-6). The *palmar digital nerves* are responsible

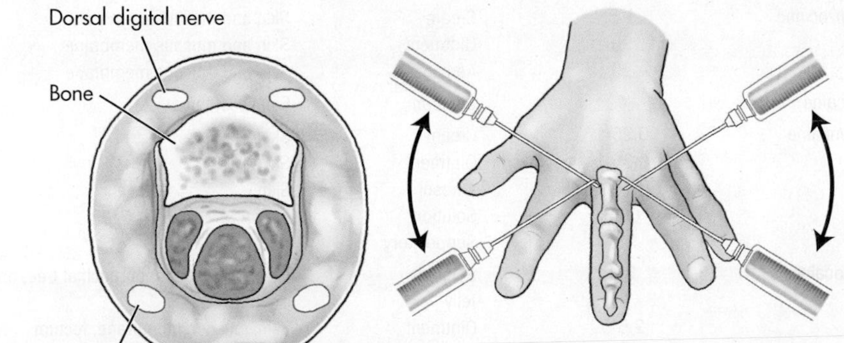

FIGURE 2-5 Anatomy and injection technique for digital nerve block. **A,** Four digital nerves of the finger viewed as a transection through the finger. The bone is used as a landmark to find the proper plane of the dorsal digital nerve. **B,** Digital nerve block of the finger as viewed from above. The sites of the nerves are injected bilaterally. To obtain the optimal effect, after blocking the nerves, place a "ring" of anesthetic agent entirely around the digit close to the bone. Inject superiorly over the bone and inferiorly under the bone in the subcutaneous plane.

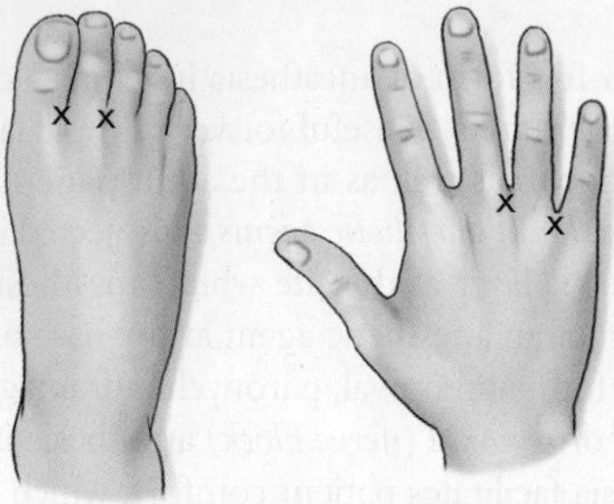

FIGURE 2-6 Digital nerve block injection sites on the hand and foot.

for distal finger and fingertip sensation and have the most extensive sensory distribution. The *dorsal digital nerves* are responsible for proximal, dorsal digit sensation and have some sensory overlap with the palmar digital nerves.

Injectable anesthetic agents vary in their onset of action, duration, and toxicity (Tables 2-4 through 2-7).

Vasoconstrictors, such as *epinephrine,* may be mixed with some agents to prolong the duration of action and to reduce bleeding. The use of vasoconstricting agents may potentiate wound infection. They should not be used in areas with terminal vasculature and should be used only with caution in patients who have peripheral vascular disease and may exhibit an exaggerated vasoconstrictor response. Vasoconstricting agents should also be avoided in areas with vascular compromise, such as on a skin flap.

Lidocaine and *mepivacaine* have an acidic pH relative to the tissue, which may cause some pain during injection. This pain can be reduced by buffering the pH with

TABLE 2-4 Topical Anesthetic Preparations

ANESTHETIC	CONCENTRATION (%)	FORM	TISSUE
Benzocaine	1-5	Cream	Skin and mucous membrane
	20	Ointment	Skin and mucous membrane
	20	Aerosol	Skin and mucous membrane
Cocaine	4	Solution	Ear, nose, throat
Dibucaine	0.25-1	Cream	Skin
	0.25-1	Ointment	Skin
	0.25-1	Aerosol	Skin
	0.25	Solution	Ear
	2.5	Suppository	Rectum
Lidocaine	2-4	Solution	Oropharynx, tracheobronchial tree, nose
	2	Jelly	Urethra
	2.5-5	Ointment	Skin, mucous membrane, rectum
	2	Viscous solution	Oropharynx
	10	Suppository	Rectum
	10	Aerosol	Gingival mucosa
Tetracaine	0.5-1	Ointment	Skin, rectum, mucous membrane
	0.5-1	Cream	Skin, rectum, mucous membrane
	0.25-1	Solution	Nose, tracheobronchial tree

Data from Elsevier Gold Standard Drug Database. Clinical Pharmacology. www.clinicalpharmacology.com. Last accessed November 21, 2014.

TABLE 2-5 Local Anesthetic Agents and Their Effects

LOCAL ANESTHETIC AGENT	EFFECTS	USES
Lidocaine (Xylocaine) without epinephrine	Can cause vasodilatation; ½- to 1-hour duration, depending on site and vascularity.	Contaminated wounds; on fingers, nose, penis, toes, and earlobes; if vascular disease is present or patient is immunocompromised; if there are cerebrovascular or cardiovascular risks; for nerve blocks
Lidocaine (Xylocaine) with epinephrine	Causes vasoconstriction; longer duration	Highly vascular areas to improve visualization of field; in general, do not use on fingers, nose, penis, toes, and earlobes although skilled surgeons may do so.
Bupivacaine (Marcaine)	Longer duration	Nerve blocks

TABLE 2-6 Local Anesthetic Agents Commonly Used in Office Settings

LOCAL ANESTHETIC AGENT	ONSET (MIN)	DURATION (HR)	EQUIVALENT CONCENTRATION (%)
Lidocaine (Xylocaine)	1	½-1	1
Lidocaine with epinephrine	1	2-6	1
Mepivacaine (Carbocaine)	3-5	¾-1½	1
Dibucaine (Nupercainal)	15	3-4	0.25
Dibucaine with epinephrine	15	6	0.25
Bupivacaine (Marcaine)	5	2-4	0.25
Bupivacaine with epinephrine	5	3-7	0.25
Etidocaine (Duranest)	3-5	3-7	0.5

TABLE 2-7 Maximum Doses of Commonly Used Local Anesthetic Agents

ANESTHETIC AGENT	CONCENTRATION (%)	MAXIMUM DOSE
Lidocaine (Xylocaine)	1	4.5 mg/kg; not to exceed 300 mg (30 ml in adults)
Lidocaine (Xylocaine)	1 with epinephrine	7 mg/kg; not to exceed 500 mg (50 ml in adults)
Bupivacaine (Marcaine)	0.25	3 mg/kg; not to exceed 175 mg (50 ml in most adults)
Bupivacaine (Marcaine) with epinephrine	0.25	3 mg/kg; not to exceed 225 mg

DiBiase M: Local anesthesia. In Dehn RW, Asprey DP, editors: *Essential clinical procedures*, ed 3, St Louis, 2013, Elsevier, p 238.
Data from Elsevier Gold Standard Drug Database. Clinical Pharmacology. www.clinicalpharmacology.com. Last accessed November 21, 2014.

sodium bicarbonate as follows: 1 ml of sodium bicarbonate (1 mEq/ml solution) to 10 ml of a 1% concentration of anesthetic (lidocaine or mepivacaine).

INDICATIONS

Anesthetic agents are indicated for any procedure that might cause pain that could be eliminated with some type of anesthesia. They are also used to relieve pain from trauma (lacerations or fractures).

Topical anesthesia is useful in the repair of superficial lacerations, especially in children. It may be used before a digital nerve block, venipuncture, lumbar puncture, or other procedures that involve needle injection, such as venipuncture, arterial puncture, shave biopsy, punch biopsy, chemical peels, cryotherapy of venereal warts, removal of embedded foreign body, circumcision, and adjunctively in vasectomy, dermabrasion, and laser resurfacing. Ice or ethyl chloride may be used for skin tag clipping or abscess incision and drainage. Eutectic mixture of local anesthetic (EMLA) is used before procedures on intact skin only.

Local anesthesia is used for laceration repair, biopsies, incision, and drainage of an abscess, some types of wart removal, and any procedure that may produce localized pain.

Digital nerve blocks are used when a larger area of anesthesia is necessary, in areas where local anesthesia is difficult to apply, or when local anesthesia may not be effective because of infection or edema. Diagnostic nerve blocks are also used to isolate pathology when the extent of injury is unclear.

2

CONTRAINDICATIONS

Local Anesthesia

- Known hypersensitivity to any of the agents.
- Use anesthetics with vasoconstrictors (e.g., lidocaine with epinephrine) with extreme care or refer to specialist if required in areas with terminal vasculature, including fingers, toes, nose, ears, and penis.
- History of central nervous system symptoms or cardiovascular reactions associated with previous lidocaine or epinephrine use or toxicity.
- Avoid epinephrine use in patients who have a skin flap with marginal blood flow or viability.
- Do not use epinephrine in patients taking monoamine oxidase inhibitors.
- Epinephrine may increase the risk of infection in contaminated wounds because of diminished blood flow.
- Do not use EMLA products in patients who have advanced liver disease or those who are at risk for methemoglobinemia.
- Products that contain lidocaine should be used carefully on mucous membranes because increased absorption increases risks for lidocaine toxicity.
- LMX4 and LMX5 are not effective on the soles and palms because they increase skin thickness and block absorption and vascularity of the area, promoting rapid clearance.

PRECAUTIONS

- Gloves and eye/face protection should be worn when any anesthetic agent is injected.
- Assess for prior allergic reactions to anesthetic agents. Allergic reactions to local anesthetic agents of the amide class, such as lidocaine, bupivacaine, and mepivacaine, are less frequent than reactions to the older ester solutions, such as procaine and tetracaine. There is no cross-reactivity between the two groups, so a patient who is allergic to procaine (an ester) often can tolerate an amide anesthetic such as lidocaine.
- Local anesthetic agents often contain lidocaine and can cause excitatory phenomena in the central nervous system, which may lead to seizures. They may also cause cardiovascular reactions, such as hypotension and bradycardia. These reactions are usually the result of inadvertent injection into a blood vessel; aspiration of the syringe before injection of the agent can prevent this. If blood is aspirated, the needle should be withdrawn and aspiration repeated before injection. Many local anesthetic agents are compounded and thus the exact amount of lidocaine may vary dramatically; therefore, toxicity is a real concern.
- It is important to keep track of the total anesthetic dose administered because toxic effects are often dose related.

• If the patient reports pain, the inadequate anesthesia may be caused by the drug not having had sufficient time to diffuse into the tissue. Avoid injecting into an area of infection or suspected cancerous tumor; inject around the site in a wheel fashion. Overinjection of anesthesia may swell or distort the tissue, making lesion removal or approximation of edges for wound closure difficult.

PATIENT PREPARATION

The procedure should be explained to the patient, including risks and benefits, possible complications, and alternatives to the procedure. The patients should be given an opportunity to ask questions about the procedure.

The patient should be positioned comfortably and instructed not to move during the injection.

TREATMENT ALTERNATIVES

Sedation may be needed for some patients who cannot cooperate with the procedure, especially with some pediatric patients.

If the patient is allergic to the anesthetic agent or agents, there are several alternatives that may be useful. If the allergy is known to be to an ester agent (procaine), an amide agent may be substituted. For small wounds or simple procedures, with a cooperative patient, no anesthesia may be needed. Ice placed over the area may provide sufficient anesthesia for some brief procedures as well (e.g., skin tag clipping). Diphenhydramine (Benadryl) can be diluted to a 1% solution (50 mg diluted with 4 ml of normal saline) and injected as a local anesthetic agent. Subcutaneous injection of normal saline may also provide sufficient anesthesia for minor procedures.

EQUIPMENT

TOPICAL ANESTHESIA

Chemical Options for Intact Skin:

- EMLA (eutectic mixture of local anesthetics) (lidocaine and prilocaine) as occlusive covering disc
- LM 4/LMX5 - LM 4 (4% liposomal lidocaine) LMS 5 (5% liposomal lidocaine)
- Lidoderm patch (often used in pain reduction with postherpetic neuralgia)
- BLT triple anesthetic gel (20% Benzocaine, 6% Lidocaine, 4% Tetracaine) (May be used in children older than 3 years)
- S-Caine Patch/S-Caine Peel (mix of 70 mg lidocaine and 70 mg tetrocaine base)

Chemical Options for Nonintact Skin:

- LET/LAT (Lidocaine, Epinephrine/Adrenalin, Tetracaine) used primarily for scalp and facial lacerations
- Topicaine (4% or 5% Lidocaine Gel) OTC product used for minor skin cuts or abrasions
- Sterile cotton balls and/or 2 × 2 gauze
- Disposable clean gloves

LOCAL ANESTHESIA

- Local anesthetic agent, for example, lidocaine, marcaine with epinephrine or BLT (Benzocaine, Lidocaine, Tetracaine which is a compounded mixture and takes 45 to 60 minutes for effective anesthesia); Quadri-Caine (10% lidocaine, 4% tetracaine, 5% prilocaine, and 1% bupivacaine in an emollient cream; produces onset anesthesia within 15 minutes)
- Sodium bicarbonate as a buffer

- 18-gauge needle to draw up solution
- 27- to 30-gauge needle for injection
- Alcohol swabs
- Appropriate syringe (1 to 3 ml or occasionally 5 to 10 ml for large site)

DIGITAL NERVE BLOCK

- Local anesthetic agent (marcaine *without* epinephrine)
- Sodium bicarbonate as a buffer
- 18-gauge needle to draw up solution
- 27- to 30-gauge needle for injection
- Sterile field and agent for skin preparation
- Sterile gloves
- Appropriate syringe (3 to 5 ml)

2

Procedure

TOPICAL ANESTHESIA

Intact Skin:

Mechanical mechanisms:

Ice

1. For brief procedures such as skin tag removal or draining an abscess, rub the skin with ice for 10 seconds. Anesthesia lasts 2 seconds in which procedure should be completed.

Ethyl Chloride

1. Wear gloves and for short procedures, spray the site with ethyl chloride for 1 to 2 seconds and watch as the skin turns white. Anesthesia lasts 2 seconds in which the procedure should be completed.

EMLA

1. Use alcohol or skin soap to remove oils from skin.
2. Wearing gloves, apply EMLA disc or other topical products to the intact skin using soaked gauze. Wipe in and over a facial or scalp laceration. If anesthesia is desired before a procedure, achieve anesthesia 30 to 60 minutes before the procedure, and then apply an occlusive dressing. The depth of anesthesia should be 3 mm after 1 hour. Decrease application time on diseased skin to 5 to 30 minutes because penetration is more rapid.
3. S-Caine Patch/S-Caine Peel. Apply patch and then use the disposable, oxygen-activated heating element which maintains heat at 39 to 41° C in about 20 to 30 minutes and lasts for a 2-hour period to increase the delivery of topical creams preprocedurally.
4. BKT Triple Anesthetic Gel: Apply with sponge to intact skin. Anesthesia onset is about 15 minutes.
5. Lidoderm 5% patch: Cover the most painful areas (may require 1 to 3 patches) for a maximum of 12 hours. Patches may be cut to fit the size needed.

Open Skin Wounds:

1. Tropicaine: Apply a thick layer of ointment (about ⅛ inch) to affected area. Anesthesia onset is 20 minutes and lasts about 1 hour.

LET/LAT

1. Wearing gloves, apply LET/LAT or other topical products to the intact skin using soaked gauze. Wipe in and over a facial or scalp laceration. Chemical contact with a wound should be for at least 10 minutes, but no longer than 30 minutes. Action onset is within 15 to 30 minutes.

LOCAL ANESTHESIA

1. Select the appropriate anesthetic agent. Use lidocaine without epinephrine (1% or 2%); Lidocaine with epinephrine (1% or 2%), or Bupivacaine (Marcaine). Use room temperature solution whenever possible to reduce pain.
2. Wipe the top of vials with an alcohol swab and draw up the anesthetic agent with an 18-gauge needle in a 10:1 ratio with sodium bicarbonate (1 to 3 ml is usually sufficient for a biopsy). The sodium bicarbonate helps reduce pain.
3. Remove the needle and choose the smallest appropriate needle for injection (usually a 27- to 30-gauge needle, ½ to 1½ inches in length).
4. Inject the anesthetic agent slowly into the subcutaneous tissue, just deep to the dermis (Figure 2-7). Aspirate pulling back on the plunger before infiltration. If there is blood return, do not infiltrate, but reposition the needle and aspirate again to ensure it is not in a blood vessel. Repeat the above procedure until an adequate area is anesthetized for the procedure to be performed. When using anesthetic agents with vasoconstrictors, blanching of the skin is observed on injection. Take care to avoid injecting the solution while advancing the needle to the desired position. Inject only while withdrawing the needle.
5. Test the area for pain sensation before proceeding.
6. If there is marked or prolonged vasoconstriction in an area where epinephrine was used, consider rubbing nitroglycerin ointment into the skin over the area to produce vasodilation.

DIGITAL NERVE BLOCK

1. Perform a neurologic examination of the area to be anesthetized and document this in the medical record. Note any abnormalities in the examination before

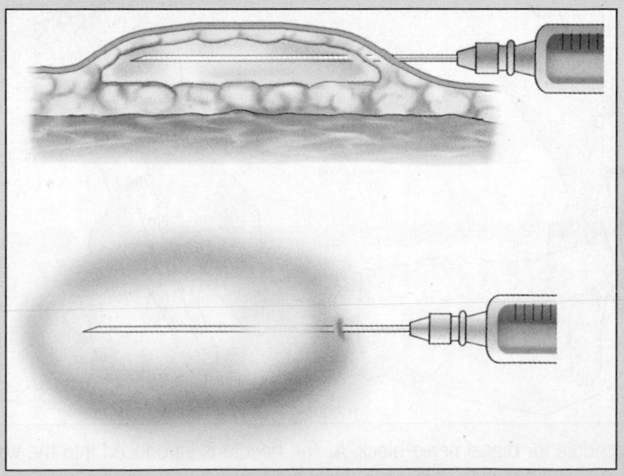

FIGURE 2-7 Subcutaneous infiltration without epinephrine. Injection is made during advance and withdrawal of needle.

2

inducing anesthesia. Review the related anatomy and remember the location and number of nerves supplying each digit.
2. Using gloves, apply topical anesthesia to the injection site (optional).
3. Wipe the top of vials with an alcohol swab and draw up the anesthetic agent with an 18-gauge needle in a 10:1 ratio with sodium bicarbonate (4 ml of 1% or 2% lidocaine *without* epinephrine).
4. Remove the needle and choose an appropriate needle for injection (usually 27- to 30-gauge needle, 1 to 1½ inches in length).
5. Clean and prepare the skin over the injection site in a sterile manner.
6. Insert the needle in the dorsal-lateral aspect of the finger or toe, just distal to the metacarpophalangeal joint until it touches bone (Figure 2-8). Aspirate for blood

2

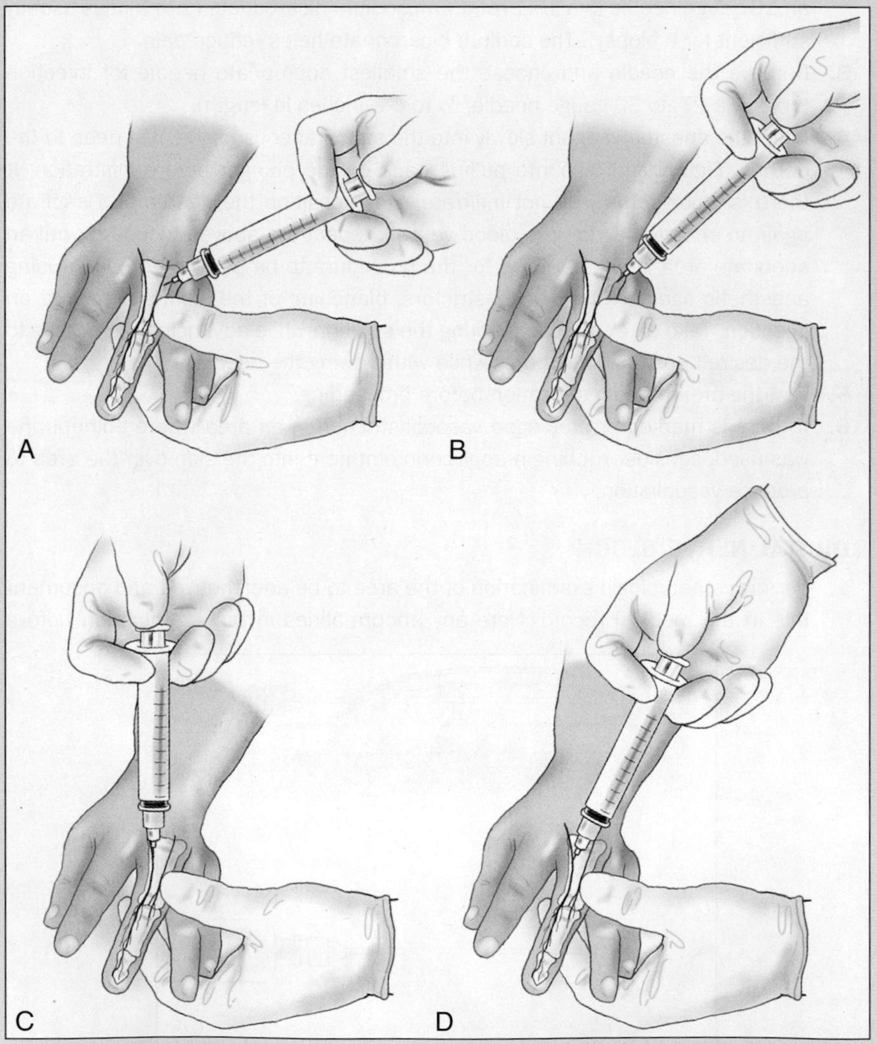

FIGURE 2-8 Procedure for digital nerve block. **A,** The needle is introduced into the webspace and advanced toward the dorsal digital nerve. **B,** After deposition of the anesthetic agent, the needle is redirected, without withdrawing it from the skin. The needle is moved toward the volar nerve, and anesthetic agent is deposited there. **C** and **D,** Repeat the same steps on the opposite side of the same digit.

(change needle position and reaspirate if needed), and then inject about 0.5 ml of anesthetic agent at this point. Advance the needle adjacent to the bone to the volar surface and, after aspiration, inject about 1 ml of the anesthetic agent around the palmar nerve.

7. Repeat the procedure on the opposite side of the digit.
8. Allow 5 to 15 minutes for anesthesia to take full effect. Test for sensation before performing the procedure.

PATIENT EDUCATION POSTPROCEDURE

Discuss with the patient the typical duration of the anesthesia and the need to protect the area from injury during this time.

COMPLICATIONS

Complications are rare, although allergic reactions may occur. Systemic absorption or injection of anesthetic agents may cause central nervous system or cardiac symptoms; if these occur, supportive care should be given. Epinephrine may cause systemic symptoms, such as arrhythmias, but this is rare. The use of epinephrine in areas with terminal vasculature can cause ischemia.

PRACTITIONER FOLLOW-UP

Follow-up is based on the procedure that is performed after anesthesia is induced.

REFERENCES AND RELATED RESOURCES

Calder K, Chung B, O'Brien C, Lalonde DH: Bupivacaine digital blocks: how long is the pain relief and temperature elevation? *Plast Reconstr Surg* 131(5):1098–1104, 2013.

Campo TM, Lafferty KA, editors: *Essential procedures for practitioners in emergency, urgent, and primary care settings*, New York, 2011, Springer.

Latham JL, Martin SN: Infiltrative anesthesia in office practice, *Am Fam Physician* 89(12):956–962, 2014.

Miller RD, Ward TA, McCulloch CE, Cohen NH: A comparison of lidocaine and bupivacaine digital nerve blocks on noninvasive continuous hemoglobin monitoring in a randomized trial in volunteers, *Anesth Analg* 118(4):766–771, 2014.

Suturing Simple Lacerations

Tom Bartol

DESCRIPTION

Lacerations are frequently seen in the primary care as well as the urgent/emergency care settings. Lacerations are seen throughout the life span. Many lacerations occur in young adult males with the majority of injuries involving the head, face, neck, and upper extremities. They are caused by trauma, blunt force, falls, sharp objects, or bites. Goals of laceration repair are to stop bleeding, promote healing, prevent infection, preserve function, and restore appearance (cosmetic). Wound closure holds wound edges together to facilitate the body's natural healing processes.

2

One of three strategies may be used for treating open wounds: (1) primary closure at the time of the presentation of the patient using sutures, staples, adhesives, or surgical tape; (2) delayed primary closure 3 to 4 days after the incident. This involves cleansing and debridement upon initial encounter, followed by delayed closure; and (3) healing by secondary intention is allowing a wound to heal without closure through the natural process of scar formation. This may be appropriate for small wounds in low tension areas as well as for larger wounds with avulsed or damaged skin that cannot be surgically closed. This is a slower process and may result in poorer cosmetic outcomes.

Skin tears are wounds caused by friction or blunt force that cause a separation in the layers of the skin on a horizontal plane. These often occur in older adults and usually on the extremities. These are different from lacerations and should not be treated with wound closure techniques used to treat lacerations.

ANATOMY AND PHYSIOLOGY

Lacerations may involve the epidermis, dermis, and subcutaneous layers or hypodermis. The epidermis and dermis can be treated as a single layer for the purposes of wound closure. The subcutaneous layer consists of adipose tissue and vascular and nerves structures. Beneath the subcutaneous layer are muscles and tendons. If a wound involves these deeper structures, it then changes from a "simple" wound to a "complex" wound. This type of wound will require subcutaneous closure or layered closure.

The majority of the strength of a skin closure is through the dermal layer. Subcutaneous closure does not provide strength of closure as much as it helps to repair underlying structures and reduce dead space. A healing wound has about 20% of its preinjury strength by 3 weeks and about 60% by 4 months.

The healing process of any wound, whether closed or healing by secondary intention, involves the process of scar formation. The final component of scar formation involves scar contraction. Areas of the body with better blood supply, such as the face, result in faster healing. The lesser trauma there is to the affected skin, the better the outcome. Better healing is also seen with less skin tension on the wound when it is closed.

CONTRAINDICATIONS

Wound closure should be based on a thorough history and assessment of the wound. The "golden period" or time from the wound occurring to closure is a concept that has generated significant research. Numerous studies since 1998 have suggested that wound closure can be safely carried out from 6 to 10 hours after the occurrence in wounds of the extremities, and 10 to 12 hours or more for wounds of the face or the scalp. These timeframes are guidelines and the decision to close wounds or not should be based on a thorough assessment of the patient. Contaminated wounds should be left open or closure should be delayed 3 to 4 days after they are cleaned, debrided, and checked for infection. Bites from humans and cats are more susceptible to infection than bites from dogs. Dog bite lacerations without signs of infection may be loosely closed for better cosmetic healing. Dog bites that are a puncture wound, not a laceration, must be evaluated and treated as a puncture wound that may involve deeper tissues and may cause a crush injury. Traditionally mammalian bite lacerations have not been closed, but more recent evidence shows closure in well irrigated, cleaned, and debrided bite lacerations may be considered.

PRECAUTIONS

All lacerations should be thoroughly inspected for damage to underlying structures, such as tendons or bones, as well as for foreign bodies such as glass, wood, or metal (also note precautions in "Anesthesia: Topical, Local, and Digital Nerve Blocks"). Devitalized tissue should be debrided before a wound is closed. Devitalized tissue can be recognized by its blue or black appearance, and it is often shredded. Simple debridement can be performed using tissue forceps and iris scissors.

Care must be taken not to traumatize healthy skin when using the tissue forceps (with teeth) or any other instrument to examine, explore, or close a wound. Trauma, even from a tissue forceps, can devitalize tissue and impair wound healing. If skin must be move around, a tissue hook (which can be fashioned from a 21-gauge needle that is bent into a hook at the tip) can be used.

2

RED FLAG

Certain types of wounds require more expertise than just knowledge of basic wound closure. Each wound should be thoroughly assessed, and the clinician must then determine his or her knowledge and comfort level in closing the wound. The following wounds require special treatment and closure, and referral should be made to a consultant, especially if the clinician is not experienced with this type of situation.

- Wounds that cannot be assessed and adequately explored
- Wounds with underlying damage to tendons, nerves, and/or blood vessels
- Wounds that require multiple layer closure (unless clinician is experienced with this type)
- Compression or crush injuries with extensive soft tissue damage
- Injection injuries caused by high-pressure equipment, such as paint guns
- Significant wounds in patients who have underlying systemic disorders that may affect wound healing, such as immunosuppression, peripheral vascular disease, or diabetes
- Wounds of the face where there is concern about cosmetic outcome
- Complex wounds with damage to tendons or nerves, or with joint penetration
- Wounds associated with fractures (i.e., open fractures)

ASSESSMENT

- Initial assessment should include assessment of the amount of bleeding and an evaluation for more serious underlying disorders. In cases of trauma, be sure to assess the patient from head to toe. A bleeding wound may distract both family and clinician from more serious conditions, such as internal injuries.
- Remember to assess airway, breathing, and circulation.
- Rings and other jewelries should always be removed from injured hands or fingers if they impair assessment and treatment, or if they impair or may potentially impair circulation as a result of swelling.
- Determine the mechanism of injury. Blunt and shearing injury can cause tissue damage and underlying injury. Bites may cause puncture wounds and even crush injuries in addition to lacerations.
- Assess the time of occurrence of the injury.

- Assess for signs and symptoms of underlying damage.
- Determine the patient's past medical history including conditions that may affect wound healing or increase the risk of infection, such as diabetes, immunodeficiency diseases, or peripheral vascular disease.
- Ascertain a history of allergies, current medications, and tetanus immunization status.
- Physical examination should include vital signs, with an assessment for signs of hypovolemia and infection (including temperature). Based on the mechanism of injury, a brief secondary examination should be made to assess for underlying injuries.
- Before closure, all wounds should be cleansed, irrigated, and explored for foreign bodies. This may be more effectively accomplished after anesthesia is induced. Further assessment depends on the type of injury and on the findings of the initial examination.
- Determine the location, length, and depth of the wound, and the presence of infection.
- Assess for neurovascular status distal to the injury.
- Clean wounds in nonimmunocompromised patients do not require prophylactic antibiotics. Patients who have wounds that are obviously infected or contaminated should receive prophylactic antibiotics and consideration should be given to delayed closure. Irrigation and debridement are essential.

2

PATIENT PREPARATION

Consent

Informed consent should be obtained. The procedure should be explained to the patient, including the risks and benefits, possible complications, and alternatives to the procedure. The patients should be given an opportunity to ask questions about the procedure. Discuss the fact that scarring may occur.

Position the patient comfortably so that the wound can be easily accessed for cleaning, exploration, irrigation, and closure. Place the affected area in a dependent position if feasible.

Anesthesia

Administer local anesthesia or a digital block as outlined in previous section.

Explore and Irrigate

Once anesthetized, thoroughly explore the wound for depth, underlying damage, and foreign bodies. Remove foreign bodies as appropriate. Exploration can be aided by using a blunt object, such as a forceps, to probe and move tissue. Irrigation with normal saline solution using copious amounts of saline and a large (20-ml) syringe with a large-bore catheter with needle removed is effective in forcing out bacteria and debris from the wound (Figure 2-9). You may use an IV saline solution with a pressure bag. Do not use a bulb syringe or an IV bag without pressure because they do not deliver adequate pressure for irrigation. Do ***not*** irrigate or soak wounds in hydrogen peroxide, povidone iodine, or other solutions. Always use water or normal saline solution. Devitalized areas can then be débrided. If skin edges do not approximate well, undermining with the use of blunt dissection with an iris scissor can increase skin mobility (Figure 2-10). Tetanus prophylaxis can be administered if indicated (see "Wound Care").

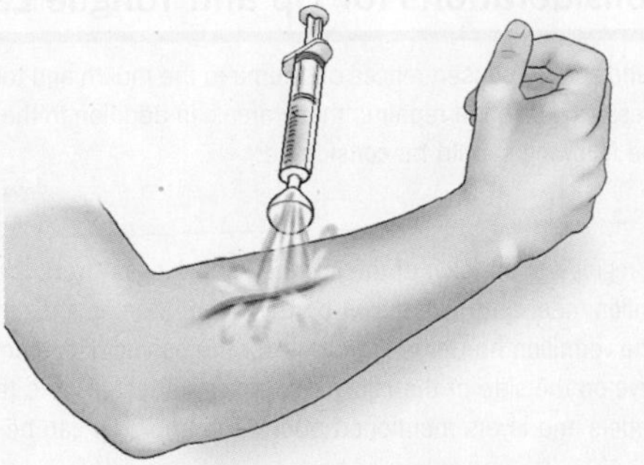

FIGURE 2-9 Technique for wound irrigation. Hold shield close to the wound.

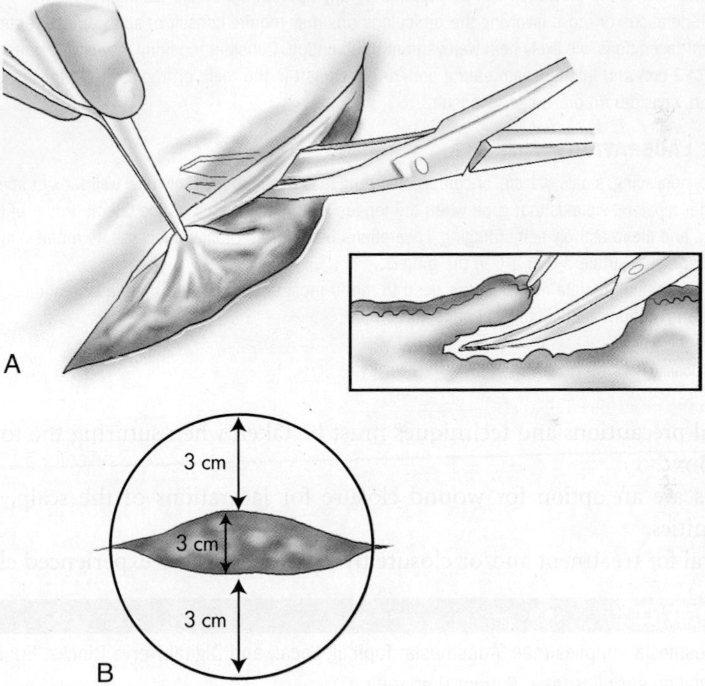

FIGURE 2-10 Undermining tissue. **A,** Use scissors for dissection at the dermal superficial fascia level. Tissue spreading with forceps providing lateral tension is preferable to cutting the sharp edges. **B,** The zone of undermining is illustrated.

TREATMENT ALTERNATIVES

- Small wounds or avulsed skin may be left open to heal by secondary intention. Even larger wounds will heal by secondary intention should the patient decline closure, although it may take longer and poorer cosmetic outcomes may occur.
- For appropriate wounds, tissue adhesives may be used to close the wound.
- Scalp wounds can sometimes be closed using a hair apposition technique (HAT). Hair on either side of the wound is twisted together and tissue adhesive is applied to secure the twist. If there is significant bleeding, this technique may not work well because hemostasis is more difficult to achieve.

BOX 2-1 Special Considerations for Lip and Tongue Lacerations

As a result of the cosmetic and speech consequences of trauma to the mouth and tongue, special consideration should be made when addressing laceration repair in these areas. In addition to the other information provided in the laceration section, the following should be considered:

LIP LACERATIONS

- There are three distinct regions of the skin of the lip: the oral mucosa (wet), the vermilion (dry), and the skin. The skin and vermilion meet at the vermilion border where there is a distinct red line and white line.
- Accurate matching of the vermilion border is important for the cosmetic outcome of lip lacerations. A block of the mental nerve on the side of the injury can provide anesthesia to the lower lip without disrupting the many borders and layers mentioned above. The upper lip can be numbed by performing an infraorbital block.
- If the vermilion border is involved in the laceration, this should be approximated first with a nonabsorbable 6-0 suture, followed by the wet-dry border.
- The remainder of the laceration can be repaired by any appropriate suture technique.
- Large lacerations or those involving the orbicularis oris may require consult or surgical intervention.
- Intraoral lacerations will likely heal well without intervention. Consider repairing intraoral lesions that are large (>2 cm) and interfere with eating and/or get caught in the teeth or trap food. If Stenson's duct is involved, consider an oral surgery consult.

TONGUE LACERATIONS

- Simple, nongaping, small, <1 cm, uncomplicated tongue lacerations will likely heal well without intervention.
- Consider repairing wounds that gape when the tongue is at rest, wounds on the lateral border of the tongue, and those actively hemorrhaging. Lacerations bisecting the tongue necessitate repair with sutures. Use absorbable suture 3-0 or 4-0 in the tongue.
- There are conflicting data regarding the need to repair most uncomplicated tongue lacerations.
- Partial amputations require surgical consultation.

Box courtesy of Joanne Rolls.

- Special precautions and techniques must be taken when suturing the tongue and lips (Box 2-1).
- Staples are an option for wound closure for lacerations of the scalp, trunk, or extremities.
- Referral for treatment and/or closure by surgeon or other experienced clinician.

EQUIPMENT

- Anesthesia supplies (see "Anesthesia: Topical, Local, and Digital Nerve Blocks, Equipment")
- Irrigation supplies (see "Patient Preparation")
- Suture tray
  - Sterile 2 × 2 or 4 × 4 gauze sponges (at least 8 to 10)
  - Needle holder
  - Iris scissors
  - Tissue forceps
  - Curved mosquito clamp
  - Skin hook or 21-gauge needle to make into skin hook
  - Sterile fenestrated drapes
- Appropriate suture materials (Boxes 2-2 and 2-3)
- Sterile gloves
- Eye and face protection
- Protective gown

BOX 2-2 Suture Selection

- Choose sutures on the basis of their basic characteristics of tissue reactivity, knot holding, wick action, tensile strength, and cost. (See Table 2-8 for suture selection.)
- Suture material also can be absorbable or nonabsorbable and either monofilament or braided. The size of the sutures and needle type should also be considered.
- Tissue reactivity is an important consideration in the selection of suture material. High tissue reactivity may lead to scar and fissure formation.
- Knots are the weakest part of the suture. Proper knotting technique is essential. The different suture materials vary in their knot-holding properties.
- Nonabsorbable sutures are used for suturing superficial lacerations. Absorbable sutures are used for layered closure of deep lacerations.
- Braided sutures are stronger and hold knots better than monofilament sutures, but monofilament sutures are less likely to harbor infection.
- Suture size is indicated by the number of 0's; more 0's designate smaller sutures. For example, a 4-0 suture material is smaller than a 3-0 suture material. Smaller sutures leave less of a scar, but are not as strong as larger sutures and are harder to see to remove. (See Tables 2-8 and 2-9 for suture selection and use.)
  In general, the different suture sizes used on parts of the body are:
  - Face: 5-0 to 6-0
  - Scalp: 3-0 to 5-0
  - Extremities: 4-0 to 5-0
  - Back/Chest/Abdomen: 3-0 to 4-0

(See Table 2-9 for more specific details.)

BOX 2-3 Needle Selection

Use a cutting needle to suture skin. A three-eighths curvature is usually adequate. The manufacturers have codes for their products that denote purpose and size.

- "For skin" (FS) and "cutting" (CE) needles should be used on thick skin.
- On cosmetic areas, plastic (P), plastic skin (PS), premium (PRE), or precision cosmetic (PC) needles are recommended.
- Facial closures are often performed with a P-3 needle, whereas other areas with thicker skin require an FS-2 or FS-3 needle (Figures 2-11 and 2-12).

TABLE 2-8 Common Suture Materials

SUTURE	TYPES	MAKEUP	USE	TISSUE REACTION	ABSORPTION RATE	TENSILE STRENGTH RETENTION
ABSORBABLE						
Gut	Plain	Mammalian collagen	Superficial vessels and quick-healing subcutaneous tissues	Moderate	70 days	7-10 days
Gut	Chromic	Mammalian collagen	Versatile; also good in the presence of infection; do not use on skin because of reaction	Moderate	90 days	21-28 days
Polyglycolic acid (Dexon*)	Mono	Synthetic polymer	Buried sutures; good tensile and knot strength	Mild	40%; 7 days	20% in 15 days, 5% in 28 days

Continued

TABLE 2-8 Common Suture Materials—cont'd

SUTURE	TYPES	MAKEUP	USE	TISSUE REACTION	ABSORPTION RATE	TENSILE STRENGTH RETENTION
Polydioxanone (PDS†)	Mono	Polyester polymer	Versatile; body cavity closure, bowel	Mild	210 days	70% in 14 days, 50% in 28 days
Polyglactic acid (Vicryl†)	Braided	Coated polymer	Subcutaneous skin; buried sutures	Mild	60-90 days	60% in 14 days, 30% in 21 days
Polyglyconate (Maxon)	Mono	Polyester	Smoother knot and excellent first-throw holding	Mild	180-210 days	81% in 14 days, 59% in 28 days
NONABSORBABLE						
Cotton	Twisted fibers	Cotton fiber	Ligating some skin, but generally too reactive	Minimal	Never; encapsulated in the body	50% in 6 months, 30% in 2 years
Silk	Braided	Silkworm-spun fiber	Ligating some skin, but rarely used	Moderate	2 years	Gone in 1 year
Steel	Mono	Alloy Fe-Ni-Cr	Tendons, sternum, abdominal wall	Low	Never; encapsulated in the body	Indefinite
Nylon (Ethilon, Dermalon)	Mono	Synthetic polymer	Skin	Very low	20% a year	Loses 20% a year
Polyester (Mersilene)	Braided	Polyester	Cardiovascular, general, and plastic surgery	Minimal	Never; encapsulated in the body	Indefinite
Polypropylene (Prolene†)	Mono	Synthetic polymer	Skin, vascular, plastic surgery	Minimal	Never; encapsulated in the body	Indefinite

Adapted from Pfenninger JL, Fowler GC: *Procedures for primary care physicians,* ed 3, St Louis, 2011; Dehn RW, Asprey DP, editors: *Essential clinical procedures,* ed 3, St Louis, 2013, Elsevier, p 238.

*Dexon Plus has a synthetic coating to facilitate knot tying and passage through tissue.

†Vicryl, Prolene, and PDS are registered trademarks of Ethicon, Inc.

TABLE 2-9 Common Suture Use

	SKIN (INTERRUPTED)	SKIN (SUBCUTICULAR)	BURIED	REMOVAL
Face	5-0 or 6-0 nylon	4-0 or 5-0 Prolene	4-0 or 5-0 synthetic absorbable or 6-0 clear nylon	4-7 days
Extremities, trunk	4-0 or 5-0 nylon	3-0 or 4-0 synthetic absorbable	4-0 Prolene or 3-0 or 4-0 synthetic absorbable	7-14 days

From Pfenninger JL, Fowler GC: *Procedures for primary care physicians,* ed 3, St Louis, 2011, Mosby.

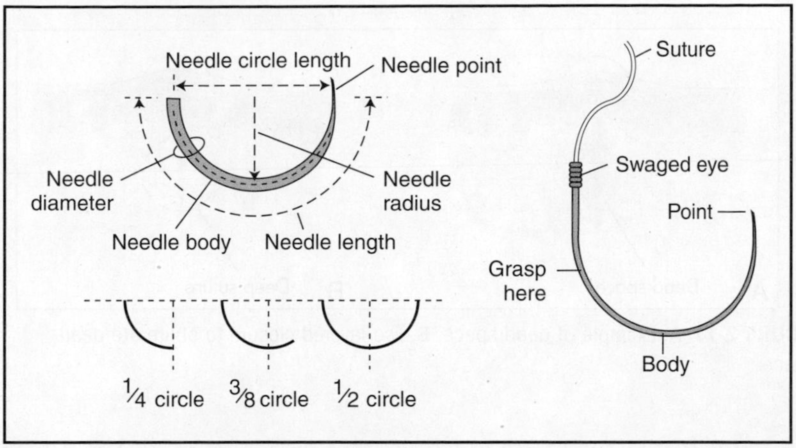

FIGURE 2-11 Anatomy of a surgical needle.

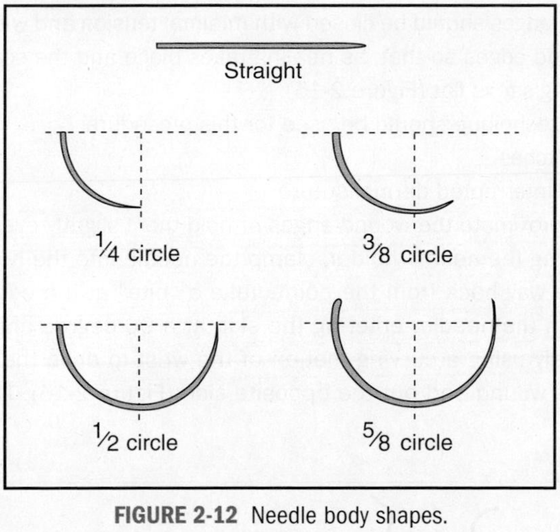

FIGURE 2-12 Needle body shapes.

Procedure

1. Prepare wound.

a. Assess wound and clean as described earlier.

b. Position patient for comfort and safety.

c. Provide anesthesia (see "Anesthesia: Topical, Local, and Digital Nerve Block").

d. Explore, irrigate, débride, and prepare wound as outlined earlier.

2. General principles

a. Wounds should be closed to eliminate dead space beneath the dermis (Figure 2-13). This prevents the accumulation of fluid and bacteria under the skin.

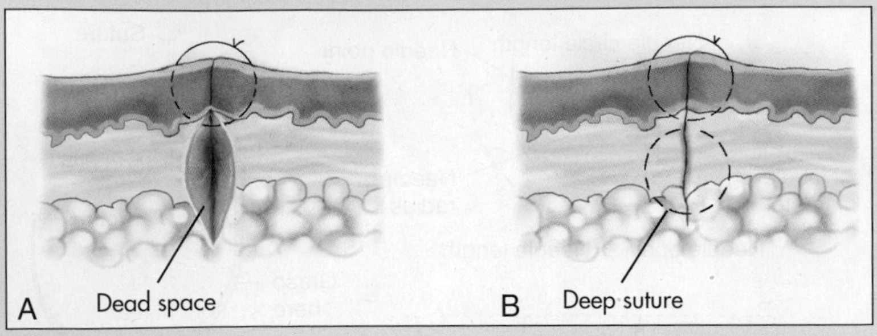

FIGURE 2-13 **A,** Example of dead space. **B,** Two-layered closure to obliterate dead space.

b. Wounds should be closed in layers—deep fascia to deep fascia, superficial fascia to superficial fascia, and dermis to dermis—approximating each layer as the wound is closed if indicated (Figure 2-14).

c. Wound edges should be closed with minimal tension and with slight eversion of wound edges so that, as healing takes place and the scar contracts, the resulting site is flat (Figure 2-15).

d. Sterile technique should be used for this procedure.

3. Types of stitches

a. Simple interrupted dermal suture

(1) Approximate the wound edges or hold them slightly everted.

(2) Using the needle holder, clamp the needle into the holder about ⅔ of the way back from the point. Take a "bite" at the edge of the wound with the needle, entering the skin at a 90-degree angle and continuously using a curving motion of the wrist to drive the needle through the wound and out the opposite side (Figure 2-16). The stitch should

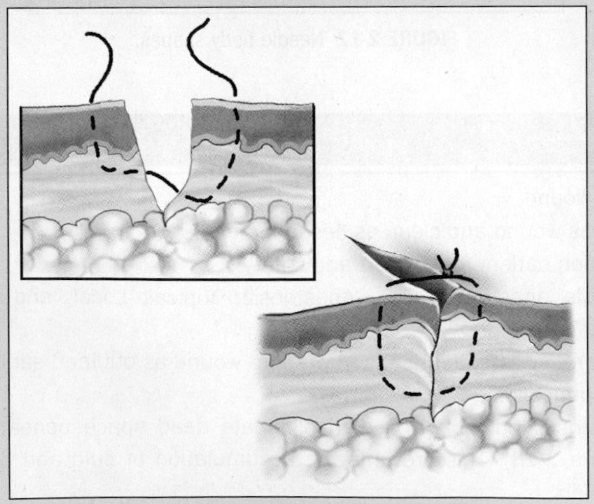

FIGURE 2-14 Incorrect technique causes mismatch of layers.

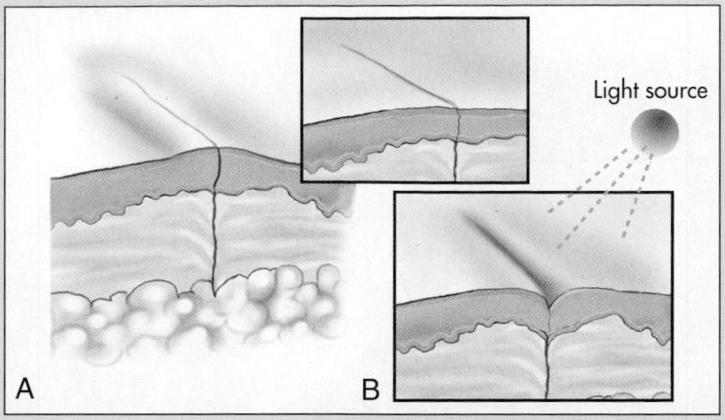

FIGURE 2-15 Wound edge eversion. **A,** Correct technique allows for a slight rise of the wound edges above the skin plane. These edges contract and flatten out at the skin plane as healing takes place. **B,** Wound edges that are not properly everted contract beneath the skin and allow light to cause unsightly shadows.

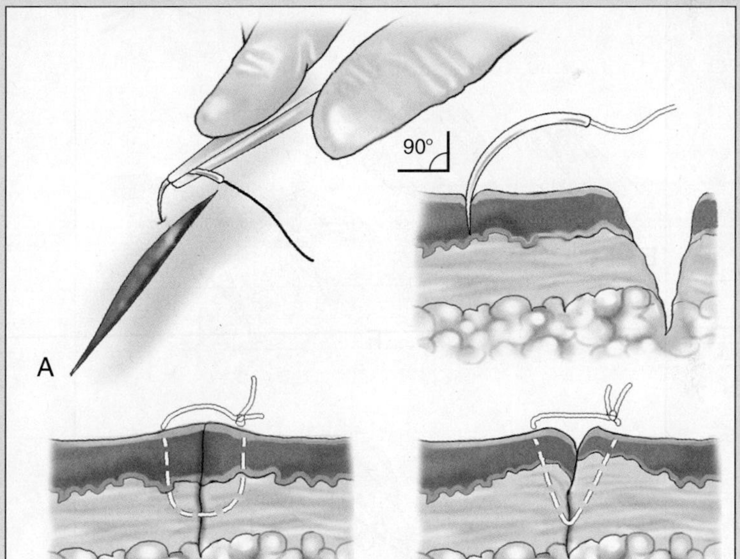

FIGURE 2-16 Technique for proper wound-edge eversion. **A,** The suture needle is introduced at a 90-degree angle to the epidermis. **B,** Theoretically the proper configuration of the suture should be square or bottle shaped. This is difficult to accomplish, but the figure illustrates the correct principle. **C,** The incorrect technique of needle placement and suture configuration leads to wound edge inversion, causing "pitting" of the scar as it develops.

be as wide as it is deep. Check to see that the wound is symmetrically approximated before tying. The suture is tied using an instrument tie (Figure 2-17). When tying the suture, pull tightly enough to approximate the wound edges and slightly evert them. If there is excessive skin tension, it may be necessary to remove the stitch to further

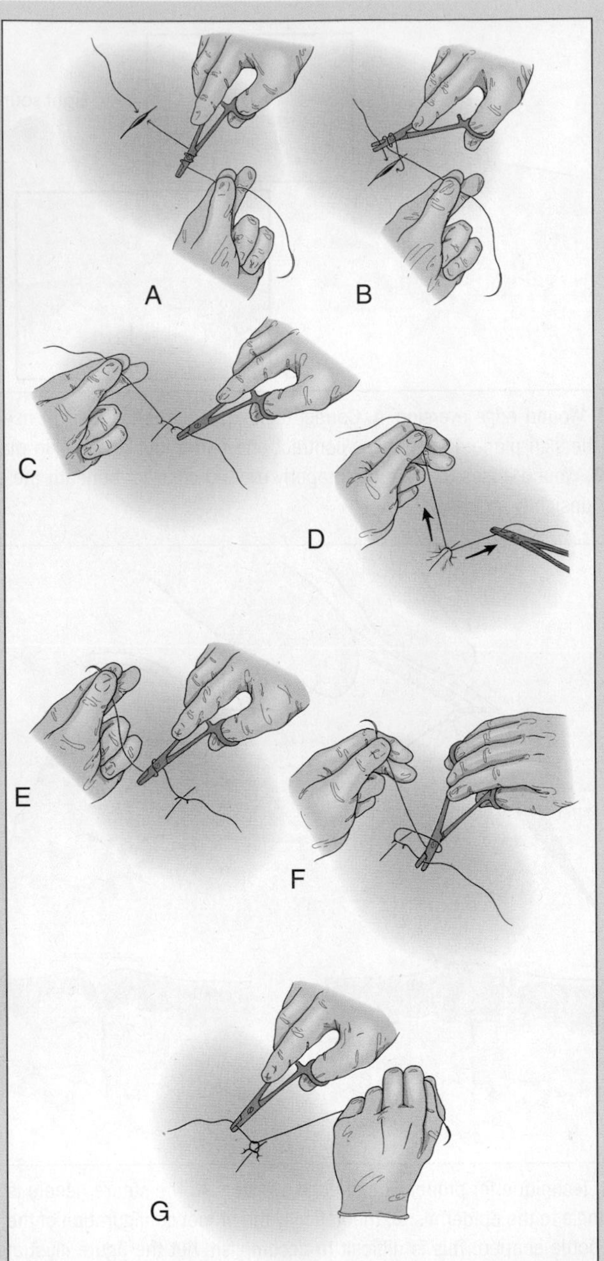

FIGURE 2-17 Instrument tie. Manipulate the needle end of the suture using the nondominant hand and the needle holder with the dominant hand. The suture enters the far side and exits the near side of the wound. **A,** Lay the needle holder on the suture on the near side and wrap the suture around the needle holder twice. **B,** Reach back with the needle holder and grab the free suture end. **C,** Cross hands and pull back the free end toward the near side and bring the needle end of suture to the far side. **D,** Raise both suture ends and cinch the first throw. **E,** Lay the needle holder on the suture on the far side and loop once. **F,** Reach back and take the free suture end. **G,** Cross hands to create a square knot. This pattern is repeated four or five times.

undermine the skin. Continue to place sutures to close the wound, spacing them a distance equal to the distance between the entrance and exit sites of each suture.

b. Subcutaneous suture (for deeper, layered closures) (Figure 2-18)
   (1) An absorbable suture is used for subcutaneous sutures.
   (2) The knot is buried or inverted to aid in the approximation of the skin edges.
   (3) Begin the stitch in the bottom of the wound, coming out through the dermis, then entering the dermis from the opposite side, and then coming out deep beneath the epidermis. Use an instrument tie, but do not use a locking wrap on your first tie, and use only two or three knots. This reduces the "bulk" from the knots beneath the skin.

c. Vertical mattress suture (Figure 2-19)
   (1) This suture is a strong stitch that helps evert wound edges.

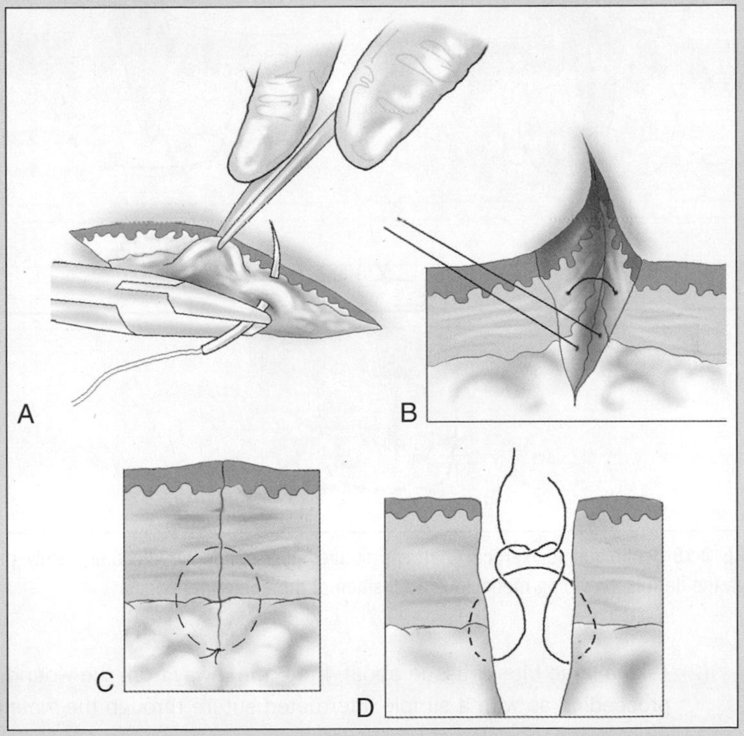

FIGURE 2-18 Technique for placing a deep suture. **A,** Begin suture placement by sending the needle deep into the wound to the superficial level. **B,** Then send the needle superficial to deep on the opposite side of the wound. The leading and trailing sutures come out on the same side of the cross-suture. **C,** This same-side technique allows for the knot to be tied deep and away from the wound surface. **D,** If the same side-technique is not followed, the knot is forced to the wound surface by the cross-suture and may protrude out of the wound.

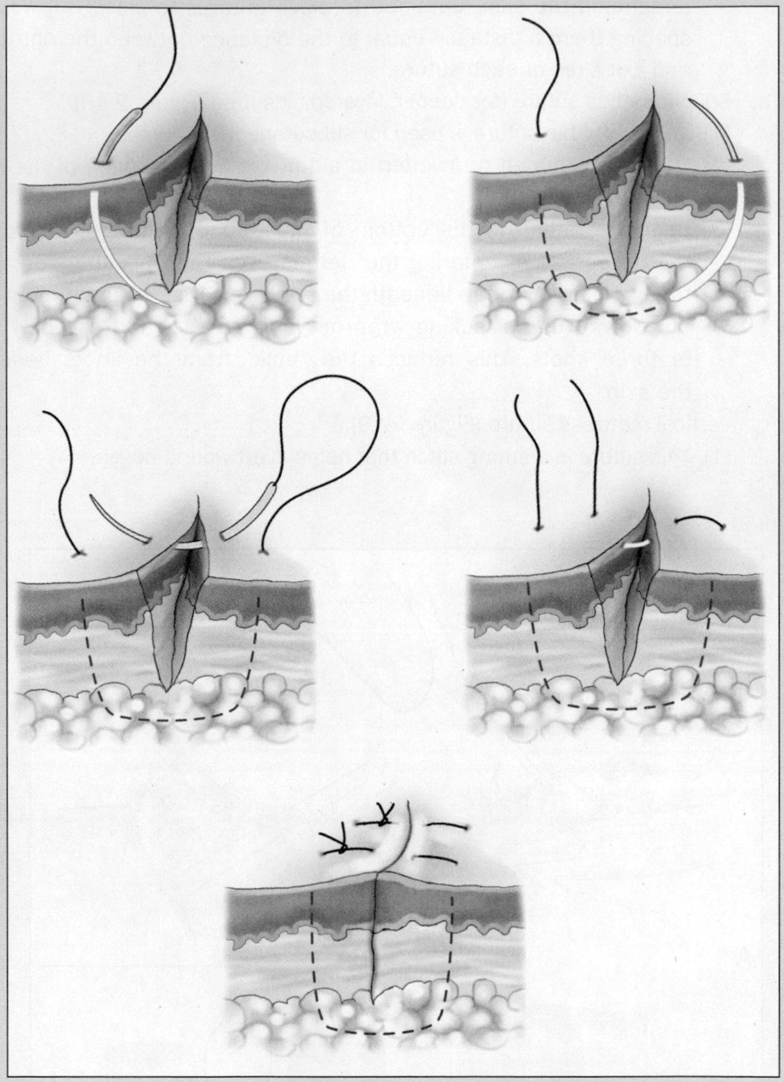

FIGURE 2-19 Technique for vertical mattress suture. The second needle bite barely passes through the dermis, providing meticulous apposition of the epidermal edges.

(2) Take a large bite of tissue about 4 to 6 mm away from the wound edge, proceeding as with a simple interrupted suture through the wound and out the opposite side of the wound.
(3) Reverse the needle and take a small bite 1 to 2 mm from the wound edge where the needle just exited, and through the wound, exit with a small bite on the opposite side of the wound, just 1 to 2 mm from the edge.
(4) Tie the suture using an instrument tie.
(5) Employ general wound care and apply the dressing as appropriate.

PATIENT EDUCATION POSTPROCEDURE

- Instruct the patient in proper wound care (see "Wound Care"). Provide the patient specific instructions regarding follow-up care and suture removal (see "Suture Removal").
- If the wound was very dirty or was caused by a crushing injury, or there are other concerns about wound healing or infection, schedule appropriate follow-up before the time of the suture removal for reevaluation.
- Instruct the patient to elevate the injured area, if appropriate, to reduce tissue swelling and thus tension on the wound edges. Ice can be applied intermittently to wounds on the head or face to reduce swelling.
- If the wound is over a joint, splinting should be used to reduce tension and improve wound healing.

COMPLICATIONS

- Bleeding and hematoma formation (some degree of this is normal)
- Infection
- Skin necrosis
- Wound dehiscence
- Unfavorable features of scars

PRACTITIONER FOLLOW-UP

- The patient should schedule follow-up for the suture removal as outlined in the next section.
- If signs of infection develop, the patient should be advised to return for follow-up.
- If incomplete healing has taken place at the time of follow-up, sutures may be left in place for a few additional days, or every other suture may be removed and then reinforced with wound tapes.

■ CPT BILLING

The repair of wounds may be classified as Simple, Intermediate, or Complex.

Simple repair is used when the wound is superficial; involving primarily epidermis, or subcutaneous tissues without significant involvement of deeper structures, and requires simple one layer closure. This involves local anesthesia. Wound closure utilizing adhesive strips as the sole repair material should be coded using the appropriate E/M code.

Intermediate repair includes the repair of wounds that, in addition to the above, require layered closure of one or more of the deeper layers of subcutaneous tissue and superficial (non-muscle) fascia, in addition to the skin (epidermal and dermal) closure. Single layer closure of heavily contaminated wounds that have required extensive cleaning or removal of particulate matter also constitutes intermediate repair.

Complex repair includes the repair of wounds requiring more than layered closure, such as scar revisions, traumatic lacerations or avulsions, extreme undermining, stents or retention sutures.

The repair wound(s) should be measured and recorded in centimeters, whether curved, angular, or stellate.

When multiple wounds are repaired, add the lengths of those in the same classification and from all anatomic sites that are grouped together into the same code descriptor. Do not add lengths of repair from different groups of anatomic sites (e.g., face and extremities) or from different classifications (simple and intermediate).

When more than one classification of wound is repaired, list the more complicated as the primary procedure and the less complicated as the secondary procedure, using modifier 59 – Distinct Procedural

Service. New codes added by Medicare in January 2015 further define modifier 59 with XE, XP, XS, or XU subsets.

Decontamination and/or debridement is considered a separate procedure only when gross contamination requires prolonged cleansing, when appreciable amounts of devitalized or contaminated tissue are removed, or when debridement is carried out separately without intermediate primary closure.

Simple exploration of nerves, blood vessels, or tendons exposed in an open wound is also considered part of the essential treatment of the wound and is not a separate procedure unless appreciable dissection is required.

12001–Simple repair of superficial wounds of scalp, neck, axillae, external genitalia, trunk and/or extremities (including hands and feet); 2.5 cm or less ■ **12001 - 12007**–Simple repair of superficial wounds of scalp, neck, axillae, external genitalia, trunk and/or extremities (including hands and feet); 2.6 cm to over 30 cm ■ **12011**–Simple repair of superficial wounds of face, ears, eyelids, nose, lips and/or mucous membranes; 2.5 cm or less ■ **12013 - 12018**–Simple repair of superficial wounds of face, ears, eyelids, nose, lips and/or mucous membranes; 2.6 cm to over 30 cm ■ **12020**–Treatment of superficial wound dehiscence; simple closure ■ **12021**–Treatment of superficial wound dehiscence; simple closure, with packing ■ **12031**–Repair, intermediate of wounds of scalp, axillae, trunk and/or extremities (including hands and feet); 2.5 cm or less ■ **12032 - 12037**–Repair, intermediate of wounds of scalp, axillae, trunk and/or extremities (including hands and feet); 2.6 cm to over 30 cm ■ **12041**–Repair, intermediate, wounds of neck, hands, feet and/or external genitalia; 2.5 cm or less ■ **12042 - 12047**–Repair, intermediate, wounds of neck, hands, feet and/or external genitalia; 2.6 cm to over 30 cm ■ **12051**–Repair, intermediate, wounds of face, ears, eyelids, nose, lips and/or mucous membranes; 2.5 cm or less ■ **12052 - 12057**–Repair, intermediate, wounds of face, ears, eyelids, nose, lips and/or mucous membranes; 2.6 cm to over 30 cm ■ **13100**–Repair, complex, trunk; 1.1 cm to 2.5 cm ■ **13101**–Repair, complex, trunk; 2.6 cm to 7.5 cm ■ **13102**–Repair, complex, trunk, each additional 5 cm or less. List separately, in addition to code for primary procedure. ■ **13120**–Repair, complex, scalp, arms, and/or legs; 1.1 cm to 2.5 cm (For 1.0 cm or less, see simple or intermediate repair) ■ **13121**–Repair, complex, scalp, arms, and/or legs; 2.6 cm to 7.5 cm ■ **13122**–Repair, complex, scalp, arms, and/or legs; each additional 5 cm or less. List separately, in addition to code for primary procedure. ■ **13131**–Repair, complex, forehead, cheeks, chin, mouth, neck, axillae, genitalia, hands and/or feet; 1.1 cm to 2.5 cm ■ **13132**–Repair, complex, forehead, cheeks, chin, mouth, neck, axillae, genitalia, hands and/or feet; 2.6 cm to 7.5 cm ■ **13133**–Repair, complex, forehead, cheeks, chin, mouth, neck, axillae, genitalia, hands and/or feet; each additional 5 cm or less. List separately, in addition to code for primary procedure. ■ **13151**–Repair, complex, eyelids, nose, ears and/or lips; 1.1 cm to 2.5 cm ■ **13152**–Repair, complex, eyelids, nose, ears and/or lips; 2.6 cm to 7.5 cm ■ **13153**–Repair, complex, eyelids, nose, ears and/or lips; each additional 5 cm or less. List separately, in addition to code for primary procedure. ■ **13160**–Secondary close of surgical wound or dehiscence, extensive or complicated.

REFERENCES AND RELATED RESOURCES

Brown D, Jaffe J, Henson J: Advanced laceration management, *Emerg Med Clin N Am* 25(1):83–99, 2007.

DeBoard RH, et al: Principles of basic wound evaluation and management in the emergency department, *Emerg Med Clin N Am* 25:23–39, 2007.

Forsch R: Essentials of skin laceration repair, *Am Fam Physician* 78(8):945–951, 952, 2008.

Patil PD, Panchabhai TS, Galwankar SC: Managing human bites, *J Emerg Trauma Shock* 2(3): 186–90, 2009.

Quinn JV, Polevoi SK, Kohn MA: Traumatic lacerations: what are the risks for infection and has the 'golden period' of laceration care disappeared? *Emerg Med J* 31:96–100, 2014.

Ricci NA, Rizzolo D: Laceration repair: avoiding infection, optimize healing, minimize scarring, *JAAPA* 24(9):28–33, 2011.

Rui-feng C, et al: Emergency treatment of facial laceration of dog bite wounds with immediate primary closure: a prospective randomized trial study, *BMC Emerg Med* 13(Suppl 1):52, 2013.

2

Stephen-Haynes J: Skin tears: achieving positive clinical and financial outcomes, *Br J Community Nurs* (Suppl):S6, S8, S10 passim, 2012.
Tejani C, et al: A comparison of cosmetic outcomes of lacerations on the extremities and trunk using absorbable versus nonabsorbable sutures, *Acad Emerg Med* 21:637–643, 2014.
Zehtabchi S, et al: The impact of wound age on the infection rate of simple lacerations repaired in the emergency department, Injury, *Int HJ Care Injured* 43:1793–1798, 2012.

Suture Removal

Tom Bartol

DESCRIPTION

Nonabsorbable sutures must be removed once the wound has adequately healed. Sutures should be removed as soon as possible once the wound has adequate strength to prevent dehiscence. The longer the sutures are left in place, the greater the risk for infection and the more likely there will be less optimal cosmetic effects.

ANATOMY AND PHYSIOLOGY

After a wound has been closed, barring interference from infection or other complications, wound healing begins to take place by primary intention. Neovascularization takes place; it is evident by day 3 and is most active by day 7. Neovascularization results in a red appearance around the wound and is often seen upon suture removal. Granulation tissue is formed as a result of neovascularization. Fibroblasts then begin to produce collagen fibrils that give strength to the wound. To prevent excessive collagen formation, collagen lysis also occurs. The delicate balance between collagen formation and lysis results in a vulnerable period about 7 to 10 days after the injury when the wound is most prone to dehiscence. The wound will have 5% of its original tensile strength at 2 weeks and 35% at 1 month, with full tensile strength not achieved for several months. At the time of suture removal, the wound is still quite fragile and may have to be reinforced after the sutures are removed. Suturing produces small puncture wounds around the original wound, which can cause keratinized epithelial plugs that leave visible scars on the skin. These scars are more likely to form the longer sutures are left in place.

INDICATIONS

Suture removal should take place at varying times based on the type of wound, age of the patient, and location of the wound (Table 2-10).

CONTRAINDICATIONS

There are none.

PRECAUTIONS

If wound healing is not adequate, sutures may be left in place longer, or every other interrupted suture may be removed with the remainder removed at a later time. Alternatively, sutures may be removed and the wound reinforced with wound tapes. Each wound must be evaluated individually.

TABLE 2-10 Recommended Intervals for Removal of Percutaneous (Skin) Sutures

LOCATION	DAYS TO REMOVAL
Scalp	6-8
Ear	4-5
Face	4-5
Hand*	8-10
Arm/leg*	8-10
Fingertip	10-12
Chest/abdomen	12-14
Back	8-10
Foot	12-14

*Add 2-3 days for joint extensor surfaces.

From Pfenninger JL, Fowler GC: *Procedures for primary care physicians,* ed 3, St Louis, 2011, Mosby.

2

ASSESSMENT

- The wound should be assessed for granulation and healing and for signs of infection or dehiscence.
- Assess for conditions that may delay wound healing, such as peripheral vascular disease, diabetes, or immunocompromised conditions.

PATIENT PREPARATION

The procedure should be explained to the patient, and questions should be answered. Some patients (especially children) may be anxious or afraid because of pain experienced during wound closure.

TREATMENT ALTERNATIVES

There are no alternatives if nonabsorbable cutaneous sutures have been placed. Leaving sutures in place may lead to infection, increased scarring, and/or a foreign body reaction.

EQUIPMENT

- Gloves
- Forceps
- Suture scissors
- Wound tapes

Procedure

1. Cleanse the area with soap and water if it is not clean. If sutures are crusted over, or are covered with granulation tissue, wash the area with warm water to remove crusts before removing the sutures.
2. Lift the suture with the forceps by gently pulling on the knot.
3. Using the suture scissors, cut the suture at skin entry on the side opposite the knot so as to minimize contamination by allowing the exposed suture to pass back through the wound (a No. 11 scalpel blade may be useful for cutting a very small suture).
4. Gently pull out the suture with the forceps.
5. Apply wound tape if reinforcement is needed.
6. Determine need for further dressing changes.

PATIENT EDUCATION POSTPROCEDURE

- Remind the patient that the wound is still healing and does not have full tensile strength for several months, so the area should be treated gently.
- If wound tapes are applied, these will fall off on their own, usually in a couple of days.
- The patient should continue to keep the wound clean and observe for signs of infection. A dressing is usually not required. If there are signs of infection or wound dehiscence, the patient should return for follow-up.
- Sunscreen should be used to protect the healing wound and resulting scar from prolonged exposure to the sun.

COMPLICATIONS

Infection may occur in sutured wounds. Wound dehiscence can occur after suture removal. Should wound dehiscence occur, the wound should be left to heal by secondary intention. Care must be taken during suture removal to prevent pieces of suture from remaining in the wound. Be sure to cut each suture in just one place (Figure 2-20).

PRACTITIONER FOLLOW-UP

No follow-up is needed unless complications occur.

■ CPT BILLING

Suture removal is part of global billing for the procedure; there is no separate billing code for removal. If the sutures were placed at another office or clinic, the clinician should just bill for the appropriate office visit.

REFERENCES AND RELATED RESOURCES

DeBoard RH, et al: Principles of basic wound evaluation and management in the emergency department, *Emerg Med Clin N Am* 25:23–39, 2007.

Forsch RT: Essentials of skin laceration repair, *Am Fam Physicians* 78:945–951, 2008.

Ricci NA, Rizzolo D: Laceration repair: avoiding infection, optimize healing, minimize scarring, *JAAPA* 24(9):28–33, 2011.

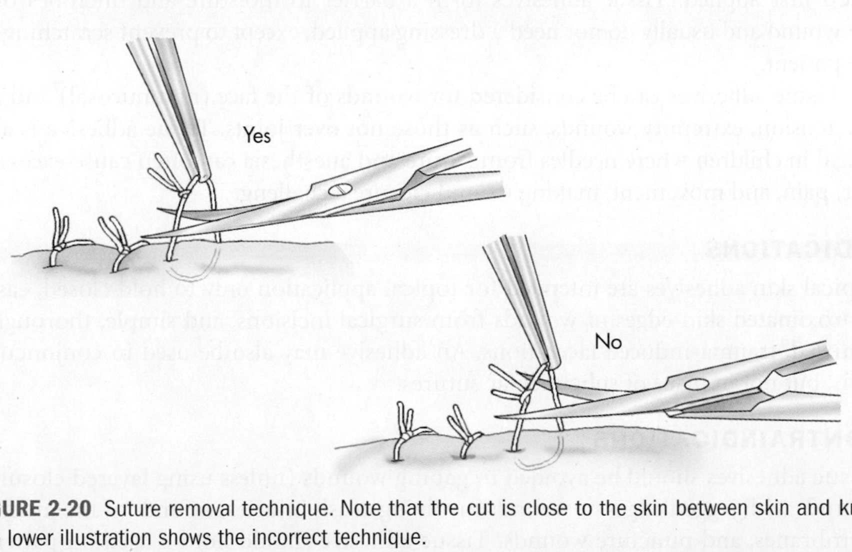

FIGURE 2-20 Suture removal technique. Note that the cut is close to the skin between skin and knot. The lower illustration shows the incorrect technique.

Wound Closure with Tissue Adhesive

Tom Bartol

DESCRIPTION

Tissue adhesive or cyanoacrylates were approved by the FDA in 1998. The adhesives are a type of glue that dries quickly and holds the wound closed for healing. It can be an alternative to suturing for some wounds and often causes less pain and is quicker to apply than sutures. These liquids form an adhesive bond within about 30 seconds of application, resulting in a relatively painless closure of certain types of simple lacerations. Tissue adhesives can be considered for closing small (<5 cm), low tension, nonmucosal wounds. They do not require anesthesia unless needed for wound exploration and irrigation. Adhesive removal is not required because the epithelium sloughs off with the adhesive after about 5 to 10 days. It can be used as part of a layered closure after placement of subcuticular sutures.

There are several cyanoacrylate tissue adhesives available, including n-d-2-cyanoacrylate (e.g., Histoacryl and PeriAcryl) and 2-octyl-cyanoacrylate (e.g., Dermabond and Surgiseal).

ANATOMY AND PHYSIOLOGY

Cyanoacrylates are a class of wound adhesives first described in 1949 (see initial section on dermatologic procedures in Chapter 1). They polymerize in an exothermic reaction on contact with a fluid or basic substance, forming a strong bond. Butyl cyanoacrylate (e.g., Histoacryl, Indermil, GluStich, and LiquiBand) forms rapid bonding (in about 15 seconds), but the bonds are more brittle. Octyl cyanoacrylate (e.g., Dermabond or SurgiSeal) is a long-chain cyanoacrylate that contains plasticizers that are a bit slower to bond (requiring about 30 seconds), but form a strong, more flexible bond. Its three-dimensional breaking strength is about 50% of a 5-0 monofilament suture when first applied. Tissue adhesives form a barrier to moisture and microbes over the wound and usually do not need a dressing applied, except to prevent scratching by the patient.

Tissue adhesives can be considered for wounds of the face (nonmucosal) and for low tension, extremity wounds, such as those not over joints. Tissue adhesive is also useful in children where needles from suture and anesthesia can often cause excessive fear, pain, and movement, making wound closure a challenge.

INDICATIONS

Topical skin adhesives are intended for topical application only to hold closed, easily approximated skin edges of wounds from surgical incisions, and simple, thoroughly cleansed, trauma-induced lacerations. An adhesive may also be used in conjunction with, but not in place of subcuticular sutures.

CONTRAINDICATIONS

Tissue adhesives should be avoided in gaping wounds (unless using layered closure), wounds with jagged edges or wounds involving crush injuries, wounds of the mucous membranes, and puncture wounds. Tissue adhesive should not be used on patients who have a known hypersensitivity reaction to cyanoacrylate (e.g., Super Glue) or formaldehyde. Tissue adhesives are contraindicated any time wound closure with other methods would be contraindicated, such as in cases of active infection or a dirty wound. Wounds over high tension areas, such as the joints, should not be closed with tissue adhesive. They are also contraindicated for use across mucocutaneous junctions or on skin that may be regularly exposed to bodily fluids or dense, natural hair. Large wounds should not be closed with tissue adhesives. Clinical judgment is necessary, but wounds smaller than 4 to 5 cm in length are ideal. Depending on skin tension and location, wounds up to 10 cm may, in some cases, be closed with tissue adhesives.

PRECAUTIONS

Use caution when applying tissue adhesives around the eyes. Petroleum jelly may be used as a barrier to block the adhesive from entering the eye, or a gauze pad may be used to protect the patient from inadvertent adhesive seepage to unwanted areas. Position the patient with the area to be repaired at a level lower than the eye so that runoff of adhesive travels away from the eye. Tissue adhesive should not be put directly into a wound. If the wound is wet due to blood or other fluids, it will not adhere, so the wound must be dry before application.

ASSESSMENT

- Assessment should be made as for any other wound (see "Wound Care, Assessment").
- Before closure, all wounds should be cleansed, irrigated, and explored for foreign bodies as indicated based on the extent of the wound and the mechanism of injury. Anesthesia may be helpful or necessary in carrying this out, depending on the depth and extent of the wound.
- Further assessment is dependent on the type of injury and on the findings from the initial examination.

PATIENT PREPARATION

1. Informed consent should be obtained for the procedure. The procedure should be explained to the patient, including risks and benefits, possible complications, and alternatives to the procedure.
2. Inform the patient that the area may feel warm as the chemical reaction of the adhesive takes place. The patient should be given an opportunity to ask questions about the procedure. Discuss the fact that scarring may occur.
3. Position the patient comfortably so that the wound can be easily accessed for cleansing, exploration, irrigation, and closure.
4. Irrigation with normal saline solution using copious amounts of saline and a large (20-ml) syringe with a large-bore needle is effective in forcing out bacteria and debris from the wound.
5. Devitalized areas can then be débrided.
6. Tetanus prophylaxis can be administered if indicated (see "Wound Care").

TREATMENT ALTERNATIVES

- Standard wound closure (suturing or stapling)
- Wound tape (Steri-Strip) closure
- Wound left open to heal by secondary intention

EQUIPMENT

- Anesthesia supplies if needed (see "Anesthesia: Topical, Local, and Digital Nerve Blocks, Equipment")
- Irrigation supplies
- Topical skin adhesive
- Eye and face protection

Procedure

1. Assess the wound as described (Figure 2-21).
2. Cleanse and explore the wound as indicated (see "Wound Care, Procedure").

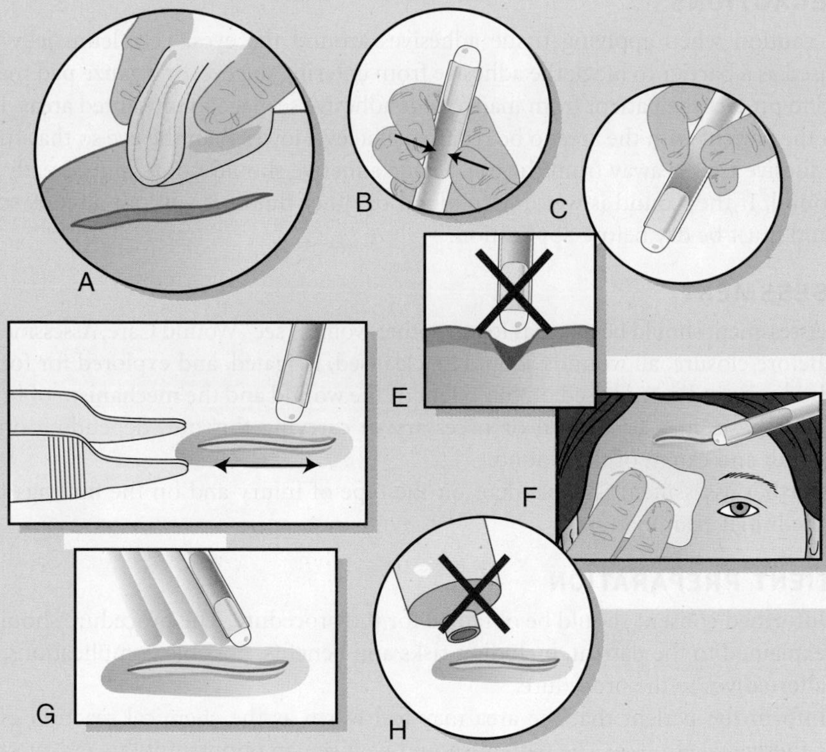

FIGURE 2-21 Procedure for application of topical skin adhesive. **A,** Cleanse and débride the wound. **B,** Remove applicator from packaging and hole with the top pointed upward. Apply pressure at the midpoint of the ampule, crushing the inner glass ampule. **C,** Invert applicator and gently squeeze to express the liquid through the applicator tip. Use the adhesive immediately. **D,** To prevent inadvertent run-off of adhesive, position the wound in a horizontal plane. Approximate the wound edges with forceps or gloved fingers. Use gentle brushing strokes to apply a thin film of liquid adhesive to the approximated wound edges. The adhesive should extend at least ½ cm on each side of the apposed wound edges. **E,** Avoid seepage into the wound because it may delay healing. **F,** To avoid getting adhesive in the eye when closing a facial wound, position the patient so that any runoff is away from eye and hold the eye closed with a gauze pad. **G,** Gradually build three or four thin layers of adhesive that are evenly distributed over the wound. Maintain approximation of the wound edges until the adhesive sets and forms a flexible film (about 1 minute). **H,** Do not apply ointments or medications on top of the adhesive.

2

3. Anesthesia usually is not needed when using tissue adhesive. As it dries it produces a very warm, hot sensation. Use of a topical anesthetic in children is recommended. Topical anesthesia may be considered, but the area must be completely dry before tissue adhesive is applied. If subcutaneous sutures are going to be placed first as a layered closure, anesthesia should be used.
4. Explore, irrigate, débride, and prepare wound as outlined earlier. Wound edges and surrounding skin should be completely dry before the application of tissue adhesive and must approximate without tension.
5. If subcutaneous sutures are needed, they should be placed as instructed in "Suturing Simple Lacerations."
6. Manually approximate the wound edges with sterile forceps or gloved fingers.
7. Apply tissue adhesive as directed in the instructions for the specific type of tissue adhesive that you are using, gently applying the liquid to the wound edges and to at least 5 mm of skin beyond the wound edges. Try to avoid placement of the tissue adhesive into the wound.

RED FLAG

The adhesive is sticky and dries quickly. Be sure gauze or gloves do not come into contact with the adhesive on the patient's skin because they will stick to the wound.

8. Allow to dry for about 30 to 60 seconds.
9. Apply in three to four layers with 30- to 60-second drying time between each layer, each extending 5 to 10 mm beyond the wound edge.
10. Maintain manual approximation of the wound edges for 60 seconds after application of the last layer.
11. Do not apply ointments or medications on top of the tissue adhesive because they may weaken the polymerized film and lead to wound dehiscence.
12. A dressing is usually not needed, but may be applied for protection after the adhesive is completely dry (not tacky; about 5 minutes after application).

PATIENT EDUCATION POSTPROCEDURE

- Patients should be instructed not to pick at the adhesive because it may disrupt adhesion. A dressing may be applied to discourage picking at the wound, but is not needed to keep the wound clean because the tissue adhesive forms a protective barrier.
- Inform patients that the adhesive will slough off naturally in about 5 to 10 days.
- Keep the area dry because water will reduce the strength of the adhesive. Patients should not swim until the adhesive has sloughed off naturally.

COMPLICATIONS

- Unintended bonding to gloves, sponges, or other body parts may occur. If it occurs, it can sometimes be released using an antibiotic ointment to soften the bond.
- Should infection occur, the adhesive may have to be peeled off using an antibiotic ointment or by soaking in water.
- If wound dehiscence occurs, the wound should be reevaluated.

PRACTITIONER FOLLOW-UP

No follow-up is necessary unless complications, such as wound infection or dehiscence, occur.

■ CPT BILLING

Wound closure utilizing topical skin adhesive as the sole repair material should be coded with the appropriate E/M code.

REFERENCES AND RELATED RESOURCES

Coulthard P, et al: Tissue adhesive for closure of surgical incisions, *Cochrane Database Syst Rev* 12(5):CD004287, 2010.

Doraiswamy NV, et al: Which tissue adhesive for wounds? *Injury Int J Care Injured* 34:564–567, 2003.

Lewis S, et al: Wound healing outcomes after laceration repair with adhesive, *Emerg Nurs* 18(10):18–21, 2011.

Package insert for DERMABOND topical skin adhesive, Piscataway, NJ, Ethicon, Johnson & Johnson.

Ricci NA, Rizzolo D: Laceration repair: avoiding infection, optimize healing, minimize scarring, *JAAPA* 24(9):28–33, 2011.

Singer AJ, et al: Evaluation of a new high-viscosity octycyanacrylate tissue adhesive for laceration repair: a randomized clinical trial, *Acad Emerg Med* 10(10):1134–1137, 2003.

2

Staple Insertion and Removal

Marilyn Winterton Edmunds

DESCRIPTION

Wound stapling is an alternative wound closure technique to suturing. The cosmetic result may be compromised by staples that leave large puncture wounds. Stapling is much quicker to perform than suturing. Staples are placed using commercially available skin-stapling devices, and removal is performed with a special staple removal tool. There are various types of devices available with different types of staples.

INDICATIONS

- Useful in the repair of long, straight lacerations of the scalp, trunk, and extremities or the torso. Areas should be where scarring is not a concern.
- Useful in repairing wounds or attaching skin grafts where the edges are relatively straight and can be easily approximated. Avoid use where there is skin tension.

CONTRAINDICATIONS

- Highly traumatized tissue, such as occurs with crush or tearing injuries
- Wounds without adequate blood supply
- Any other wound that should not be closed

PRECAUTIONS

- Avoid use in areas of the body where computed tomography scanning or magnetic resonance imaging may be needed.
- Stapling is not recommended in hand or facial lacerations.
- A staple removal tool, provided by each manufacturer, must be used to remove staples. The use of other instruments may cause increased pain and/or damage to the wound.

ASSESSMENT

- Initial assessment should include extent of bleeding and an assessment for more serious underlying disorders. A bleeding wound may distract both family and clinician from more serious conditions, such as internal injuries.
- Remember to assess for airway, breathing, and circulation.
- Obtain a history to determine the mechanism of injury, the time of occurrence, symptoms of underlying damage, and tetanus immunization status.
- Determine the patient's past medical history, including conditions that may affect wound healing or increase the risk of infection, such as diabetes, immunodeficiency diseases, or peripheral vascular disease.
- Ascertain a history of allergies and current medications.
- Physical examination should include vital signs, including an assessment for signs of hypovolemia and infection (including temperature). Based on the mechanism of injury, a brief secondary examination should be made to assess for underlying injuries.
- Before closure, all wounds should be cleansed, irrigated, and explored for foreign bodies. This may be more effectively accomplished after anesthesia is induced.
- Further assessment is dependent on the type of injury and on the findings from the initial examination.

PATIENT PREPARATION

1. The procedure should be explained to the patient, including risks and benefits, possible complications, and alternatives to the procedure. The patient should be given an opportunity to ask questions about the procedure. Discuss the fact that scarring may occur.
2. Position the patient comfortably so that the wound can be easily accessed for cleansing, exploration, irrigation, and closure.
3. Irrigation with normal saline solution using copious amounts of saline and a large (20-ml) syringe with a large-bore needle is effective in forcing out bacteria and debris from the wound.
4. Devitalized areas can then be débrided. If skin edges do not approximate well, undermining using blunt dissection with iris scissors can increase skin mobility.
5. Tetanus prophylaxis can be administered if indicated (see "Wound Care").

TREATMENT ALTERNATIVES

- Suturing
- Wound tape
- Topical skin adhesive
- Wound left open to heal by secondary intention

EQUIPMENT

- Anesthesia supplies (see "Anesthesia: Topical, Local, and Digital Nerve Block, Equipment")
- Irrigation supplies (see "Suturing Simple Lacerations, Patient Preparation")
- Sterile 2 × 2 gauze sponges (8 to 10 or more)
- Iris scissors
- Tissue forceps
- Staple kit with insertion device, removal tool, and staples (Figure 2-22)
- Sterile gloves
- Eye and face protection
- Protective gown

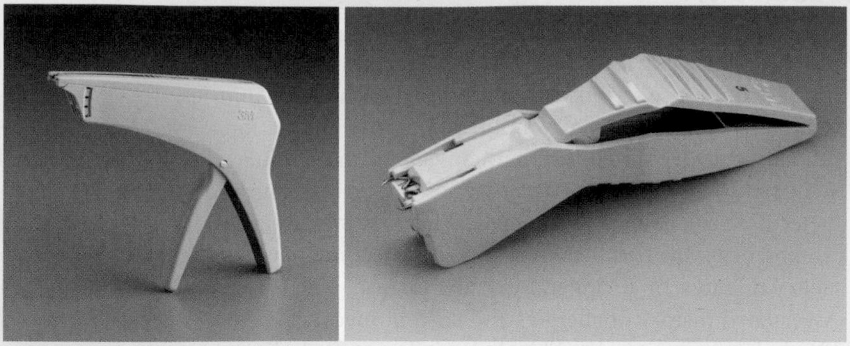

FIGURE 2-22 Examples of wound-stapling devices. (Photos courtesy of 3M Infection Prevention Division.)

Procedure

STAPLE INSERTION

1. Prepare the wound.
   a. Assess the wound (see "Wound Care").
   b. Cleanse the wound (see "Wound Care").
   c. Using sterile gloves, provide anesthesia (see "Anesthesia: Topical, Local, and Digital Nerve Block").
   d. Explore, irrigate, débride, and prepare the wound as outlined earlier.
   e. Prepare and drape the wound.
2. If the wound is gaping or has tissue loss, it might be necessary to undermine the edge of the wound and, using buried absorbable sutures, close the deeper layers.
3. Evert and approximate the wound edges gently using a forceps or skin hook. If an assistant is available, it is helpful to have that person evert and approximate the wound edges in front of the stapler, slightly elevating the skin while another operates the stapler (Figure 2-23).

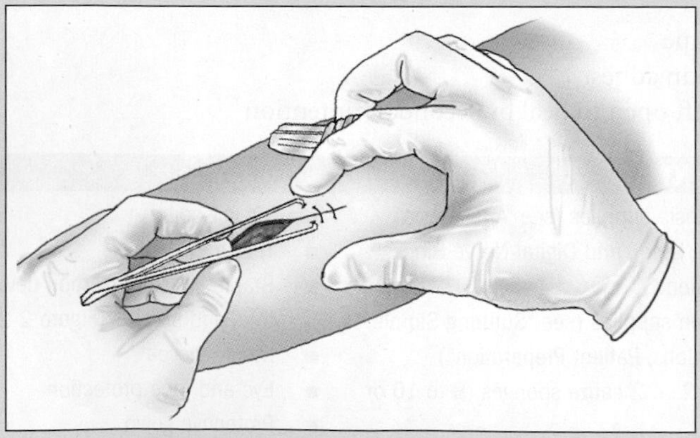

FIGURE 2-23 Use of forceps to approximate and evert wound edges for stapling.

4. Start at one end of the wound and point the stapler toward the other end of the wound. Following the stapler guide arrow, place the stapler on the skin over the wound without applying excessive force. Only light pressure is needed; too much pressure will cause the staple to penetrate too deeply.
5. Gently squeeze the trigger or handle so the staple penetrates the tissue (Figures 2-24 and 2-25). Do not release the trigger, but pull up carefully on

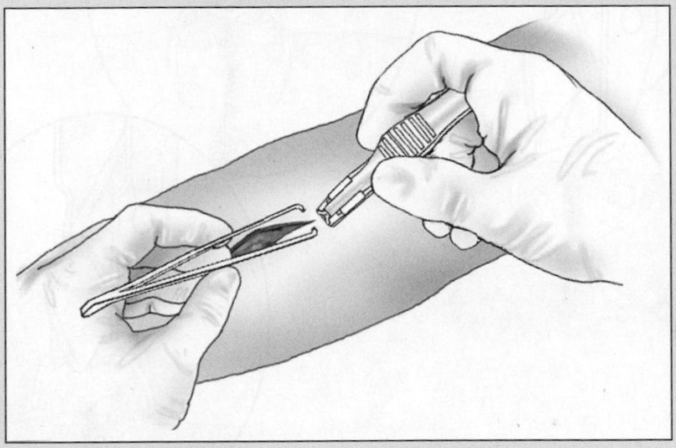

FIGURE 2-24 Place stapler gently on the skin. Indenting the skin with too much pressure causes staples to be placed too deeply.

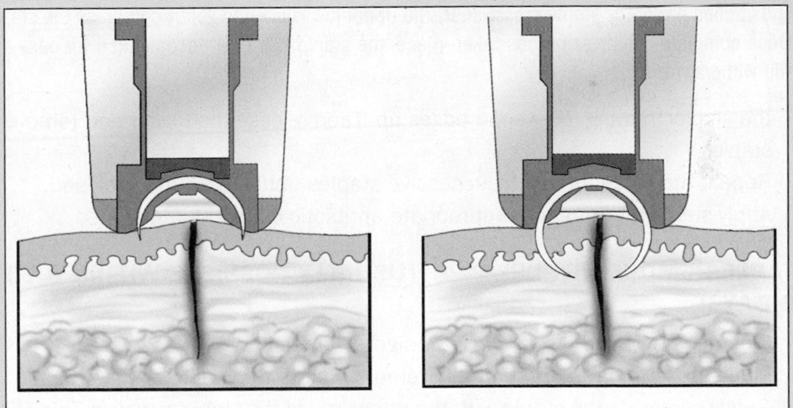

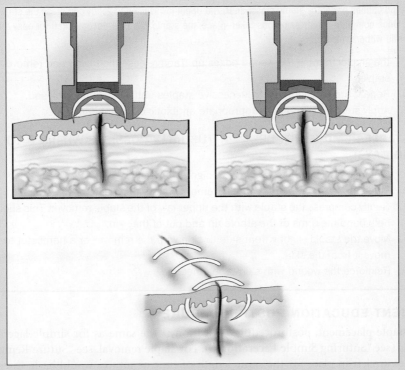

FIGURE 2-25 During triggering, the staple is reconfigured to approximate wound edges.

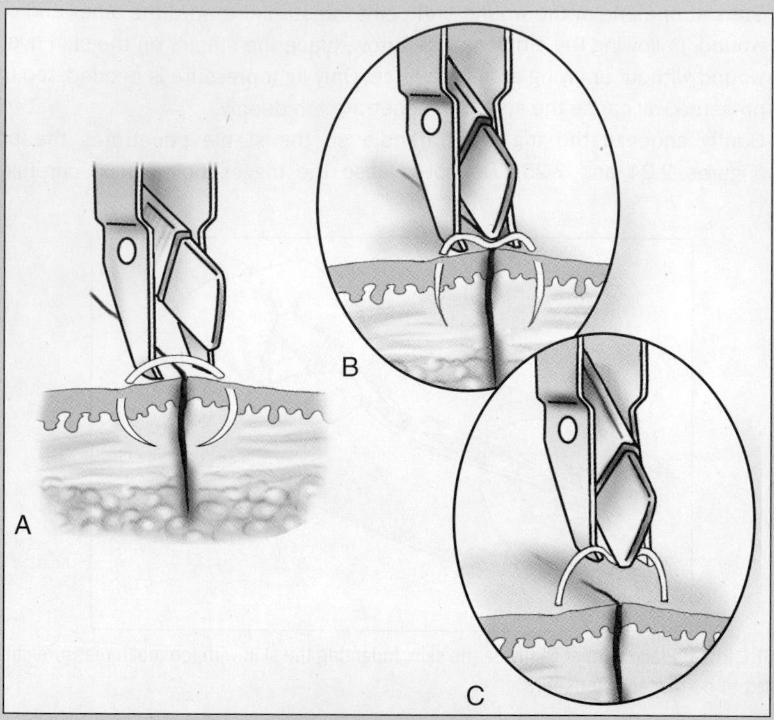

FIGURE 2-26 Procedure for removal of staples. **A,** The lower jaws of the staple-removing device are positioned under the staple crossbar. **B,** The upper jaw is used to gently compress the staple. **C,** Once complete compression has taken place, the staple has been reconfigured for easy and gentle withdrawal.

the stapler, moving the wound edges up. Then release the trigger and remove the stapler.

6. Repeat the procedure with successive staples until the wound is closed.
7. Apply sterile dressing and appropriate antibiotic ointment if indicated.

STAPLE REMOVAL (FIGURE 2-26) (USUALLY POSSIBLE WITHIN 8 TO 10 DAYS)

1. Cleanse the wound. Assess for any signs of infection.
2. Place the lower jaws of the staple remover under the staple.
3. Gently compress the staple with the upper jaw of the staple remover. This should help bend the arms of the staple up and out of the skin.
4. Move the staple slightly from side to side with the remover or a hemostat to remove it from the skin.
5. Reinforce the wound with skin tape if needed.

PATIENT EDUCATION POSTPROCEDURE

For staple placement, postprocedure education is the same as for simple laceration repair (see "Suturing Simple Lacerations"). For staple removal, see "Suture Removal." Staples are left in place for the same length of time as sutures would be in the same anatomic location.

REFERENCES AND RELATED RESOURCES

Jolley J: Surgical staples for scalp laceration repair: A quick and easy solution, *Adv Nurs Pract* 17(7):37–38, 2009.

Lammers RL: Principles of wound management. In JR Roberts, UJR Hedges, editors: *Clinical procedures in emergency medicine*, ed 5, Philadelphia, 2010, Saunders Elsevier.

Skin Lesion Removal

Tom Bartol

DESCRIPTION

Skin lesion removal is a common office procedure that can help both remove a lesion (therapeutic) and develop a diagnosis (assessment). There are many methods or techniques for lesion removal or biopsy and the technique should be based on the size of the lesion, the suspected clinical diagnosis, and the location of the lesion. In some cases it is desired to remove a lesion completely and other cases a portion of a lesion is removed for biopsy. Common office procedures used for lesion removal and/or biopsy include (1) punch removal or biopsy; (2) excisional removal (with or without biopsy), which is usually performed using a fusiform technique; (3) incisional biopsy; and (4) shave biopsy.

Punch removal can be used to remove a lesion completely if the lesion can be contained within the punch size available (up to 12 mm if this punch is available, but more commonly up to 6 mm). The punch can also be used to remove a portion of a lesion for biopsy to help determine further treatment. Incisional biopsy removes part of a lesion, but not the whole lesion.

Excisional removal is typically performed by fusiform excision. This has long been termed "elliptical" excision in the past, but because the ends of the incision have points and are not curved, it is technically fusiform or tangent-to-circle, not a true ellipse. Unlike the punch biopsy or the incision biopsy, the fusiform excision allows for biopsy and diagnosis and complete removal or excision through one procedure.

Incisional biopsy is not therapeutic and uses a scalpel to remove a portion of a lesion, usually a lesion too large to completely excise, to make a diagnosis and determine further treatment.

A shave removal uses a shaving technique and does not remove the lesion to the base of the dermis. This technique can be used for biopsy and diagnosis and/or for the therapeutic removal of some benign lesions.

ANATOMY AND PHYSIOLOGY

Skin lesions are removed for a variety of reasons. Some may be removed because they are suspicious for malignancy. Removal is a means of biopsy and, if completely excised, of treatment for some types of skin cancer. Certain lesions may be removed for cosmetic reasons. If the removal is for purely cosmetic reasons and the lesion is not suspicious, the patient might want to first check insurance coverage to see whether the procedure will be covered. Sometimes a lesion or part of a lesion or rash is removed and sent for pathologic examination to assist in diagnosing and treating a skin condition, such as an inflammatory dermatosis. Lesions, such as warts, may be removed because they cause pain or affect activities of daily living. Some lesions, such as an abscess, are opened or drained to facilitate the healing process.

A basic knowledge of dermatologic diagnoses is essential for the clinician who performs biopsies. The clinician must use differential diagnoses to determine which technique should be used. If the clinician has no idea of a differential diagnosis for a lesion or rash, it is best not to perform a biopsy and instead to refer the patient to a consultant. Some of the lesions or conditions that may require removal and/or biopsy are inflammatory dermatosis, pigmented lesions, basal cell carcinoma, squamous cell carcinoma, melanoma, angiomas, dermatofibromas, acrochordons (skin tags), verruca (warts), and epidermal inclusion cysts (sebaceous cyst). This section is designed not to provide comprehensive knowledge of these lesions and their diagnosis, but rather to provide introductory and summary information about various types of skin lesions.

Inflammatory dermatoses or certain skin rashes may have biopsy samples taken to assist in making a diagnosis and in providing treatment. These lesions should be sampled only if the clinician has one or more differential diagnosis for the rash or lesion. If the clinician has no differential diagnosis for the lesion, consultation is more appropriate. Even a phone call to a dermatologist may help to determine a differential diagnosis and plan for assessment and treatment. The biopsy of an inflammatory dermatosis should be a full-thickness biopsy, often performed best with a punch or an incisional biopsy and not a shave biopsy, which is only a partial thickness removal. Select a site for biopsy that has primary inflammatory changes, but is free of crusting, erosion, infection, or ulceration (secondary changes).

Pigmented lesions, if suspicious, should be fully excised if practical. Normal adjacent skin tissue should be included at the border. If the lesion is highly suspicious for melanoma, additional excision may be necessary, even if the lesion is completely excised.

Basal cell carcinoma is a surface epithelial tumor. It usually has a small central depression and raised pearly borders, although the appearance may vary. This type of cancer only rarely metastasizes, and excision is usually curative. *Squamous cell* carcinoma lesions usually appear crusted and may occur at the base of an actinic keratosis. These lesions are usually found in sun-exposed areas. Other pigmented lesions include *actinic keratoses, seborrheic keratoses, lentigo,* and *nevi.*

Acrochordons, or skin tags, are benign pedunculated lesions that usually occur on the eyelids, neck, axillae, or groin. These lesions may appear flesh-colored or hyperpigmented and vary in size from less than 1 mm to more than 10 mm. They are easily removed using electrosurgery, cryotherapy, or excision with sharp tissue scissors or scalpel.

Verruca are benign epithelial tumors caused by viruses, and they occur on the skin and mucous membranes. They are mildly contagious and have an incubation period of 1 to several months (average, 2 to 18 months). These lesions are sharply demarcated with a rough surface and typically from 2 to 10 mm in diameter. Despite the type of treatment, verruca commonly recur, with recurrence rates of 30% or higher. There are many over-the-counter preparations that work effectively on warts, although cryotherapy or electrosurgery may be necessary. Most verruca resolve spontaneously over time, but it may take years for some to resolve.

The *epidermal inclusion cyst,* also known as an epidermal cyst or a sebaceous cyst, is a superficial, freely mobile, subcutaneous lesion. The lesion is usually nontender, although it may become enlarged and inflamed, and may exude thick white fluid at times. This lesion is benign and, if not inflamed or infected, requires no treatment. Recurrence is common, and similar cysts may occur in other parts of the body (Table 2-11).

TABLE 2-11 Surgical Diagnosis and Management of Common Skin Lesions

LESION / PROCEDURE	PUNCH BIOPSY	SHAVE BIOPSY	SHAVE REMOVAL	FUSIFORM EXCISION	INCISIONAL BIOPSY	CAUTERY/CURETTEMENT	CRYOTHERAPY	ELECTROSURGERY (RADIOFREQUENCY)	85% TRICHLOROACETIC ACID	LASER ABLATION	RADIATION	FLUOROURACIL 5% OR MASOPROCOL 10%	OTHER
Achrochordon (Skin tags)		X*	X*				X	X					
Cancer, basal cell	X	X		X	X	X*	X	X		X	X	X	
Cancer, squamous cell	X			X*	X	X		X		X	X	X	
Condyloma acuminata	X	X	X	X§		X	X	X	X	X		X†	X
Dermatofibroma	X	X	X	X*	X		X	X		X			
Hemangiomas, cherry	X§	X	X				X	X		X			
Keratoacanthoma	X	X	X	X*	X	X	X	X		X		X	
Keratosis, actinic	X	X	X	X	X	X	X	X	X			X	
Keratosis, seborrheic	X	X	X*	X§	X	X	X	X					
Lentigo	X	X	X		X		X*		X				
Lentigo maligna	X			X*	X								
Lipomas				X	X								
Melanoma	X			X*	X								X
Molluscum contagiosum	X§	X	X			X	X	X	X				X
Pyogenic granuloma	X	X	X	X	X	X	X	X	X	X			

Continued

TABLE 2-11 Surgical Diagnosis and Management of Common Skin Lesions—cont'd

LESION / PROCEDURE	PUNCH BIOPSY	SHAVE BIOPSY	SHAVE REMOVAL	FUSIFORM EXCISION	INCISIONAL BIOPSY	CAUTERY/CURETTEMENT	CRYOTHERAPY	ELECTROSURGERY (RADIOFREQUENCY)	85% TRICHLOROACETIC ACID	LASER ABLATION	RADIATION	FLUOROURACIL 5% OR MASOPROCOL 10%	OTHER
Nevi, acquired	X		X‡	X	X		X‡	X‡		X			
Nevi, atypical	X			X*	X								
Nevi, giant congenital	X			X	X					X‡			
Paronychia													X
Rashes	X												X
Sebaceous hyperplasia	X	X	X	X§		X	X	X					
Sebaceous cysts				X									X
Telangiectasias								X		X			X
Warts (Verrucae vulgaris)	X	X	X		X§	X	X	X	X	X			X
Warts, plantar	X	X	X			X	X	X	X	X			X
Xanthalasma		X	X	X		X		X		X			X

From Pfenninger JL, Fowler GC: *Procedures for primary care physicians*, ed 3, St Louis, 2011, Mosby.

*Procedure of choice.

†Not approved by the Food and Drug Administration.

‡An exception; to be used only on lesions that are confirmed as benign.

§To be used only if cancer is a possibility or the nature of lesion unknown.

Basic Biopsy Steps

1. Provide anesthesia.
2. Label specimen container(s) with the patient's name, patient's date of birth, date of procedure, and site of lesion.
3. Cleanse and drape the biopsy area.
4. Remove the lesion.
5. Control bleeding using the most appropriate technique.
6. Close the wound.

DOCUMENTATION OF PROCEDURE

The following should be clearly noted in the chart:

- Date of procedure
- Biopsy site
- Lesion description (size, characteristics, etc.)
- Informed consent
- Procedure
- Follow-up

Lesion Excision (Fusiform)

Tom Bartol

DESCRIPTION

An excisional removal is a full-thickness biopsy technique that involves removing the whole lesion, usually by making a fusiform incision. This procedure has long been termed an "elliptical" excision, but because the ends of the incision have points and are not curved, it is now referred to as a fusiform excision. This technique is useful for removal of benign or malignant lesions. The typical fusiform excision has a length-to-width ratio of 3:1 that results in points at the ends of the long access. For many lesions, complete excision is curative.

ANATOMY AND PHYSIOLOGY

Fusiform excisions should be made with the long axis of the excision parallel to the skin tension lines to reduce tension on the wound edges, which results in a more satisfactory cosmetic outcome. When planning a fusiform excision, sometimes the orientation may vary based on location and tension during activity. Using a pinching method with the thumb and forefinger, the clinician can determine the direction of greatest skin laxity to help determine orientation of the fusiform excision (see Figures 2-2 and 2-3).

INDICATIONS

- Diagnosis and treatment of suspicious skin lesions
- Removal of lesions that are causing problems because of their size or location
- Lesions that a patient wants removed for cosmetic reasons

CONTRAINDICATIONS

- Infection at the site of the proposed biopsy
- Patient has a bleeding disorder (coagulopathy) of sufficient consequence that hemostasis would be difficult
- Relative contraindication: History of keloids or hypertrophic scar formation

PRECAUTIONS

- If the patient has an allergy to anesthetics, alternative agents may need to be used.
- Systemic disorders that may affect wound healing, such as immunosuppression conditions, peripheral vascular disease, or diabetes.
- For cosmetic reasons, patients who have lesions on the face should be given the option to see a plastic surgeon if the clinician is not comfortable with excision in these areas.

ASSESSMENT

- Obtain a history to determine differential diagnoses, such as how long the lesion has been present and whether it has been changing or bleeding.
- Inquire about previous or recent sun exposure.
- Determine the patient's past medical history, including conditions that may affect wound healing or increase the risk of infection, such as diabetes, immunodeficiency diseases, or peripheral vascular disease.
- Ascertain a history of allergies and current medications.
- Physical examination should include size, symmetry, color, border characteristics, and character of the lesion.
- Determine the direction of the skin tension lines and tension on the skin so that the orientation of the excision can be determined (see Figures 2-2 and 2-3).

PATIENT PREPARATION

Explain the procedure to the patient, including risks and benefits, possible complications, and alternatives to the procedure. Give the patient an opportunity to ask questions about the procedure. Discuss the fact that scarring may occur. Using a skin pen or permanent marker, it may be helpful to draw the incision lines on the patient's skin before administering local anesthesia, especially for subcutaneous lesions and cysts, because they may be more difficult to visualize and palpate after administering the anesthesia subcutaneously.

Position the patient comfortably so that the site can be easily accessed.

TREATMENT ALTERNATIVES

- No biopsy
- Punch biopsy (depending on lesion)
- Shave biopsy (depending on lesion)
- Referral to a dermatologist (for evaluation and possible excision/biopsy), surgeon, or plastic surgeon (for removal/biopsy)

EQUIPMENT

- Anesthesia supplies (see "Anesthesia: Topical, Local, and Digital Nerve Block")
- Antiseptic solution (e.g., povidone-iodine) and swabs
- Suture tray containing:
  - Sterile 4 × 4 gauze sponges (8 to 10 or more)
  - Needle holder
  - Iris scissors
  - Tissue forceps
  - Curved mosquito clamp
  - Skin hook or 21-gauge needle that can be bent into a needle hook
  - Sterile fenestrated drape
  - No. 15 blade and handle
- Appropriate suture materials (see Tables 2-8 and 2-9)
- Specimen container (with formalin)
- Dressing supplies (sterile gauze, antibiotic ointment, tape, etc.)
- Sterile gloves
- Eye and face protection
- Protective gown

Procedure

1. With a skin marker, draw an outline of the excision. In most cases the excision should be parallel to the skin tension lines and fusiform in shape that comes to a point at each end at about a 30-degree angle and is about three times as long as it is wide (Figure 2-27).
2. Provide local anesthesia (see "Anesthesia: Topical, Local, and Digital Nerve Block").
3. Cleanse the area using antiseptic solution (see "Skin Preparation").
4. Place fenestrated drape over the area to be excised.
5. Using sterile technique and a No. 15 blade, make a fusiform incision through the dermis—first from one side and then from the other. Hold the scalpel like a pencil with the blade perpendicular to the skin and, as the incision progresses, use more of the belly of the blade. Incise deeply enough to reach the subcutaneous tissue. A suture may be placed in one end of the ellipse that is excised to identify the orientation of the specimen after removal. (After the procedure, be sure to document the orientation of the "tag" placed on the specimen.)
6. Using the scalpel or iris scissors, separate the lesion from the subcutaneous tissue. Handle the specimen gently with a tissue forceps or skin hook and place in the specimen container.
7. Obtain hemostasis with direct pressure if needed.
8. Close the wound (see "Suturing Simple Lacerations"). If there is a gap between tissue margins or there is pronounced skin tension on the margins, the subcutaneous tissue on both sides of the margin can be undermined using iris scissors or scalpel to reduce the skin tension (Figure 2-28). This requires 3 mm of undermining for every 1 mm of desired tissue relaxation. Use subcutaneous sutures, if needed, to eliminate dead space and reduce skin tension.
9. Dress the wound with a sterile dressing.

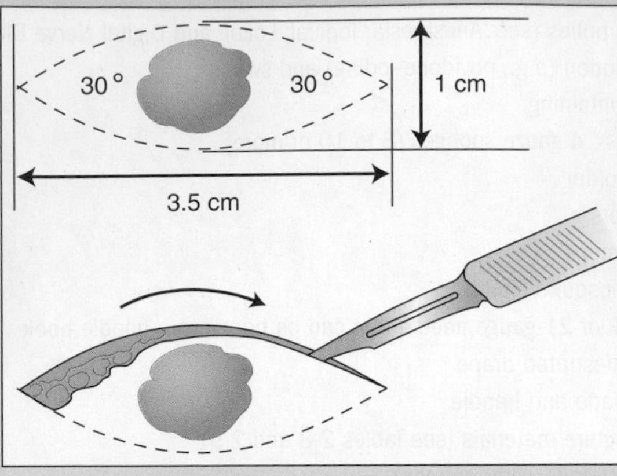

FIGURE 2-27 Elliptical excision biopsy technique.

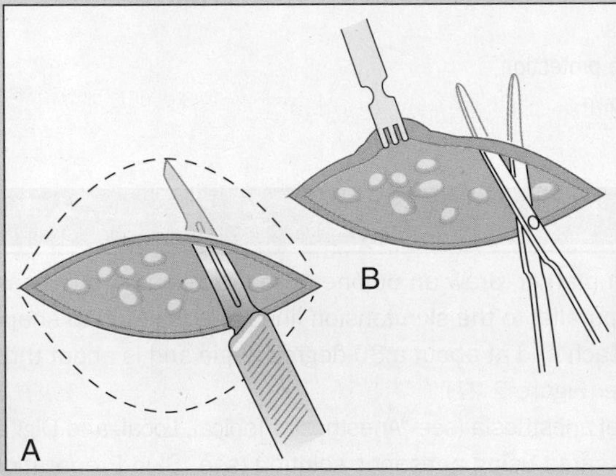

FIGURE 2-28 Subcutaneous undermining to release tension on wound margins with scalpel (**A**) and with scissors (**B**). This also aids in eversion of the edges during closure.

PATIENT EDUCATION POSTPROCEDURE

Instruct the patient in proper wound care (see "Wound Care"). Provide the patient with specific instructions regarding follow-up care and suture removal (see "Suture Removal").

COMPLICATIONS

- Bleeding
- Infection
- Scarring and keloid formation (can be minimized by reducing skin tension during closure)

PRACTITIONER FOLLOW-UP

- The patient should schedule follow-up for suture removal as outlined earlier.
- If signs of infection develop, the patient should be advised to return for follow-up.
- If incomplete healing has taken place at the time of follow-up, sutures may be left in place for a few additional days, or every other suture may be removed and reinforced with surgical tapes.

- The pathology report and further treatment are discussed at follow-up. Malignant lesions may require a second procedure if margins were not clear, or if melanoma was diagnosed by the biopsy. A phone call to the dermatopathologist can often be very helpful in clarifying the diagnosis and treatment if they are not clear to you from the pathology report.

■ CPT BILLING

Excision (including simple closure) of benign lesions of the skin includes local anesthesia. Excision is defined as full thickness removal of a lesion, including margins, and includes simple (non-layered) closure when performed. Code selection is determined by measuring the greatest diameter of the apparent lesion plus that margin required for complete excision (lesion diameter plus the most narrow margins required equal the excised diameter). The closure of defects created by incision, excision, or trauma may require intermediate or complex closure, and this should be reported separately.

11400–Excision, benign lesion, including margins, except skin tag (unless listed elsewhere) of trunk, arms or legs; excised diameter 0.5 cm or less ■ **11401 - 11406**–Excised diameters 0.6 cm to over 4.0 cm ■ **11420**–Excision, benign lesion, including margins, except skin tag (unless listed elsewhere) of scalp, neck, hands, feet, genitalia; excised diameter 0.5 cm or less ■ **11421 - 11426**–Excised diameters 0.6 cm to over 4.0 cm ■ **11440**–Excision, benign lesion, including margins, except skin tag (unless listed elsewhere) of face, ears, eyelids, nose lips, mucous membranes; excised diameter 0.5 cm or less ■ **11441 - 11446**–Excised diameters 0.6 cm to over 4.0 cm ■ **11450 - 11471**–Excision of skin and subcutaneous tissue for hidradenitis with simple or intermediate or complex repair, depending on location

Malignant Lesions

Excision (including simple closure) of malignant lesions of skin (e.g., basal cell carcinoma, squamous cell carcinoma, and melanoma) includes local anesthesia. For destruction of malignant lesions, see destruction codes (17260-17286).

Excision is defined as full thickness (through the dermis) removal of a lesion including margins, and includes simple closure when performed. Report separately each malignant lesion that is excised. Code selection is determined by measuring the greatest clinical diameter of the apparent lesion plus that of the margin required equal the excised diameter. This measurement is made before the actual incision.

The closure of defects created by incision, excision, or trauma may require intermediate or complex closure. Repair by intermediate or complex closure should be reported separately.

Removal of skin tags by any method, including scissoring or any sharp method, ligature strangulation, electrosurgical destruction, or combination of treatment modalities as well as chemical destruction or electrocauterization of wound, with or without local anesthesia.

11200–Removal of skin tags, multiple fibrocutaneous tags, any area; up to and including 15 lesions ■ **11201**–Each additional 10 lesions, or part thereof (List separately in addition to code for primary procedure.)

REFERENCES AND RELATED RESOURCES

Affleck AG, Colver G: Skin biopsy techniques. In Robinson JK, Hanke CW, Siegel DM, Fratila A, editors: *Surgery of the skin: procedural dermatology*, ed 2, Philadelphia, 2010, Elsevier Mosby.

Habif TP: *Clinical dermatology: a color guide to diagnosis and therapy*, ed 5, Philadelphia, 2009, Elsevier Mosby, Chap 27.

Musso SZ, Stefania P, Bertero M: *Skin biopsy procedures: how and where to perform a proper biopsy.* http://cdn.intechopen.com/pdfs-wm/22579.pdf. Posted 2011. Accessed September 30, 2014.

Nischal U, Nischal KC, Khopkar U: Techniques of skin biopsy and practical considerations, *J Cutan Aesthet Surg* 1(2):107–111, 2008.

Pfenninger JL, Fowler GC: *Procedures for primary care physicians*, ed 3, St Louis, 2011, Mosby.

Son D, Harijan A: Overview of surgical scar prevention and management, *J Korean Med Sci* 29(6):751–757, 2014.

Tadiparthi S, Panchani S, Iqbal A: Biopsy for malignant melanoma–are we following the guidelines? *Ann R Coll Surg Engl* 90:322–325, 2008.

Punch Removal

Tom Bartol

DESCRIPTION

A punch biopsy is used for full-thickness removal and biopsy of a lesion of 10 mm or less in diameter, or for a biopsy of a large lesion for diagnostic purposes (e.g., inflammatory dermatosis).

Punches are available in sizes from 2 to 12 mm in diameter. When a punch is performed to make a diagnosis of a skin condition, biopsy samples should be taken of the more recently developing areas and a small border of normal skin should be included. For a biopsy without excision of nonfacial lesions, a 4-mm punch is usually adequate. Punch biopsies that are smaller than 3 mm may be more difficult for the pathologist to diagnose because key features may be missing.

INDICATIONS

- To remove an appropriate-size skin lesion that is causing discomfort or concern
- To obtain a specimen for pathologic evaluation if suspicious for malignancy
- To clarify diagnosis of dermatoses or other skin conditions after differential diagnoses have been focused

CONTRAINDICATIONS

- Infection at the biopsy site (unless performed as part of an incision and drainage)
- No differential diagnoses or suspected diagnoses
- Severe bleeding disorders

PRECAUTIONS

- Select the site based on the type of lesion. Sometimes it is helpful to perform more than one biopsy of a lesion at different sites. For blistering lesions, biopsy the newest-forming vesicles. Biopsy bullae near the edge to include a small part of normal skin. Nonbullous, large lesions should be biopsied at the site that has the most abnormal color, is the thickest, or is near the edge, depending on the lesion characteristics.

  When doing a punch where the skin and subcutaneous tissue is thin and overlying a bone, such as the shin, scalp, or forehead, use caution so as to not to hit the periosteum, which can be painful.
- If the patient has an allergy to anesthetic agents, alternative agents may have to be used.

ASSESSMENT

- Obtain a history to determine how long the lesion has been present and if it has been changing or bleeding.
- Inquire about previous or recent sun exposure.
- Determine the patient's past medical history, including conditions that may affect wound healing or increase the risk of infection, such as diabetes, immunodeficiency diseases, or peripheral vascular disease.
- Ascertain a history of allergies and current medications.

- Physical examination should include size, symmetry, color, border characteristics, and character of the lesion.
- Determine the direction of the skin tension lines so that the skin can be stretched perpendicularly to the tension lines during the punch biopsy (see Figures 2-2 and 2-3).

PATIENT PREPARATION

Informed consent should be obtained for the procedure. The procedure should be explained to the patient, including risks and benefits, possible complications, and alternatives to the procedure. The patient should be given an opportunity to ask questions about the procedure. Discuss the fact that scarring may occur.

Position the patient comfortably so that the site can be easily accessed.

TREATMENT ALTERNATIVES

- No biopsy
- Excision biopsy
- Shave biopsy (depending on lesion)
- Referral to a dermatologist or surgeon

EQUIPMENT

- Anesthesia supplies (see "Anesthesia: Topical, Local, and Digital Nerve Block")
- Antiseptic solution (e.g., povidone-iodine solution) and swabs
- Suture tray containing:
  - Sterile 4 × 4 gauze sponges (8 to 10 or more)
  - Needle holder
  - Iris scissors
  - Tissue forceps
  - Sterile fenestrated drape
  - Punch of appropriate size
  - 21-gauge needle for gently manipulating and moving specimen
- Appropriate suture materials if indicated
- Specimen container containing formalin
- Dressing supplies (sterile gauze, antibiotic ointment, tape, etc.)
- Sterile gloves
- Eye and face protection

Procedure

1. Provide local anesthesia (see "Anesthesia: Topical, Local, and Digital Nerve Blocks").
2. Cleanse the area using antiseptic solution (see "Skin Preparation").
3. Place fenestrated drape over the area to be excised.
4. Apply tension with thumb and index finger of nondominant hand perpendicular to the skin tension lines (Figure 2-29). This causes the resulting biopsy site to be more oval shaped on release, which facilitates a more cosmetically pleasing closure.
5. Place the punch over the lesion and, while applying gentle pressure, rotate the punch cutting through the skin to the subcutaneous tissue. A slight decrease in resistance will be felt when the subcutaneous tissue has been reached (Figure 2-30).

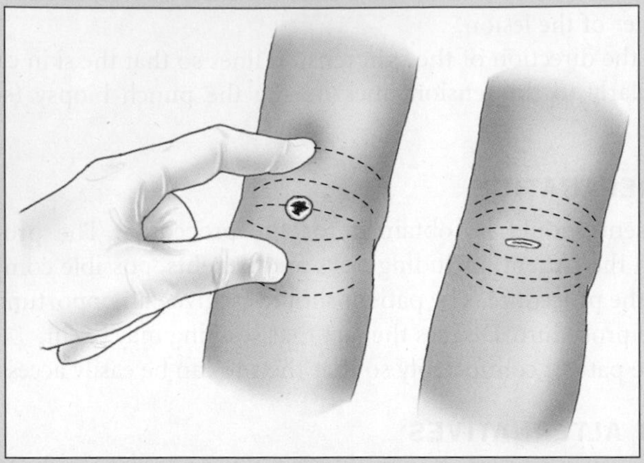

FIGURE 2-29 Proper stretching of skin tension lines before punch biopsy. On release, the usual result is to make the circular biopsy sample more elliptical and the outcome more cosmetically pleasing.

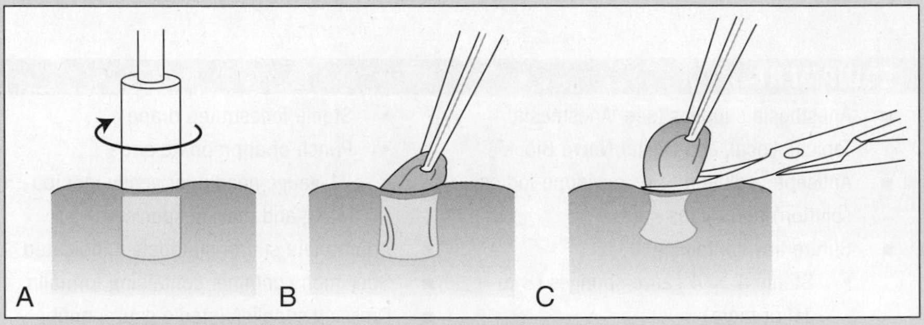

FIGURE 2-30 Punch biopsy technique. **A,** Twisting the punch. **B,** Picking up the loosened piece. **C,** Cutting with scissors.

6. Remove the punch. Gently lift the specimen with a needle or *very* gently with a tissue forceps so as to prevent a crushing artifact, and then cut it at the base using sharp iris scissors.
7. Place the specimen in the container with formalin.
8. Apply pressure to obtain hemostasis.
9. Usually 2- or 3-mm punches do not require sutures and can be closed using wound tapes. Larger punches usually require a single suture for closure. Suture the wound closed as discussed in "Suturing Simple Lacerations," closing parallel to skin tension lines. A vertical mattress suture is useful for closing a punch biopsy site.
10. Apply antibiotic ointment and dressing as indicated.

PATIENT EDUCATION POSTPROCEDURE

Instruct the patient in proper wound care (see "Wound Care"). Provide the patient with specific instructions regarding follow-up care and suture removal if indicated (see "Suture Removal").

COMPLICATIONS

- Bleeding
- Infection
- Scarring and keloid formation

PRACTITIONER FOLLOW-UP

- The patient should schedule follow-up for suture removal as outlined earlier if sutures were placed.
- If signs of infection develop, the patient should be advised to schedule a follow-up visit.
- If incomplete healing has taken place at the time of follow-up, sutures may be left in place for a few additional days, or every other suture may be removed, and then the wound can be reinforced with Steri-Strips.
- The pathology report is discussed at a follow-up visit, and further treatment, if necessary, can be arranged.

■ CPT Billing

During certain procedures in the integumentary system, such as excision, destruction, or shave removals, the removed tissue is often submitted for pathologic evaluation. The obtaining of tissue for pathology during the course of these procedures is a routine component of such procedures. This obtaining of tissue is not considered a separate biopsy procedure and is not separately reported. The use of a biopsy procedure code indicates that the procedure to obtain tissue for pathologic evaluation was performed independently, or was unrelated or distinct from other procedures/services provided at that time. Such biopsies are not considered components of other procedures when performed on different lesions or different sites on the same date, and are to be reported separately.

11100—Biopsy of skin, subcutaneous tissue and/or mucous membrane (including simple closure), single lesion ■ **11101**—Each additional lesion (list separately, in additional to primary code). Use 11101 in conjunction with 11100.

REFERENCES AND RELATED RESOURCES

Affleck AG, Colver G: Skin biopsy techniques. In Robinson JK, Hanke CW, Siegel DM, Fratila A, editors: *Surgery of the skin: procedural dermatology*, ed 2, Philadelphia, 2010, Elsevier Mosby.

Musso SZ, Stefania P, Bertero M: *Skin biopsy procedures: how and where to perform a proper biopsy*. http://cdn.intechopen.com/pdfs-wm/22579.pdf. Posted 2011. Accessed September 30, 2014.

Nischal U, Nischal KC, Khopkar U: Techniques of skin biopsy and practical considerations, *J Cutan Aesthet Surg* 1(2):107–111, 2008.

Pickett H: Shave and punch biopsy for skin lesions, *Am Fam Physician* 84(9):995–1002, 2011.

Son D, Harijan A: Overview of surgical scar prevention and management, *J Korean Med Sci* 29(6):751–757, 2014.

Shave Removal Biopsy

Tom Bartol

DESCRIPTION

A shave removal biopsy is a technique for the removal of elevated skin lesions. Full-thickness removal is not accomplished with this procedure. Should biopsy results identify a cancerous lesion, further treatment and excision are necessary.

INDICATIONS

- To remove a skin lesion that is causing discomfort or concern
- Removal of actinic keratosis and other benign lesions
- To obtain a specimen for pathologic evaluation

CONTRAINDICATIONS

- Lesions known to be suspicious or are highly suspicious for melanoma
- Infection at the biopsy site
- No differential diagnoses or suspected diagnoses for lesion

PRECAUTIONS

If the patient has an allergy to anesthetics, alternative agents may have to be used (see "Anesthesia: Topical, Local, and Digital Nerve Blocks").

There may be excessive bleeding in patients using anticoagulants or with bleeding disorders.

ASSESSMENT

See "Skin Lesion Removal."

- Obtain a history to determine how long the lesion has been present and whether it has been changing or bleeding.
- Inquire about previous or recent sun exposure.
- Determine the patient's past medical history, including conditions that may affect wound healing or increase the risk of infection, such as diabetes, immunodeficiency diseases, or peripheral vascular disease.
- Ascertain a history of allergies and current medications.
- Physical examination should include size, symmetry, color, border characteristics, and character of the lesion.

PATIENT PREPARATION

Informed consent should be obtained for the procedure. The procedure should be explained to the patient, including risks and benefits, possible complications, and alternatives to the procedure. The patient should be given an opportunity to ask questions about the procedure. Discuss the fact that scarring may occur.

Position the patient comfortably so that the site can be easily accessed.

TREATMENT ALTERNATIVES

- No biopsy
- Chemical or electrical cautery
- Excision biopsy
- Punch biopsy
- Referral to a dermatologist or surgeon

EQUIPMENT

- Anesthesia supplies (see "Anesthesia: Topical, Local, and Digital Nerve Block")
- Antiseptic solution (e.g., povidone-iodine solution) and swabs
- Sterile 4 × 4 gauze sponges (8 to 10 or more)
- Double-edged razor blade or No. 15 surgical blade and handle

- Tissue forceps
- Sterile fenestrated drape
- Specimen container (containing formalin)
- Dressing supplies (sterile gauze, antibiotic ointment, tape, etc.)
- Sterile gloves
- Eye and face protection for provider

Procedure

1. Cleanse the area using antiseptic solution.
2. Place fenestrated drape over the area to be shaved.
3. Provide local anesthesia (see "Anesthesia: Topical, Local, and Digital Nerve Block"). As the local aesthetic agent is injected, the lesion will be slightly elevated.
4. Roll the skin between the thumb and forefinger to create a flat cutting surface and a tamponade effect on the surrounding blood vessels.
5. With a No. 15 blade held parallel or at a slight angle down toward the skin, shave the lesion flush with or slightly beneath the surrounding skin (Figure 2-31). An alternative method, sometimes called "saucerization," is performed using a double-edge shaving razor held between the thumb and index finger to form a curve (Figure 2-32). The curve of the blade is used to shave off the lesion.

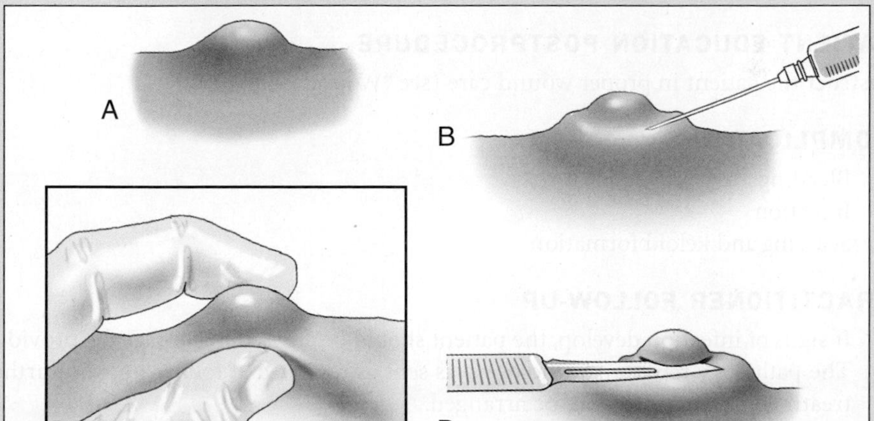

FIGURE 2-31 Shave biopsy technique. **A,** Color the lesion to define it clearly. **B,** Inject a local anesthetic agent to elevate the lesion. **C,** Roll the skin between the thumb and forefinger to create a flat, cutting surface and a tamponade effect on the surrounding blood vessels. **D,** With a No. 15 blade held parallel to the skin or at a slight downward angle, shave the lesion flush with or slightly beneath the surrounding skin.

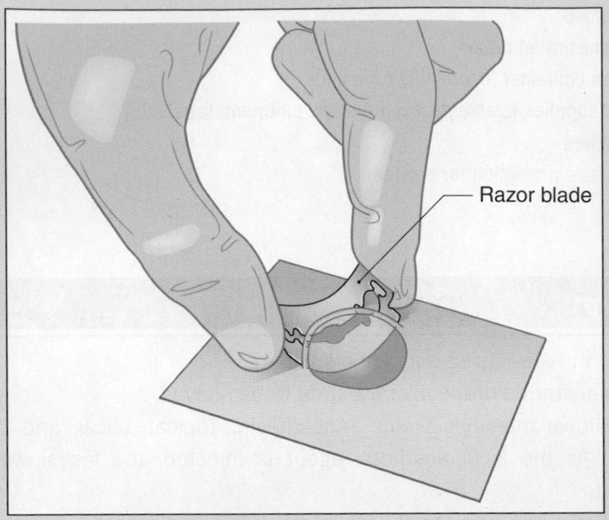

FIGURE 2-32 Saucerization biopsy. Razor blade bent to accommodate depth of lesion. (Adapted from Nouri K, Leal-Khouri S: *Techniques in dermatologic surgery,* Philadelphia, 2003, Mosby.)

6. Place the specimen in the container with formalin.
7. Control bleeding with direct pressure, or use chemical or electrical cautery, as needed.
8. No suturing is needed. The wound is left to heal by secondary intention.
9. Apply antibiotic ointment and dressing, as indicated.

PATIENT EDUCATION POSTPROCEDURE

Instruct the patient in proper wound care (see "Wound Care").

COMPLICATIONS

- Bleeding
- Infection
- Scarring and keloid formation

PRACTITIONER FOLLOW-UP

- If signs of infection develop, the patient should be advised to contact the provider.
- The pathology report, if pathology was sent, is reviewed at follow-up, and further treatment, if necessary, can be arranged.

■ CPT BILLING

Shaving of epidermal or dermal lesions is the sharp removal by transverse incision or horizontal slicing to remove epidermal and dermal lesions without a full thickness dermal excision. This includes local anesthesia, with chemical or electrocauterization of the wound. The wound does not require suture closure.

11300–Shaving of epidermal or dermal lesion, single lesion, trunk, arms or legs; lesion diameter 0.5 cm or less ■ **11301** – **11303**–Lesion diameters 0.6 to over 2.0 cm ■ **11305**–Shaving of epidermal or dermal lesion, single lesion, scalp, neck, hands, feet, genitalia; lesion diameter 0.5 cm or less ■ **11306 – 11308**—Lesion diameters 0.6 to over 2.0 cm ■ **11310**—Shaving of epidermal or dermal lesion, single lesion, face, ears, eyelids, nose, lips, mucous membranes; lesion diameter 0.5 cm or less ■ **11311 – 11313**—Lesion diameters 0.6 to over 2.0 cm

REFERENCES AND RELATED RESOURCES

Habif TP: *Clinical dermatology: a color guide to diagnosis and therapy*, ed 5, Philadelphia, 2009, Elsevier Mosby.

Musso SZ, Stefania P, Bertero M: *Skin biopsy procedures: how and where to perform a proper biopsy*. http://cdn.intechopen.com/pdfs-wm/22579.pdf. Posted 2011. Accessed September 30, 2014.

Nischal U, Nischal KC, Khopkar U: Techniques of skin biopsy and practical considerations, *J Cutan Aesthet Surg* 1(2):107–111, 2008.

Pickett H: Shave and punch biopsy for skin lesions, *Am Fam Physician* 84(9):995–1002, 2011.

Son D, Harijan A: Overview of surgical scar prevention and management, *J Korean Med Sci* 29(6):751–757, 2014.

Tadiparthi S, Panchani S, Iqbal A: Biopsy for malignant melanoma—are we following the guidelines? *Ann R Coll Surg Engl* 90:322–325, 2008.

Wart Removal

Kent D. Blad and Sabrina Jarvis

2

DESCRIPTION

Wart removal can be accomplished in a variety of ways, yet recurrence rates with all treatments can be high. Common treatments in the primary care setting include chemical destruction, cryotherapy, and electrosurgery (see Box 2-4 for available treatments). Procedures discussed in this text are wart removal by chemical destruction and cryotherapy.

Warts are caused by the human papillomavirus (HPV) and often resolve spontaneously, although it may take months to years for spontaneous resolution.

ANATOMY AND PHYSIOLOGY

Warts (verrucae) are common, benign epithelial tumors that are viral in origin and occur on the skin or mucous membrane. All warts are mildly contagious and have an incubation period (after inoculation) of 1 month to several months (average, 2 to 18 months).

BOX 2-4 Types of Treatments Available for Common Warts

1. Chemical destruction examples (not all-inclusive):
   a. Salicylic acid solutions
   b. Cantharidin
   c. Silver Nitrate
2. Cryotherapy with liquid nitrogen
3. Curettage with electrodesiccation
4. Surgical or laser excision – refer patient to a specialist
5. Intralesional injection (bleomycin) – refer patient to a specialist
6. Immunotherapy with medications (e.g., imiquimod) – usually refer patient to a specialist

Common warts (verrucae vulgaris) are almost universal in the population, and most do not become malignant. These light gray, yellow, brown, or grayish-black tumors are sharply demarcated, rough surfaced, round or irregular, firm, and 2 to 10 mm in diameter. They appear most frequently on sites subject to trauma (e.g., fingers, elbows, knees, face, and scalp), but may spread elsewhere.

Periungual warts are common warts that occur around the nail plate.

Plantar warts (verrucae plantaris) are common warts on the sole of the foot; they are flattened by pressure and surrounded by cornified epithelium. They may be exquisitely tender and can be distinguished from corns and calluses by their tendency to pinpoint bleed when the surface is pared away. *Mosaic warts* are plaques of myriad small, closely set, plantar warts.

Filiform warts are long, narrow, small growths usually seen on the eyelids, face, neck, or lips. *Flat warts* are smooth, flat, yellow-brown lesions that occur more commonly in children and young adults, most often on the face and along scratch marks through autoinoculation. Warts of unusual shapes (e.g., pedunculated or resembling a cauliflower) are most frequent on the head and neck, especially on the scalp and bearded region.

As with most viral infections, warts occur more commonly in children, and they go away when immunity develops. In young children, warts may last just a few months; in older children, they may last about 1 year; and in adults, they may last for months to years. Most warts go away spontaneously and heal without scars. Research suggests that some warts will disappear when covered with duct tape for several days.

Warts may behave differently in different locations. Warts around the fingernails and on the palms and soles are particularly long lived and stubborn. Warts on the bearded area of men who shave are particularly troublesome because shaving often spreads them, as does the shaving of legs in women. In the same way, picking at or chewing of warts on the hands may spread them, especially under the fingernails. Warts caused by HPV may grow profusely on the genitalia of adults and can be passed between sexual partners.

INDICATIONS

All treatments work through tissue destruction, with the goal being to destroy the virus-containing epidermis and preserve as much uninvolved tissue as possible. The type and aggressiveness of therapy depend on the type of wart, its location, and the patient's cooperation and immune status. The least painful methods should be used initially, especially in young children. More destructive therapies should be reserved for areas where scarring is not a consideration or for recalcitrant lesions.

A major point to remember when treating warts is that the virus is microscopic, and although after treatment the skin may look normal, the virus is often still present in the remaining tissue. Unless that tissue is also removed, the warts will recur a few months later. Therefore, all treatments should be attempts to remove several layers of skin beyond the first signs of normal tissue. Such therapy may take several weeks or even months, but patience and perseverance are essential. Patients should never be guaranteed that the initial removal of a wart is the definitive treatment.

Plantar warts should be treated with nonscarring methods if at all possible because a scar on the sole of the foot can be quite painful and is irreversible. Therefore, only severe, recalcitrant plantar lesions should be considered for possible treatment with curettage and desiccation or excision. These patients should be referred to a podiatrist.

Periungual warts usually require no treatment if they are not painful. Patients should be instructed to stop nail and cuticle biting. Warts on the proximal nail fold must be treated gently to avoid permanent injury to the underlying nail bed; this results in permanent nail deformity.

CONTRAINDICATIONS

- Uncertain diagnosis
- History of an adverse reaction to the treatment method
- Chemical treatments contraindicated in pregnancy
- Cellulitis
- Allergy to treatment
- Noncompliance

PRECAUTIONS

- Avoid surgical excision of plantar warts.
- Use caution when removing warts from a patient who has diabetes or who is immunocompromised.
- Usually no more than five warts are removed at any one time.

ASSESSMENT

- Obtain a history to determine how long the lesion has been present and if it has been changing or bleeding.
- Determine the patient's past medical history, including conditions that may affect wound healing or increase the risk of infection, such as diabetes, immunodeficiency diseases, or peripheral vascular disease.
- Ascertain a history of allergies and current medications.
- Physical examination should include size, symmetry, color, border characteristics, and character of the lesion.
- Examine the area closely to determine wart morphology, evidence of trauma, or infection.

PATIENT PREPARATION

The procedure should be explained to the patient, including risks and benefits, possible complications, and alternatives to the procedure. The patient should be given an opportunity to ask questions about the procedure. Discuss the fact that scarring may occur.

Position the patient comfortably so that the site can be easily accessed.

TREATMENT ALTERNATIVES (See Box 2-4)

Imiquimod *(S)*-26308,*(R)*-837(1-(2-methylpropyl)-1*H*-imidazo[4,5**c**]quinolin-4 amine), an immune response modifier, is approved as a 5% cream (Aldara, 3M Pharmaceuticals) for the treatment of genital and perianal warts. The innate immune response is activated primarily from induction of interferon-alpha and other cytokines in the skin. Imiquimod also stimulates cellular acquired immunity, which is important for controlling viral infections and tumors.

Chemical Destruction Using Topical Keratolytics

Salicylic acid and cantharadin 0.7% are two common topical keratolytics that are used to treat warts.

PATIENT PREPARATION

The chemical treatment of warts causes the epithelium to swell, soften, macerate, and then desquamate. Treatment may become progressively more painful because wart tissue macerates and the chemical reaches more sensitive epidermal and dermal tissue.

Inform patients about the high rate of recurrence; they may need multiple treatments.

EQUIPMENT

Salicylic Acid (available mostly as OTC meds)

- White bandage tape (not paper tape)
- Adhesive bandage with center cut out to fit around wart
- Salicylic acid preparation
  - Salicylic acid preparations are available in various strengths. Stronger preparations are usually reserved for thicker areas (e.g., palms, soles, and extremities), and weaker strengths are usually reserved for the digits of younger children. DuoFilm, Compound W (salicylic acid 6.7% and lactic acid 16.7%), or Occlusal-HP (salicylic acid 17%) allow for easy application on multiple sites and is useful for common plantar and palmar warts. DuoPlant (salicylic acid 27%) is a stronger concentration that is useful for thicker lesions. Mediplast (salicylic acid 40%) is especially useful for plantar warts and is best applied to the wart and a few millimeters of surrounding normal skin. Keralyt, Cuplex (salicylic acid 6% to 11%), or salicylic acid 20% to 40% plaster (self-adhesive corn plaster) can be used on plantar warts.

Cantharidin 0.7%

- Cantharidin 0.7%
- Clear tape
- Triple antibiotic ointment

Silver Nitrate

- Silver nitrate sticks
- Adhesive bandage

Procedure

SALICYLIC ACID

This procedure can be taught so that the patient can perform it at home. Follow universal precautions.

1. Soak the affected area in warm water for 5 to 10 minutes.
2. Put on a bandage with the center cut out around the wart to prevent maceration of the surrounding skin.
3. Cover the wart with the chemical solution and allow it to dry. The compound turns white when it is dry. Blowing on it or using a fan makes it dry faster. Apply at bedtime.
4. Cover with white bandage tape to seal out the air. This macerates the wart skin and causes the acid solution to penetrate much better. Do not use paper tape or

tape with holes in it that breathes. It is not harmful to get the tape wet as long as it stays in place.

5. Remove the tape after 48 to 72 hours. Peel off as much of the wart skin as possible. A small knife, emery board, or razor blade may be used to remove any remaining wart tissue.
6. Do not retreat the wart for 24 hours or the medicine may sting and irritate the affected area. The wart is very sensitive just after peeling.
7. Repeat the process until the entire wart is removed and only pink skin is left on the affected area.
8. When the wart appears to be gone, check at least weekly for any early recurrence. The earlier a recurrence is seen and treatment is initiated, the easier it will be to clear the wart permanently.
9. To obtain maximum benefit, it may be necessary to continue treatment for as long as 3 months. Contamination of the surrounding skin causes irritation, and there is often discomfort before the wart is cured.

CANTHARIDIN 0.7%

Cantharidin is an extract of the blister beetle and may be useful in conjunction with salicylic acid preparations or between treatments. If the patient is very responsive, he or she may need only one treatment, followed by the application of a salicylic acid preparation. Follow universal precautions.

1. Apply cantharidin carefully to the individual lesions, following the same guidelines used for salicylic acid.
2. Cover with clear tape.
3. Blistering will occur within 2 to 24 hours after which the tape should be removed and the medication washed off with soap and water.
4. Apply triple antibiotic ointment to the exposed areas twice daily.
5. Blistering may be very uncomfortable, and the chemotoxic response varies among patients; some have swelling with pain, and others have no response at all. The application itself is painless.

SILVER NITRATE

Follow universal precautions.

1. Soak wart in warm water.
2. Pare away lesion as much as possible.
3. Apply silver nitrate at the end of the stick. Do not apply for longer than a few seconds.
4. Repeat weekly until resolved.
5. Application may darken tissue, but will resolve.

Cryotherapy

Cryotherapy is the use of cold as a destructive medium. Cryogenic materials include carbon dioxide (≈78.5° C), liquid nitrous oxide (≈89.5° C), and liquid nitrogen (≈195.6° C). Liquid nitrogen is considered to be the most useful because of its low temperature, easy availability, low cost, and safety. Liquid nitrogen evaporates very quickly on exposure to room air, so it is stored in metal Dewar containers.

Liquid nitrogen is effective for warts on the face, around the eyes, nose, and mouth, including the mucosa. It is safe to use in children and in pregnant women; however, the treatment may be too painful in small children who have multiple warts.

Common warts (verrucae vulgaris) and plantar warts (verrucae plantaris) are usually treated using liquid nitrogen-soaked cotton-tipped applicators. A spray tip adapter can be used to treat mosaic warts, flat warts, and condylomata acuminata.

Cryotherapy is especially useful for warts that have failed to respond to 3 months of topical treatment and for facial warts. Cryotherapy is rarely successful with just one treatment because of the depth of the wart; however, repeated treatments may be successful.

PATIENT PREPARATION

During the treatment, the patient may feel no pain or, at the most, a burning sensation.

Moderate to severe throbbing pain occurs after the treatment and usually lasts from several minutes to many hours, depending on the location and size of the affected area.

If hyperkeratosis is present, 10% salicylic ointment should be applied to the wart for several days before the treatment.

EQUIPMENT

- Liquid nitrogen, in either a Styrofoam container or a metal Thermos-type container with a spray applicator
- Sterile cotton-tipped applicators, if nitrogen is in a Styrofoam container; the diameter of the cotton-tipped applicator should be more or less the same as the diameter of the lesion. Standard cotton swabs usually have to be loosened or have additional cotton rolled onto the swab for a better matrix to hold the liquid.

Procedure

COTTON-TIP METHOD:

Follow universal precautions.

1. Dip the prepared cotton tip into the liquid nitrogen.
2. Press the tip firmly against the lesion. Hold the applicator perpendicularly against the lesion until a white frozen halo (the "ice ball") appears and extends 2 to 3 mm beyond the base of the lesion. Pressure on the swab increases the depth of the penetration.
3. The time of freezing varies, depending on the type of wart and its depth, diameter, and location. It may vary from a few seconds (15 to 30 seconds) for verrucae plana to about 90 seconds for verrucae plantaris.
4. Directly after the treatment, the treated area first becomes pale, and then turns red. After a few minutes, a swelling occurs, which may last for several hours. Serous or blood-filled blisters form later. The blister should cover the whole lesion with a several-millimeter margin around it; however, it should not extend significantly beyond the frozen area.

5. Do not remove the roof of the blister because this may lead to infection of the uncovered area. The blister covering serves as protection from organisms and eliminates the need for a bandage.
6. After a few days, the blister dries up, and a scab forms that lasts for 1 or 2 weeks. The lesion is usually healed within 3 weeks.
7. Recommend a follow-up visit to determine whether viable wart tissue remains at the base of the healed blister. If the remaining wart tissue is found, follow-up treatment is needed.

SPRAY METHOD:

1. Use changeable nozzles adapted to the shape and diameter of the lesions. The nozzle should be held closely to the skin to prevent spraying the surrounding areas.
   a. An otoscope cover can easily be cut to the size of the wart to create a target area.
   b. Freeze plantar warts with use of the spray method for a few seconds (very superficially), enough to bring an inflammatory reaction, but not to produce blisters.
   c. Mosaic warts should be frozen superficially, but sufficiently, to produce blisters (15 to 30 seconds).
   d. For condylomata acuminata, the period of freezing lasts from a few seconds for small lesions to between 20 and 30 seconds for large lesions. Avoid spraying numerous lesions during a single procedure because this leads to swelling. Condylomata acuminata disappear more rapidly than do ordinary warts; therefore, reexamine the patient after 7 to 14 days.
   e. Repeat spray method 2 to 3 times during a single visit.
   f. Multiple applications may be necessary.

COMPLICATIONS

Chemical Destruction and Cryotherapy

- Infection can occur.
- The lesion can recur.
- There are some reports in the literature of fever that lasts for 2 to 3 days, of hypertrophic scars in patients who have a tendency to develop keloids, and of neuropathy caused by treatment that is reversible within a period of several weeks to months.

PRACTITIONER FOLLOW-UP/REFERRAL

Chemical Destruction and Cryotherapy

Consider referring patients when warts do not respond to treatment, when they are excessively numerous, or when they are on the face or in areas that may result in disfiguration from scarring.

Spontaneous regression occurs in as many as two thirds of warts within 2 years; however, new warts may appear while others are regressing.

2

RED FLAGS

- Allergic reactions
- Infection
- Blistering
- Scarring
- Unresolved lesion
- Unresolved pain
- Unresolved bleeding
- Increase in size and number of warts

CPT BILLING

Destruction means the ablation of benign, premalignant, or malignant tissues by any method, with or without curettement, including local anesthesia, and not usually requiring closure. Any method includes electrosurgery, cryosurgery, laser, and chemical treatment.

17110—Destruction of benign lesions other than skin tags or cutaneous vascular proliferative lesions; up to 14 lesions. ■ **17111**—15 or more lesions. These codes should not be used together.

Genital lesions have their own codes and are not included with the above codes.

56501—Destruction of lesion(s), vulva, simple (e.g., laser, electrosurgery, cryosurgery, chemosurgery) ■ **54050**—Destruction of lesion(s), penis (e.g., condyloma, papilloma, molluscum contagiosum, herpetical vesicle), simple; chemical ■ **540555**—Destruction of lesion(s), penis (e.g., condyloma, papilloma, molluscum contagiosum, herpetical vesicle), simple; electrodesication ■ **54056**—Destruction of lesion(s), penis (e.g., condyloma, papilloma, molluscum contagiosum, herpetical vesicle), simple; cryosurgery ■ **54057**—Destruction of lesion(s), penis (e.g., condyloma, papilloma, molluscum contagiosum, herpetical vesicle), simple; laser surgery ■ **54058**—Destruction of lesion(s), penis (e.g., condyloma, papilloma, molluscum contagiosum, herpetical vesicle), simple; surgical excision

REFERENCES AND RELATED RESOURCES

Pfenninger J, Fowler G: *Pfenninger and Fowler's procedures for primary care*, ed 3, Philadelphia, 2011, Elsevier.

Usatine RP, Smith MA, Chumley H, Mayeaux Jr EJ: *The color atlas of family medicine*, ed 2, New York, 2013, McGraw-Hill.

Abscess Incision and Drainage

Kent D. Blad and Sabrina Jarvis

DESCRIPTION

An *abscess* is the result of an infection that forms a localized collection of pus surrounded by inflamed tissue. *Furuncles* (abscesses formed in a hair follicle or sweat gland) and *paronychia* (abscess of the nail) are examples of specific types of abscesses.

ANATOMY AND PHYSIOLOGY

The most common causative agent of the infection is *Staphylococcus aureus,* although *Streptococcus* and other bacteria, including anaerobes, can be a cause. Warm compresses and/or antibiotics may cause spontaneous drainage and healing of a small abscess. Larger abscesses have a walled-off cavity, and soaking and/or antibiotics are usually not effective without incision and drainage. Routine culture of drainage in healthy patients is not necessary, and in the healthy patient, routine use of antibiotics after incision and drainage is controversial. Systemic antibiotics should be considered in the presence of associated cellulitis or septic phlebitis, abscesses in an area difficult to drain, signs and symptoms of systemic illness, associated comorbidities or immunosuppression, extremes of age, and lack of response to incision and drainage.

INDICATIONS

- Presence of a fluctuant abscess that is tender and not resolving spontaneously, or with conservative treatments or any large, inflamed abscess
- To obtain a specimen for culture and sensitivity testing
- Once a collection of pus is present, antibiotics alone are usually inadequate

CONTRAINDICATIONS

- Abscesses that are not fluctuant should not be incised.
- Incision and drainage of facial abscesses are contraindicated if the abscess is located within a triangle formed by the bridge of the nose and the corners of the mouth. There is a high risk of septic phlebitis with intracranial extensions for incision and drainage in these areas. Treatment should be antibiotics and warm compresses. Referral may be necessary if treatment is not resolved.
- Coagulopathies.

PRECAUTIONS

The patient who has diabetes or immunocompromised conditions should be followed closely, and culture and sensitivity should be obtained during the incision and drainage. Consider the use of antibiotics in these patients.

ASSESSMENT

- Obtain a history to determine how long the abscess has been present and whether it has been changing or growing.
- Ask about systemic signs of infections, such as fever, chills, body aches, or swollen lymph nodes.
- Determine the patient's past medical history, including conditions that may affect wound healing or increase the risk of infection, such as diabetes, immunodeficiency diseases, or peripheral vascular disease.
- Ascertain a history of allergies and current medications.
- Ascertain a history of bleeding disorders.
- Physical examination should include size, color, and whether the abscess is fluctuant.
- Check for fever and for proximal lymphadenopathy.
- The white blood cell count may be checked if systemic signs of infection are present. If the patient has had frequent infections, testing for diabetes may be indicated.

PATIENT PREPARATION

The procedure should be explained to the patient, including risks and benefits, possible complications, and alternatives to the procedure. The patient should be given an opportunity to ask questions about the procedure. Discuss the fact that scarring may occur.

Position the patient comfortably so that the abscess can be easily accessed.

TREATMENT ALTERNATIVES

Provide conservative treatment with warm, moist soaks and antibiotics if indicated.

EQUIPMENT

- Anesthesia supplies (see "Anesthesia: Topical, Local, and Digital Nerve Block, Equipment")
- Antiseptic solution (e.g., povidone-iodine) and swabs
- Sterile 2 × 2 or 4 × 4 gauze sponges (8 to 10 or more)
- No. 11 surgical blade and handle
- Curved hemostats
- Tissue forceps
- Sterile fenestrated drape
- Sterile iodoform gauze (if packing may be needed)
- Culture swab (if indicated)
- Scissors
- Sterile cotton-tipped swabs
- Dressing supplies (sterile gauze, antibiotic ointment, tape, etc.)
- Sterile gloves
- Eye and face protection
- Protective gown

Procedure

2

Follow universal precautions.

1. Cleanse the abscess area using antiseptic solution (see "Wound Care"). Clean up to 3 inches in diameter of abscess.
2. Provide local anesthesia (see "Anesthesia: Topical, Local, and Digital Nerve Block, Equipment").
3. Place fenestrated drape over the area to be incised.
4. Using a No. 11 blade, make an incision parallel to the skin lines across the abscess to allow drainage of the cavity. Do not make the incision too small as the incision may prematurely close during healing (Figure 2-33).
5. If no spontaneous drainage occurs, apply light pressure to the surrounding skin.
6. If a culture is needed, obtain it from the abscess cavity, not from drainage on the skin.

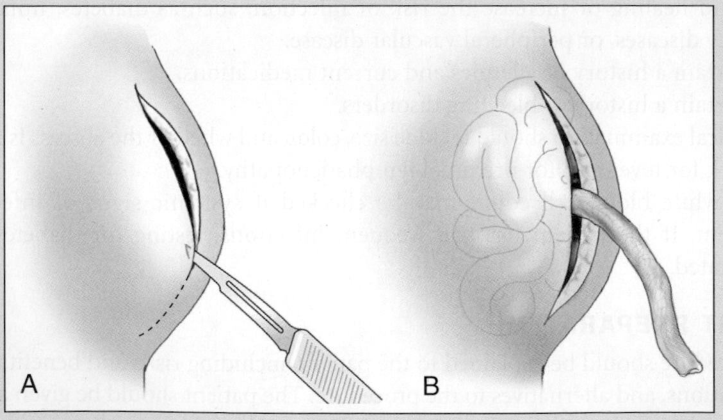

FIGURE 2-33 Incision and drainage of an abscess. Prepare and drape the area. Inject 1% to 2% lidocaine around the perimeter of the abscess, taking care not to infiltrate the abscess cavity. **A,** Make an incision sufficiently wide to allow for drainage and prevent premature closure that might result in pus being trapped and recurrence of the abscess. **B,** Place a drain. In this case gauze is used.

7. Explore the abscess cavity using a sterile cotton-tipped applicator or a curved hemostat. Break down walled-off pockets within the cavity. Abscesses are usually irregularly shaped with finger-like projections throughout that must be broken to optimize drainage and healing.
8. Apply external pressure to express all purulent material from the abscess.
9. Pack the cavity lightly with plain or iodoform packing strips, taking care not to insert too much packing, which could impede the wound healing.
10. Secure a sterile dressing over the area that will absorb oozing pus and/or blood.
11. Dress the site with antibiotic ointment, sterile gauze, and tape.

PATIENT EDUCATION POSTPROCEDURE

- The patient should expect some oozing from the site. Packing may have to be removed and replaced. While packing is present in the cavity, the area should be kept dry to prevent the introduction of bacteria or other contaminants into the cavity. Healing should progress from inside out so that the incision does not close until the abscess cavity has healed and closed. If the packing falls out, the patient should not replace it. Healing time varies from 7 to 21 days.
- If signs or symptoms of infection occur, such as recollection of pus in the abscess, increased pain, redness or swelling, fever and chills, or red streaks near the abscess, the patient should notify the clinician immediately.
- Return to clinic in 24 to 48 hours to assess site and change dressing.

COMPLICATIONS

- Cellulitis
- Bacteremia and septicemia (if inadequately treated)

PRACTITIONER FOLLOW-UP

- The patient should return for reevaluation in 24 to 48 hours, depending on the location and severity of the abscess.
- The packing may have to be removed, replaced, or partially removed, depending on whether or not it is saturated.
- Consider antibiotic treatment based on the criteria listed above.
- Provide for pain relief and discuss with patient.

RED FLAGS

- Increased swelling in the abscess area
- Increased pain in the abscess area
- Cellulitis unresolved
- Formation of fistula
- Osteomyelitis
- Gangrene

CPT BILLING

10060—Incision and drainage of abscess (carbuncle, suppurative hidradenitis, cutaneous or subcutaneous abscess, cyst, furuncle, or paronychia); simple or single ■ **10061**—Complicated or multiple ■ **10080**—Incision and drainage of pilonidal, cyst; simple ■ **10081**—Complicated ■ **10120**—Incision and removal of foreign body, subcutaneous tissues; simple ■ **10121**—Complicated ■ **10140**—Incision and drainage of hematoma, seroma or fluid collection ■ **10160**—Punctate aspiration of abscess, hematoma, bulla, or cyst

REFERENCES AND RELATED RESOURCES

Pfenninger J, Fowler G: *Pfenninger and Fowler's procedures for primary care*, ed 3, Philadelphia, 2011, Elsevier.

Usatine RP, Smith MA, Chumley H, Mayeaux Jr EJ: *The color atlas of family medicine*, ed 2, New York, 2013, McGraw-Hill.

Cyst Removal

Kent D. Blad and Sabrina Jarvis

2

DESCRIPTION

An epidermoid (sebaceous) cyst is a small, mobile, superficial cyst that contains a thick, white/yellow substance known as *keratin*.

ANATOMY AND PHYSIOLOGY

Epidermoid cysts usually occur on the face, ears, chest, or back, but may occur on any skin surface. Stratified squamous epithelium in the cyst wall produces cytokeratins. The most common source for this epithelium is the hair follicle infundibulum. The cyst often has a "head," or communication through the surface of the skin. The cysts may grow over time and spontaneously rupture, releasing the soft keratin. Many epidermoid cysts do not require removal unless they cause pain or become inflamed or infected.

The cyst often recurs, especially if the sac is not completely removed. Some patients seem prone to the development of these cysts, and they may recur in other locations.

INDICATIONS

- Inflamed or infected cysts
- Bothersome or unsightly cysts

CONTRAINDICATIONS

There are none.

PRECAUTIONS

Surgical consultation should be considered for the following situations:

- Cysts embedded in the outer table of the skull, breast, and bone
- Appearance of lesion that is suggestive of a malignancy
- Very large cysts

ASSESSMENT

- Obtain a history to determine how long the cyst has been present and whether it has been changing or growing or has become inflamed.
- Ascertain whether the patient has had prior incision and drainage of similar cysts.
- Ask about systemic signs of infections such as fever, chills, body aches, or swollen lymph nodes if the cyst is inflamed.

- Determine the patient's past medical history, including conditions that may affect wound healing or increase the risk of infection, such as diabetes, immunodeficiency diseases, or peripheral vascular disease.
- Ascertain a history of allergies and current medications.
- Physical examination should include size, mobility, and signs of inflammation.
- Check for fever and proximal lymphadenopathy if inflamed.

PATIENT PREPARATION

Informed written consent should be obtained for the procedure. The procedure should be explained to the patient, including the risks and benefits, possible complications, and alternatives to the procedure. The patient should be given an opportunity to ask questions about the procedure. Discuss the fact that scarring may occur.

Position the patient comfortably so that the abscess can be easily accessed.

TREATMENT ALTERNATIVES

- Excision of the cyst (if not infected)
- No treatment if not inflamed/infected

EQUIPMENT

- Anesthesia supplies (see "Anesthesia: Topical, Local, and Digital Nerve Block, Equipment")
- Antiseptic solution (e.g., povidone-iodine) and swabs
- Sterile 2 × 2 or 4 × 4 gauze sponges (8 to 10 or more)
- No. 11 surgical blade and handle
- Curved hemostats
- Tissue forceps
- Sterile fenestrated drape
- Sterile iodoform gauze (if packing may be needed)
- Culture swab (if indicated)
- Scissors
- Sterile cotton-tipped swabs
- Dressing supplies (sterile gauze, antibiotic ointment, tape, etc.)
- Sterile gloves
- Eye and face protection
- Protective gown

Procedure

Follow universal precautions.

1. Cleanse the area using antiseptic solution (see "Wound Care").
2. Provide local anesthesia (see "Anesthesia: Topical, Local, and Digital Nerve Block, Equipment").
3. Place fenestrated drape over the area to be incised.

TREATMENT ALTERNATIVES

Alternative 1

1. Using a No. 11 blade, make an incision in the skin, but not through the cyst. Using a blunt dissection, release the cyst from the surrounding connective tissue and remove. If the cyst is infected, it is better to proceed with incision and drainage, as discussed previously.

Alternative 2

1. Incise the cyst parallel to the skin lines with a No. 11 blade.
2. Express the contents of the cyst by applying a light pressure to the cyst margins.
3. If the shiny cyst sac comes out of the incision, grasp it, use blunt dissection to free it, and remove the sac completely. If the sac does not invert, use blunt dissection to separate the sac from the surrounding connective tissue and attempt to remove it completely if possible.

Alternative 3

1. Use a 5-mm punch to punch through the dermis and into the cyst. Express the contents of the cyst, and then use blunt dissection to separate and remove the sac from the surrounding connective tissue.
2. Depending on the wound and the procedure, pack the wound or close with suture (Figure 2-34).
3. Apply a sterile dressing, as appropriate.

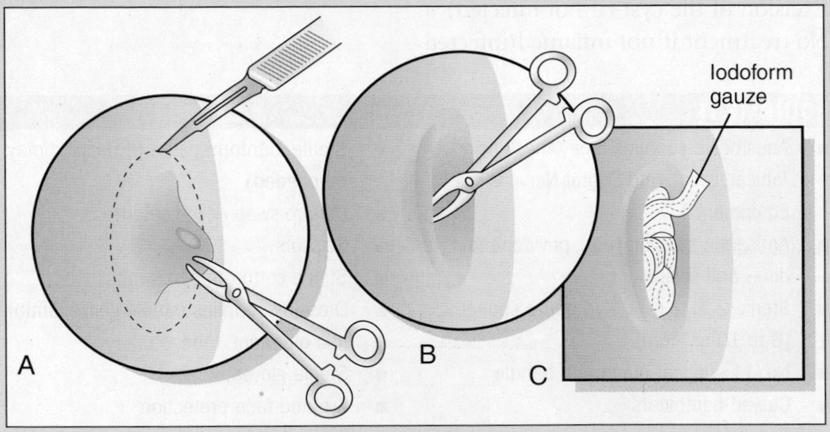

FIGURE 2-34 Sebaceous cyst removal. **A**, Cut the elastic tissue around the outer edges of the sac until released. **B**, After expressing the contents of the cyst, explore the cavity with a hemostat. **C**, Pack the wound with gauze, leaving a small tail protruding from the wound.

PATIENT EDUCATION POSTPROCEDURE

- The patient should expect some oozing from the site.
- Packing may have to be removed or replaced if it was used. While packing is present in the cavity, the area should be kept dry to prevent the introduction of bacteria or other contaminants into the cavity.
- Healing should progress from the inside out so that the incision does not close until the abscess cavity has healed and closed. If the packing falls out, the patient should not replace it, but should return to the health care practitioner. Healing time varies from 10 to 14 days.
- If signs or symptoms of infection occur, such as increased pain, redness or swelling, fever and chills, or red streaks near the abscess, the patient should notify the clinician immediately.
- If sutures were used, they will have to be removed. Advise the patient that the cyst may recur, especially if the cyst sac was not removed completely.

COMPLICATIONS

- Infection
- Scarring and keloid formation

PRACTITIONER FOLLOW-UP

Follow-up is needed only if packing was used, sutures were placed, or the patient develops signs of infection at the site.

▶ RED FLAG

Refer to surgeon if the cysts occur in the breast, bone, or in the intracranial region, or if there is a suspicion of a possible malignancy.

■ CPT BILLING

See codes under incision and drainage.

REFERENCES AND RELATED RESOURCES

Fromm L: *Epidermal inclusion cyst treatment & management*, 2014. http://emedicine.medscape.com/article/1061582-treatment.

Pfenninger J, Fowler G: *Pfenninger and Fowler's procedures for primary care*, ed 3, Philadelphia, 2010, Elsevier.

Skin Tag Removal

Kent D. Blad and Sabrina Jarvis

DESCRIPTION

Acrochordons, or skin tags, are pedunculated, benign skin lesions.

ANATOMY AND PHYSIOLOGY

These lesions are found in approximately 25% of the population. They occur most commonly in the axilla, neck, and inguinal region. They usually begin to form in the second decade of life and increase with age up to the fifth decade. Skin tags form as a small, brown- or flesh-colored lesion attached by a stalk. They may or may not grow with time. Some may aggravate the patient when they are caught on clothes or jewelry. If the lesion can be identified as an acrochordon, pathologic analysis may not be necessary.

INDICATIONS

- Skin tags that are traumatized or irritated due to clothing, jewelry, etc.
- Cosmetic (many insurance companies will not reimburse removal for cosmetic reasons)

CONTRAINDICATIONS

- Any lesion suspicious of malignancy.
- High dose of steroid therapy.
- Coagulopathies.

PRECAUTIONS

Patients who have diabetes and have a history of poor healing.

ASSESSMENT

- Obtain a history to determine how long the skin tag has been present and whether it has been changing or growing, or has become inflamed.
- Ascertain whether the skin tag is getting caught on clothing, jewelry, etc.
- Determine the patient's past medical history, including conditions that may affect wound healing or increase the risk of infection, such as diabetes, immunodeficiency diseases, or peripheral vascular disease.
- Ascertain a history of allergies and current medications.
- Ascertain a history of coagulopathies.
- Physical examination should include size, description, location, and number of skin tags.

PATIENT PREPARATION

The procedure should be explained to the patient, including the risks and benefits, possible complications, and alternatives to the procedure. Patients should be given an opportunity to ask questions about the procedure.

Position the patient comfortably so that the skin tag can be easily accessed. Discuss the use of anesthesia and the fact that it will likely be more painful than the actual procedure itself, and then ascertain the patient's desires regarding the anesthesia.

TREATMENT ALTERNATIVES

- No treatment

EQUIPMENT

ELECTROCAUTERY

- Anesthesia (optional)
- Electrocautery unit
- Chemical cautery (silver nitrate, aluminum chloride, or ferrous subsulfate)
- Dressing material

SCISSORS/BLADE EXCISION

- Antiseptic solution
- Iris scissors or No. 11 or 15 scalpel
- Forceps with teeth

CRYOTHERAPY

- Cryotherapy unit and tips
- Liquid nitrogen
- Forceps

Procedure

ELECTROCAUTERY

Follow universal precautions.

1. Provide anesthesia if desired.
2. Use a fine-tipped, electric cautery device at a low setting, and apply cautery lightly to skin at the base of the stalk.

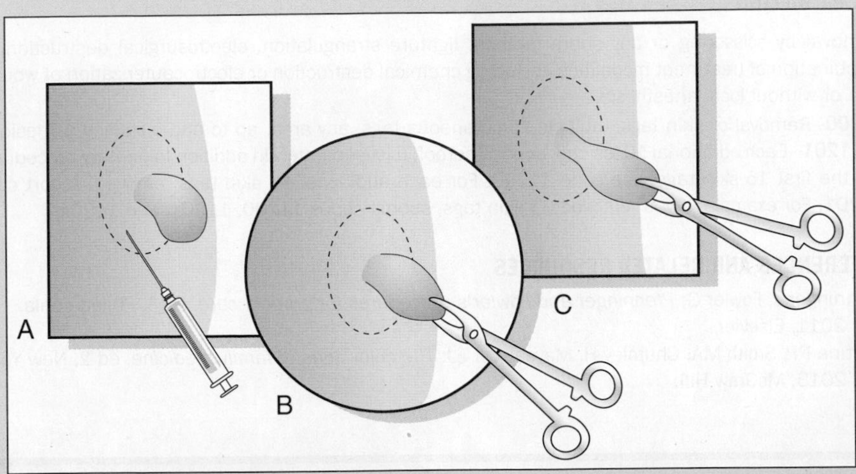

FIGURE 2-35 Skin tag removal. **A**, Infiltrate the base of the skin tag with lidocaine. **B**, Grab the skin tag at the largest part with the hemostat. C, Pull the skin tag until the stalk base is visible and clip off with scissors or blade.

SCISSORS/BLADE REMOVAL (Figure 2-35)

1. Provide anesthesia if desired.
2. Cleanse the area with antiseptic solution.
3. Grasp the skin tag with the forceps and snip or cut at the base of the stalk.
4. Use direct pressure, electrocautery, or chemical cautery to control bleeding.

CRYOTHERAPY

1. Apply liquid nitrogen on a cotton swab or the tip of the cryotherapy gun unit to the skin tag until the tag turns white. This may be repeated once.
2. If using a cryotherapy gun with tips, the cold may be conducted better if lubricating gel is first applied to the skin tag. Lubricating gel will form an ice ball.
3. Application time is usually 30 seconds for small skin tags and 45 seconds for larger skin tags.

PATIENT EDUCATION POSTPROCEDURE

After cryotherapy (and electrocautery if the lesion did not slough off), the lesion will dry and slough off in a few days. There may be slight bleeding if the skin tag was removed with a scissors or blade. This should stop with direct pressure. Review signs and symptoms of infection with the patient and recommend follow-up if they occur.

COMPLICATIONS (DEPENDING ON PROCEDURE)

- Bleeding
- Infection

PRACTITIONER FOLLOW-UP

No follow-up is necessary, unless complications develop.

CPT BILLING

Removal by scissoring or any sharp method, ligature strangulation, electrosurgical destruction, or combination of treatment modalities, including chemical destruction or electrocauterization of wound, with or without local anesthesia.

11200—Removal of skin tags, multiple fibrcutaneous tags, any area, up to and including 15 lesions.
■ **11201**—Each additional 10 lesions, or part thereof. (List separately in addition to primary procedure.)
For the first 15 skin tags, use code 11200. For each additional 10 skin tags removed, report code 11201. For example, if you removed 33 skin tags, submit codes 11200, 11201, and 11201.

REFERENCES AND RELATED RESOURCES

Pfenninger J, Fowler G: *Pfenninger and Fowler's procedures for primary care*, ed 3, Philadelphia, 2011, Elsevier.
Usatine RP, Smith MA, Chumley H, Mayeaux Jr EJ: *The color atlas of family medicine*, ed 2, New York, 2013, McGraw-Hill.

2

Care for Superficial and Partial Thickness Burns

Kent D. Blad and Sabrina Jarvis

DESCRIPTION

This section will address only superficial burns that can be managed in an outpatient setting. Treatment is designed to reduce cellular damage to tissues caused by abrasions, chemicals, electricity, gas, or heat. Burns restricted to a small area are often minor and may be treated on an outpatient basis. The following information is used to determine whether the patient should be treated in an outpatient facility or hospital setting:

▶ RED FLAGS

- Age > 60
- Burns on more than 40% of total body surface area
- Presence of inhalation injury
- Increased depth of burn
- Premorbid diseases
- Comorbid disorders (e.g., respiratory complications, etc.)
- Associated trauma
- Distribution of the burn
- Injuring agent (electricity, chemicals, etc.)
- Patient's social situation (Can they care for themselves?)

ANATOMY AND PHYSIOLOGY

Chemical burns occur when corrosive or caustic substances (e.g., lye, battery acid) come in contact with the skin. Alkali burns are more serious than acid burns because alkali produces a liquefaction necrosis that penetrates deep into the skin and burns longer than acids. Acids damage tissue through a coagulation necrosis. External chemical wounds may produce red, discolored, raw, white, soft, or mushy skin, with pain dependent on the depth of the burn.

Electrical burns result from electric current (touching faulty electrical wiring) or being struck by lightning. Lightning frequently causes swollen, charred, or reddened skin around the entrance wound and a burn pattern that resembles a tree branch. In addition, lightning and other electrical burns cause varying damage to the nervous system, cardiovascular system, and kidneys. Fifty percent of patients have ruptured tympanic membranes.

Inhalation burns result from the inhalation of smoke containing gases or certain chemicals. Many plastics contain substances that are toxic when they are burned. Symptoms are systemic: chest pain, dyspnea, light-headedness, loss of consciousness, and burning of the eyes or mouth. There may be burns of the face or only evidence of laryngeal edema. Damage to airways may be permanent.

Thermal burns are produced by fires, space heaters, explosives, firecrackers, scalding, or motor vehicle accidents and are classified by depth.

The traditional classifications of first-, second-, and third-degree burns have been replaced by a system that classifies cutaneous burns by the depth of the tissue injury and the need for surgical interventions (http://www.ameriburn.org) (Box 2-5).

- Superficial burns involve only the epidermis (e.g., sunburn, brief contact with hot burner) and, although painful, have little or no blistering or swelling.
- Superficial partial-thickness burns damage the dermis and epidermis (short exposure to flame, hot liquids, or prolonged sun exposure), producing blisters between

BOX 2-5 American Burn Association Burn Injury Severity Grading System

MINOR BURN

15% of total body surface area (TBSA) or less in adults
10% TBSA or less in children and older adults
2% TBSA or less for full-thickness burns in children or adults who are without cosmetic or functional risk to the eyes, ear, face, hands, feet, or perineum

MODERATE BURN

15% to 25% TBSA in adults who have less than 10% of full-thickness burns
10% to 20% TBSA partial-thickness burn in children under 10 and adults over 40 years of age with less than 10% full-thickness burn
10% TBSA or less full-thickness burn in children or adults without cosmetic or functional risk to eyes, ears, face, hands, feet, or perineum

MAJOR BURN

25% TBSA or greater
20% TBSA or greater in children under 10 and adults over 40 years of age
10% TBSA or greater full-thickness burn
All burns involving the eyes, ears, face, hands, feet, or perineum that are likely to result in cosmetic or functional impairment
All high-voltage electrical burns
All burn injuries complicated by major trauma or inhalation injury
All patients who are at poor risk for burn injury

TBSA: Total body surface area; burn: partial- or full-thickness; young or old: <10 or >50 years old; adults: >10 or <50 years old.
Reproduced from Hartford CE, Kealey CP: Care of outpatient burns. In Herndon DN, editor: *Total burn care,* ed 3, Philadelphia, 2007, Elsevier. Table used with the permission of Elsevier Inc.

the epidermis and dermis within 24 hours. The blisters are red, weeping, and blanch with pressure. The burn usually heals in 7 to 21 days with little or no scarring.
- Deep partial-thickness burns damage the dermis, hair follicles, and glandular tissue. The burn is painful to pressure, almost always blisters, has mottled discoloration, and does not blanch with pressure.
- Full-thickness burns destroy all dermis layers and often injure the subcutaneous tissue. Pain is often absent because nerve endings have been destroyed. Skin appears waxy, white or gray to black, and charred. Blisters do not develop and scarring can be severe.
- Fourth-degree burns damage all skin layers and underlying muscle, fascia, and may involve the bones.

INDICATIONS

The history provides information as to the onset of the burn, its location, characteristics of the burn agent (name, concentration, quantity, mechanism of action), therapeutic actions that have been taken, and whether the burn was accidental or intentional.

CONTRAINDICATIONS

- Patients who have extensive and deep second- or third-degree burns from any source should not be cared for in an outpatient setting; they should be referred to a hospital emergency department or burn center.
- Patients who have electrical burns should be referred to an emergency department for evaluation of extensive injuries.
- Patients who have tendon, muscle, or bone involvement need referral to emergency department.

PRECAUTIONS

Treatment depends on the type and severity of the burn. *Do not* act until this information is known.

- *Do not* use soap if the burn resulted from an alkali or an unknown chemical.
- Keep the patient's burned surfaces from rubbing together. Separate damaged tissue with clean gauze or towels.
- *Do not* put ice or ice water on the burn because this causes rapid tissue chilling and increases damage.
- *Do not* apply burn ointments, creams, butter, or other preparations to the burn. Many preparations trap heat inside, increase tissue damage, and delay healing. It is acceptable, but not necessary in most cases, to use an antibacterial ointment such as Neosporin on facial wounds and superficial wounds on other parts of the body. There are also commercially prepared dressings that can be applied.
- *Do not* use silver sulfadiazine on the face, in patients who have sulfonamide hypersensitivity, or who are pregnant or nursing. Because of the risk of sulfonamide kernicterus, silver sulfadiazine should not be used in infants who are younger than 2 months.

ASSESSMENT

- Determine the source of the burn.
- Determine the degree of the burn.

- Determine the degree of pain experienced by the patient.
- Determine the level of fear or anxiety of the patient.

PATIENT PREPARATION

Patients who call the office should be told to cool the wound with cool tap water or a cool (not ice) pack immediately until the pain is relieved. Neither dressing nor antibiotic ointment is essential before the patient is seen.

EQUIPMENT

Silver sulfadiazine 1% ointment is an alternative choice, even though it is usually not necessary, for superficial partial-thickness burns and is the topical antibiotic of choice around mucous membranes.

Procedure

Follow universal precautions.

SUPERFICIAL (FIRST-DEGREE) BURNS

1. Usually no treatment is required.
2. Remove from source of heat.
3. Cool the burn to dissipate the heat. Cool tap water is adequate. Ice can be detrimental.
4. Aspirin, acetaminophen, or ibuprofen may be taken to reduce mild pain and inflammation.
5. A topical corticosteroid or short course of methylprednisolone may be prescribed for severe sunburn.
6. Skin lubricants, such as aloe vera gel, may be applied.
7. There is no need to use a topical antimicrobial agent or dressing.

SUPERFICIAL PARTIAL-THICKNESS (SECOND-DEGREE) BURNS

1. Wash the area gently, but thoroughly, with bland soap and water (except for chemical burns caused by lime, sodium, or hydrofluoric acid). Remove debris from the wound.
2. Clean the wound using sterile normal saline. Antiseptic solutions should not be used.
3. Use of topical agents: no published evidence exists that shows the use of a topical agent has any positive effect on preventing infection or wound healing. If one feels that they must use a topical agent, the application of 1% silver sulfadiazine with a sterile tongue blade or a gloved hand, approximately 1⁄16-inch thick, has been used by many, but no evidence exists that validates its routine use. Alternative antimicrobial agents may be substituted.
4. If blisters are present, the recommendations vary on whether or not to remove them. The evidence gives equal attention to advantages and disadvantages of blister removal. Each individual is different; make your best clinical judgment based on risks versus benefits. If blisters are removed, lance with a small blade and cover with a nonadherent dressing (Telfa).

5. If the epidermis is intact, the wound does not require a topical agent or a dressing.
6. If the epidermis is not intact, then dressing the wound serves to absorb drainage, to protect the wound from the environment, and to decrease the wound pain. Wrap with gauze dressing (Kling) in layers, forming a soft, bulky dressing, and secure with tape or a cohesive flexible bandage. If a topical antimicrobial agent is used, then change the dressing twice daily for 5 to 7 days. If no agent is used, change the dressing daily to inspect the wound.
7. The patient may require aspirin, acetaminophen, ibuprofen, or oral narcotic analgesics for pain, or tetanus prophylaxis. There is no need for systemic antibiotics.

PATIENT EDUCATION POSTPROCEDURE

- Keep the dressing clean and dry; change the dressing every day (1 to 2 times) for the first 5 to 7 days, then as needed prn.
- Watch for signs of infection.
- Keep burn area clean.
- Obtain tetanus shot if it has been 5 or more years since the last one.

COMPLICATIONS

- Infection
- Scarring
- Pain

PRACTITIONER FOLLOW-UP

- If the burn is large and/or deep and there is a question of whether infection is a high risk, patient should be seen as soon as possible by a specialist in burn care.
- Systemic antibiotics may be necessary for second-degree burns if a secondary cellulitis develops.
- Patient may need to be seen every day for dressing change and wound assessment.

RED FLAGS

- See above referral criteria
- Suspected deep second- or third-degree burns
- Suspected tendon, muscle, or bone involvement
- Circumferential burns of the neck, trunk, or extremities
- Burns of the eyes, ears, face, feet, perineum, genitalia, or hands
- Presence of other trauma
- Conditions that impair wound healing (diabetes mellitus, cardiovascular disease, patients who are immunocompromised)

CPT BILLING

16000—Initial treatment, first degree burn, when no more than local treatment is required ■ **16020**—Dressings and/or debridement of partial thickness burns, initial or subsequent, small (less than 5% total body surface area) ■ **16025**—Dressings and/or debridement of partial thickness burns, initial or subsequent, medium (whole face or whole extremity or 5% to 10% total body surface area)

REFERENCES AND RELATED RESOURCES

Herndon D: Care of outpatient burns. In *Total burn care*, ed 4, Philadelphia, 2012, Elsevier.

Morgan E, Miser W: Treatment of minor thermal burns. In Moreira M, editor: *UpToDate*, Waltham, MA, 2014, UpToDate. Accessed December 17, 2014.

Pfenninger J, Fowler G: *Pfenninger and Fowler's procedures for primary care*, ed 3, Philadelphia, 2011, Elsevier.

Rice P, Orgill D: Classification of burns. In Jeschke M, editor: *UpToDate*, Waltham, MA, 2014, UpToDate. Accessed December 17, 2014.

SKIN SPECIMEN COLLECTION

Scrapings from the skin are used to more precisely diagnose the cause of various dermatologic conditions. How the specimen is taken and how it is preserved depend on the diagnostic suspicions of the clinician.

Scabies Scraping

Kent D. Blad and Sabrina Jarvis

2

DESCRIPTION

This is a diagnostic procedure in which the superficial skin is scraped to obtain a specimen that may be microscopically examined for scabies mites.

ANATOMY AND PHYSIOLOGY

The mite *Sarcoptes scabiei* burrows into the superficial skin, leaving burrows or pustules that contain the mites, fecal pellets, or mite eggs. This debris causes the pruritic irritation. The mite is transmitted via skin-to-skin contact, but may also be spread via fomites, such as towels, clothing, and bedding.

INDICATIONS

The procedure is performed as a diagnostic procedure when infestation is suspected. The skin eruptions mimic several other pruritic dermatoses, and accurate diagnosis is required to determine appropriate treatment. Scraping is indicated particularly when the patient or multiple family members have a known or suspected exposure to scabies and report pruritic eruptions.

CONTRAINDICATIONS

There are none.

PRECAUTIONS

- The scabies organism is transmitted easily; therefore, specimen materials should be handled using universal precautions.
- Small children may require immobilization to collect a specimen.

ASSESSMENT

- Obtain a history of skin eruptions with generalized itching, which can be severe. The pruritus is often worse at night.

- The diagnostic clue is the presence of pruritic vesicles and pustules in burrows or threadlike linear ridges ½ to 1 cm in length. The most common sites are the webs of the finger, the heels of the palm, and in wrist creases. They are also found on the feet, elbows, axilla, and buttocks. In women, they may be found on the thighs, abdomen, and nipples. In men, they may be found on the scrotum or penis. They are not usually found on the head or neck (Figure 2-36).
- Assess for secondary infection of areas that have been denuded or excoriated by scratching.

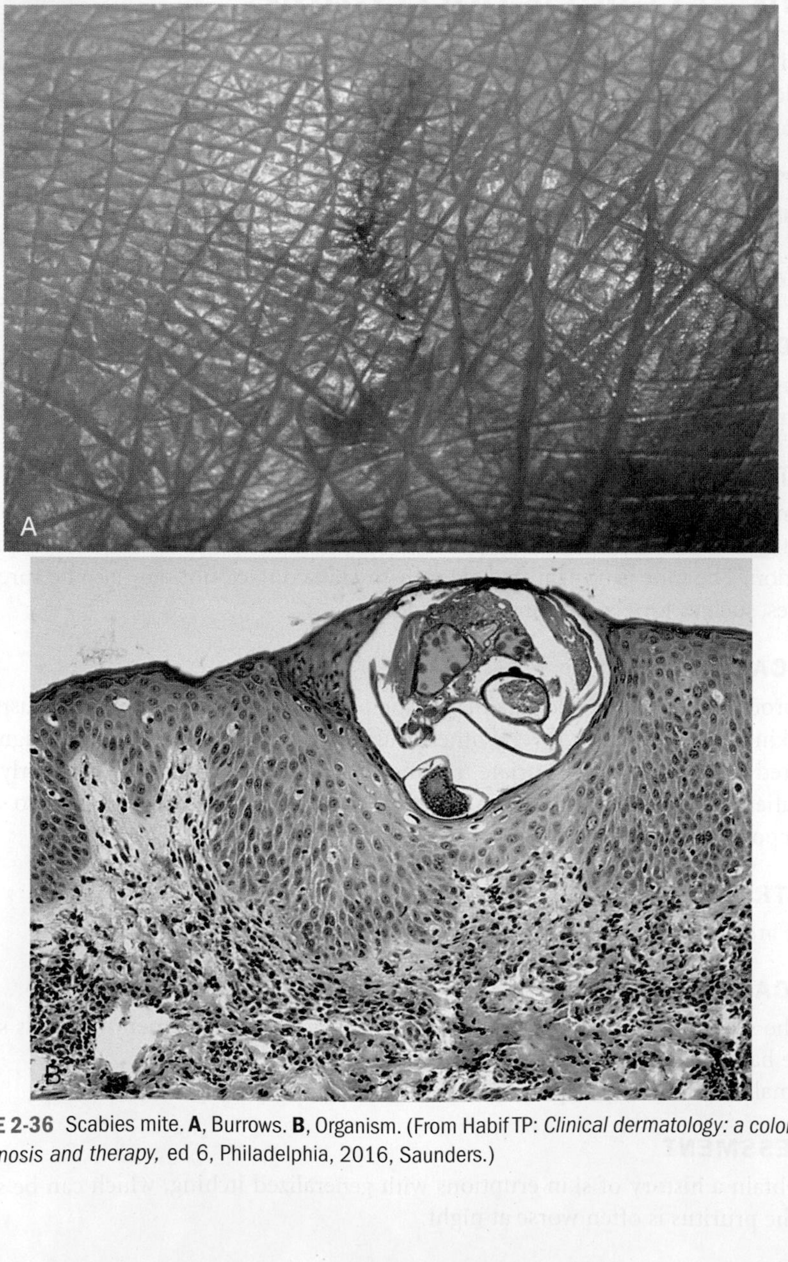

FIGURE 2-36 Scabies mite. **A**, Burrows. **B**, Organism. (From Habif TP: *Clinical dermatology: a color guide to diagnosis and therapy*, ed 6, Philadelphia, 2016, Saunders.)

PATIENT PREPARATION

The diagnosis of scabies must be confirmed by microscopic observation of the organism, ova, or feces in a specimen. The procedure is virtually painless and requires only a few minutes.

Explain procedure to the patient.

TREATMENT ALTERNATIVES

- Not relevant

EQUIPMENT

- Gloves
- Alcohol
- No. 15 scalpel blade
- Mineral oil
- Light source with strong magnification (e.g., an otoscope or procedures light)
- Blue- or green-colored marking pen
- Glass slide and coverslip
- Microscope

Procedure

Follow universal precautions.

1. Expose burrow areas with well-defined skin eruptions.
2. Position the patient comfortably; if a child, restrain if necessary.
3. Wearing gloves, the areas to be scraped are rubbed with a blue- or green-colored marker, and then the skin is dried with alcohol. The color that remains on the skin more specifically localizes the burrow.
4. Rub mineral oil over the skin eruptions, particularly on elbows or dry, scaly areas. This changes the refractory index of the superficial layers of the skin and facilitates better visibility of the erupted area. The mineral oil allows the mites and other debris obtained during the scraping to adhere to the oil and keeps the mites alive and moving.
5. Holding the scalpel blade perpendicularly to the skin, shave or vigorously scrape each burrow lesion six or seven times until all of the area colored by the marker is removed. The mite itself is often hard to find because the mites may have already left the burrow to travel to a new area. The skin reacts to the debris left in the burrow, so the entry part of the burrow usually has the greatest degree of inflammation and itching.
6. Put the scraped material from each lesion onto a separate glass slide and top with a coverslip.
7. Rub the patient's skin with alcohol. Dressing is not usually required.
8. Microscopically examine the specimens under the coverslip using the ×10 magnification objective. Look for mites, feces, or eggs; the presence confirms the diagnosis.

PATIENT EDUCATION POSTPROCEDURE

A scabicide should be prescribed when the diagnosis is confirmed. Instruct the patient or family on how the medication is to be applied, on the washing of bedding and clothing, and on the treatment of others who were exposed to the patient. Medications may require more than one application to kill eggs as they hatch.

COMPLICATIONS

- Secondary infection of lesions due to scratching

PRACTITIONER FOLLOW-UP

Usually is not necessary, unless pruritic lesions fail to resolve.

■ CPT BILLING

87220—Tissue examination by KOH slide of samples from skin, hair, or nails for fungi or ectoparasite ova or mites (scabies, for example)

REFERENCES AND RELATED RESOURCES

Center for Disease Control and Prevention: *Scabies. Resources for health professionals.* http://www.cdc.gov/parasites/scabies/health_professionals/index.html. Accessed October 25, 2014.

Heukelbach J, Feldmeier H: Scabies, *Lancet* 367:1767–1774, 2006.

Shimose L, Munoz-Price L: Diagnosis, prevention, and treatment of scabies, *Curr Infect Dis Rep* 15:426–431, 2013.

Herpes Scraping: Tzanck Smear

Kent D. Blad and Sabrina Jarvis

DESCRIPTION

The Tzanck smear is a diagnostic procedure that is used in the diagnosis of vesicular viral infections caused by herpes simplex or the herpes zoster/varicella virus.

ANATOMY AND PHYSIOLOGY

Herpes zoster is a reactivation of the varicella-zoster virus. After the initial infection of varicella (chickenpox), the virus remains in a dormant state in a dorsal root or cranial nerve ganglia. At some point later in life, the virus becomes reactivated and produces a characteristic rash.

INDICATIONS

A specimen should be collected any time infection with the herpes virus is suspected. This is important because early and aggressive therapy for herpes zoster is essential to reduce the incidence of postherpetic neuralgia.

CONTRAINDICATIONS

There are none.

PRECAUTIONS

Use universal precautions in the collection of potentially hazardous specimen materials.

The patient who has the herpes virus infection may transmit it to anyone who has not previously had chickenpox.

ASSESSMENT

- Obtain a history related to the onset of the lesions, including any tingling or other prodromal symptoms, distribution patterns, and any attempts at treatment. Pain may precede the rash; the skin lesions then erupt. The pain may persist after the rash is resolved.
- Obtain a specific history on whether the patient has had previous outbreaks of herpes. Eruptions frequently reoccur in the same site. The rash appears as coalescing vesicles on an erythematous base, presenting in patterns that follow specific dermatomes. Usually a cluster of red lesions of varying sizes progresses into edematous vesicles on an erythematous base, filled with cloudy fluid. New vesicles may continue to develop for up to 7 days. About 10 days after they appear, the vesicles dry and form scabs. Compared with varicella zoster lesions, herpes zoster lesions are unilateral, more deeply seated, more closely aggregated, and restricted to the area supplied by the dorsal root ganglia that contained the reactivated varicella zoster (Figure 2-37).

PATIENT PREPARATION

Children may require immobilization during the procedure.

Explain the procedure to the patient.

TREATMENT ALTERNATIVES

Not relevant; this is a diagnostic test.

EQUIPMENT

- Gloves
- Antiseptic cleansing pads
- No. 15 scalpel
- Gauze pads
- Glass slide
- 95% Ethanol
- One of the following nuclear stains:
  - Giemsa stain
  - Wright's stain
  - Hansel stain

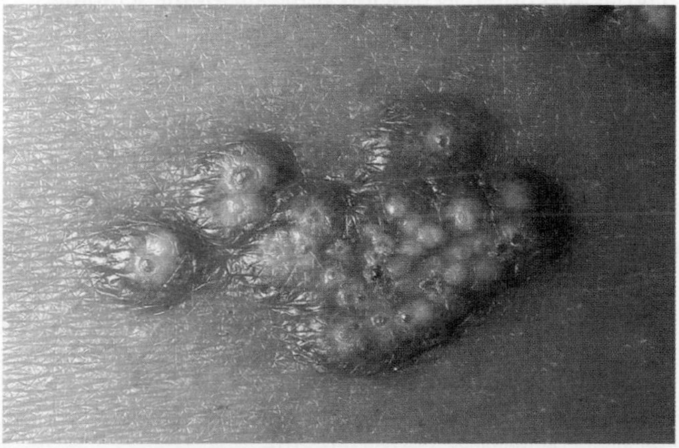

FIGURE 2-37 Herpes lesion. (From Habif TB: *Clinical dermatology: a color guide to diagnosis and therapy*, ed 5, Philadelphia, 2010, Mosby.)

2

Procedure

Follow universal precautions.

1. Place the patient in a comfortable position with the lesion visible under good lighting.
2. Choose a lesion in the early phase of development.
3. Remove the top of a vesicle with the No. 15 scalpel. Excess clear fluid should be sponged up with a gauze pad. Carefully scrape the base of the vesicle to obtain a specimen, which should be taken from the scalpel blade and thinly distributed onto a glass slide.
4. Immediately immerse these slides in 95% methanol for 5 seconds, and then air dry for 1 to 2 minutes.
5. Apply the stain to the slides following the directions for the staining material chosen.
6. Examine the entire stained slide under ×10 magnification on the microscope to obtain a general indication of what is on the slide. Then examine the slide using the oil-immersion lens, or at ×45 magnification, to look at the specific cells.
7. A positive smear shows the presence of multinucleated giant cells and giant epithelial cells. Newly infected cells have one enlarged nucleus that develops into giant cells with 2 to 12 multinucleated cells as the infection progresses.
8. Tzanck smears do not differentiate between herpes zoster and herpes simplex. Staining antibodies from vesicular fluid and identification under a fluorescent light will show the differences between these two organisms.

PATIENT EDUCATION POSTPROCEDURE

The patient should be given the results of the diagnostic test. If a herpes infection is confirmed, it should be treated with antiviral medications. Severe infections may require referral to a physician or dermatologist for aggressive therapy, including intravenous medications.

COMPLICATIONS

Secondary bacterial infection may develop at the site of the scraping.

RED FLAG

The patient should be referred to a physician for treatment if he or she is immunocompromised and to an ophthalmologist if the eyes are involved.

PRACTITIONER FOLLOW-UP

- If treatment is prescribed, the patient should follow-up with the practitioner within 2 weeks to determine the efficacy of treatment.

REFERENCES AND RELATED RESOURCES

Eryilmaz A, Durdu M, Baba M, et al: Diagnostic reliability of the Tzanck smear in dermatologic diseases, *International J Dermatology* 53:178–186, 2014.

Goldstein B, Goldstein A: Dermatologic procedures. In Dellavalle R, (Ed), *UpToDate*, Waltham, MA 2013. Accessed October 24, 2014.

Heukelbach J, Feldmeier H: Scabies, *Lancet* 367:1767–1774, 2006.
Marks Jr J, Miller J: *Lookingbill and Marks' principles of dermatology*, ed 5, New York, 2013, Elsevier Saunders.

Fungal Scraping: The KOH Test

Kent D. Blad and Sabrina Jarvis

DESCRIPTION

This procedure is used to obtain specimens of suspected fungi. Potassium hydroxide solution (KOH) 10% or 20% is an alkali solution that dissolves skin keratin and cellular debris, leaving the fungal hyphae and spores intact so they may be visually identified.

Another diagnostic test involves using the Wood's lamp, which shines an ultraviolet light. Certain fungal organisms fluoresce when viewed under the light of the Wood's lamp.

2

ANATOMY AND PHYSIOLOGY

Scaling is a common characteristic of the fungal disease process. These disorders result from infection of the skin by fungal organisms collectively called *dermatophytes.* Dermatophytes are keratinophilic (feed on keratin) and live primarily in the stratum corneum, hair, and nails. Fungal scraping of the skin is necessary to identify the causative organism.

INDICATIONS

If fungal infection is suspected, perform a scraping.

CONTRAINDICATIONS

There are none.

PRECAUTIONS

Caution needs to be taken when scraping the suspected area with the instrument. The skin should not be broken open over the pustules, and the dermis or epidermis should not be cut accidentally with the edge of the scalpel, if one is used.

ASSESSMENT

- Patients should be asked whether they have already tried treating the skin lesion with an antifungal agent because that could interfere with obtaining accurate results.
- Fungal infection can manifest itself as scaly patches or a boggy inflammatory mass, patches of hair loss, or small, scattered pustules. The physical findings and differential diagnosis vary depending on the location of the infection (Table 2-12). Children may have a fungal infection of the hair in which the hair is broken off at the skin level. This is called "black dot" tinea. The lesions may be very pruritic to the patient or barely noticeable.
- Fungal infections can sometimes produce pustules (especially around hair follicles), and the examiner may misdiagnose these pustules as bacterial in origin.

TABLE 2-12 Differential Diagnosis

NAME	DIFFERENTIAL DIAGNOSIS
Tinea capitis (scalp)	Alopecia areata Seborrheic dermatitis Pyoderma
Tinea corporis (body)	Nummular eczema Pityriasis rosea (herald patch) Psoriasis Impetigo
Tinea cruris (groin)	Intertrigo Candidiasis
Tinea pedis (feet)	Hyperhidrosis Dry skin Contact dermatitis Dyshidrotic eczema
Tinea manuum (hand)	Contact dermatitis Psoriasis
Tinea faciale (face)	Photodermatitis Lupus erythematosus Seborrheic dermatitis
Tinea unguium (nail)	Psoriasis Trauma
Tinea versicolor (trunk)	Vitiligo (white) Seborrheic dermatitis (tan or pink)

Kerions, which present as tender, edematous, erythematous lesions, may be mistaken for bacterial infections. Kerions result from a hypersensitivity reaction to the tinea capitis and are treated by treating the fungal infection. Positive fungal scrapings confirm the diagnosis. Certain tinea can gain access to the deeper tissues and cause cellulitis of the lower extremities.

PATIENT PREPARATION

This is a quick, painless, and noninvasive procedure.

TREATMENT ALTERNATIVES

To examine skin that is suspected of being infected with a fungus using the Wood's lamp, darken the room and shine the Wood's lamp onto the skin at a distance of 8 inches from the skin's surface.

EQUIPMENT

- Alcohol preparations
- No. 15 scalpel or glass slide
- One glass microscope slide and one plastic coverslip
- Microscope with ×10 objective
- KOH 10% or 20% solution. If the solution contains dimethyl sulfoxide (DMSO), then heating is not required
- Alcohol lamp, lighter
- Hemostats (scalp), tongue blade (mouth), nail clippers (nail)

Procedure

Follow universal precautions.

1. Cleanse the skin by scrubbing it with a gauze pad soaked in 70% alcohol.
2. Position the patient in a good light with the lesion visible. Hold a glass slide next to the lesion. Scrape the edge of the lesion where there are fine scales, using either a scalpel or another glass slide. Avoid collecting thick scales. If there is hair loss, sample the short, broken hairs with the scalpel, or use the hemostats to pluck 5 to 10 hairs. If the nail is involved, scrape thin pieces of the nail.
3. Scrape the scales onto the slide, using the scalpel blade to gather the scales without overlapping to the center of the slide.
4. Place 1 or 2 drops of 10% KOH solution on the skin or hair samples. (Use 20% KOH if examining nails.) **Warning:** KOH is very caustic, so avoid contact with the skin and eyes. It may cause permanent damage to microscope objectives and other equipment.
5. Place a coverslip over the specimen. Use plastic coverslips so that loose scales are picked up by the electrostatic charge to the underside.
6. Gently heat the slide over the heat source for 10 to 20 seconds. An alcohol lamp is preferable because it does not leave any black carbon on the undersurface of the slide. Avoid boiling the slide contents; the bottom of the slide should feel quite warm to the touch. Heat serves to speed the chemical reaction of KOH, dissolving the keratin of the scales. Allow skin scrapings to stand for about 5 minutes; hair must sit for 15 to 30 minutes; and nails must sit for 30 minutes (Figure 2-38).
7. Place the slide on the microscope and examine it under low light at ×10 magnification. The refractive quality of the fungus hyphae is more pronounced under the low light. Scan the entire field for the thin, long, branched forms of the hyphae, which may or may not be accompanied by spores. When an object is found that looks suspicious, examine it under a higher power magnification (×250 magnification) to look for internal structures, such as vacuoles. Cell walls have an irregular linearity, whereas threads appear uniform and lack internal structure.

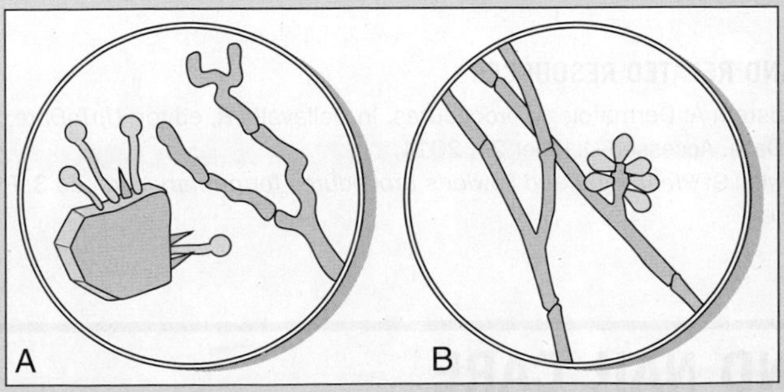

FIGURE 2-38 Characteristic appearance of hyphae, seen under magnification. **A,** *Trichophyton verrucosum.* **B,** *Trichophyton interdigitale.*

INTERPRETATION OF RESULTS

- A positive KOH test occurs when hyphae are visualized.
- A positive Wood's lamp test occurs when the skin fluoresces.
  - Tinea capitis—yellow green to pale green
  - Tinea versicolor—golden yellow
  - Dermatophytosis in the hair shaft—green to yellow
  - Erythrasma (caused by *Corynebacterium minutissimum*)—coral red
- Other substances may also fluoresce, such as tetracycline, fluorescein dye, and many cosmetics.

PATIENT EDUCATION POSTPROCEDURE

- Instruct the patient on how to use the antifungal medication that is prescribed.
- Instruct the patient on hygiene that discourages further fungal infections (keep skin clean and dry, avoid walking on locker room floors in bare feet, use cotton socks and underwear, etc.).

COMPLICATIONS

Fungal infections can result in secondary bacterial infections, but this is rare.

PRACTITIONER FOLLOW-UP

- If the KOH test is positive, treatment with oral or topical antifungal agents is necessary.
- The practitioner may reevaluate the patient in 2 or 3 days by telephone to see whether there has been improvement, or the patient can be instructed to call the office if the signs and symptoms are not improving.
- If the infection does not improve in a few days (or a few weeks in the case of tinea capitis), the patient should come back for reevaluation of the diagnosis.
- If the KOH test is inconclusive, the practitioner may elect to perform a fungal culture.

RED FLAGS

- Infection is resistant to treatment.
- Moderate to severe infections in immunocompromised patients.

CPT BILLING

87220–Tissue exam by KOH slide of samples from skin, hair, or nails for fungi or ectoparasite ova or mites

REFERENCES AND RELATED RESOURCES

Goldstein B, Goldstein A: Dermatologic procedures. In Dellavalle R, editor: *UpToDate*, Waltham, MA, 2013, UpToDate. Accessed October 24, 2014.

Pfenninger J, Fowler G: *Pfenninger and Fowler's procedures for primary care*, ed 3, Philadelphia, 2011, Elsevier.

FOOT AND NAIL CARE

Often health care professionals in the primary care setting must provide routine patient foot care. Patients who have medical conditions, such as diabetes and peripheral vascular disease, require meticulous and careful foot care in order to minimize trauma and the risk of infection and amputation.

This section includes common procedures for caring for nails, corns, and calluses. This includes procedures for treating nail problems, such as subungual hematomas, ingrown toenails, nail avulsions, and paronychias. Each of these is discussed separately.

Toenail Care in the At-Risk Patient

Kent D. Blad and Sabrina Jarvis

DESCRIPTION

This procedure describes the routine care of nails, particularly toenails, in patients who have diabetes and chronic diseases that impair circulation. Foot infections and their direct sequelae are the complications that most frequently lead to hospitalization in these patients. The consequences of foot ulceration include extensive suffering, prolonged functional disability, increased risk of amputation, and associated mortality.

ANATOMY AND PHYSIOLOGY

The nail is composed of the eponychium, nail bed, nail plate, and hypoychium epithelial structures. The nail body grows out from the nail root, which is hidden by the cuticle.

See Figure 2-39 for an illustration of the nail bed anatomy.

INDICATIONS

The health care provider performs routine foot examinations in patients who have neuropathy and lower extremity impaired circulation to help detect early signs of nail and foot infection or injury that could lead to serious complications requiring hospitalization and risk of amputation. The provider should perform nail and foot care if these patients are physically unable to perform their own care.

CONTRAINDICATIONS

- Existing and severe circulatory problems
- Infected foot ulcers

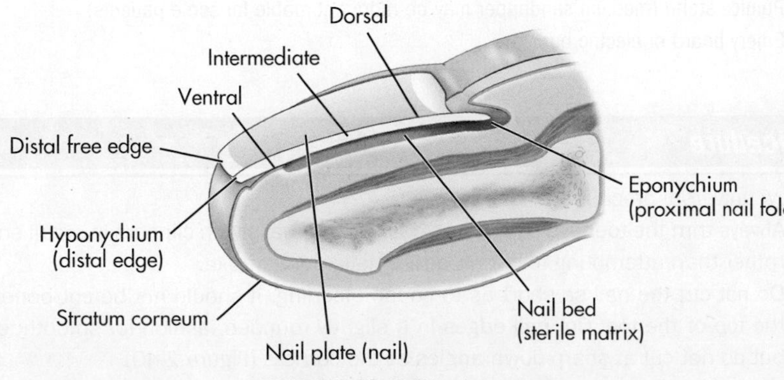

FIGURE 2-39 Nail bed anatomy.

2

PRECAUTIONS

Neuropathy, vascular insufficiency, and an altered response to infection make the patient who has diabetes susceptible to nail and foot infections and injury. The health care provider must take care to minimize risk of injury during the nail procedure. For example, if the patient is unable to hold still, an electric burr should not be used because of burn risk.

If the patient's nails are very damaged or deformed, refer the patient for podiatry consultation. Any ulcers or foot injuries should be referred to the wound management team or appropriate specialist.

ASSESSMENT

- Focused history should include information on diabetes, glucose control, smoking and peripheral vascular disease, prior foot ulcers, and any concerns or changes in the lower extremities suggestive of neuropathy and peripheral artery disease.
- Perform a lower extremity neurovascular examination assessing tactile sensation level (with 10-g monofilament), vibratory sensation (128-Hz tuning fork), motor function, ankle reflexes, skin color and temperature, capillary refill, pedal pulses, nail structure, and foot health. The examination should include a detailed assessment of the sole of the foot and areas between the toes, looking for any pressure areas, calluses or corns, blisters, bruises, ulcerations, and breaks in the skin. Inspect the nails for length, thickness, discoloration, and damage.
- Perform a musculoskeletal examination assessing for any foot deformities, such as Pes cavus and hammer or claw toe.
- Inspect socks and observe shoes for proper fit.

PATIENT PREPARATION

Unless inflammation or infection is present, it is preferable to soak the feet in warm water or to wrap the feet in a warm, damp washcloth for about 10 minutes before the procedure to help soften the nails.

Instruct the patient that the procedure should not hurt.

EQUIPMENT

- Nail clippers or scissors—concave nail clippers of the plier type (available in medical supply stores)
- Pumice stone (medium sandpaper may be more affordable for some patients)
- Emery board or electric burr

Procedure

Follow universal precautions.

1. Always trim the toenails straight across. Cut the nails with clippers in small snips rather than attempting to cut an entire nail in one stroke.
2. Do not cut the nail so short as to cause bleeding. It should not be cut beneath the top of the toe. Cut nail edges in a slightly rounded fashion for smoothness, but do not cut at sharp-down angles at the corners (Figure 2-40).

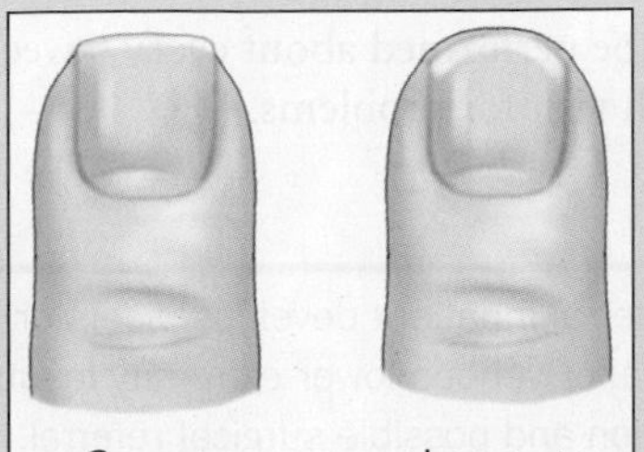

FIGURE 2-40 Proper nail care prophylaxis. Trim the nail flat, but not too short.

3. File any remaining sharp edges with an emery board. Smooth the edges and thin the undersides of the thickened nails with a sanding board or electric burr. Thick, fungal nails are best managed with thinning and shaping.
4. Buff calluses or corns lightly with a pumice stone or sandpaper to prevent cracking and breaks in the skin integrity.
5. Do not disturb the cuticles because they provide barriers against infection.

PATIENT EDUCATION POSTPROCEDURE

All individuals who have diabetes should learn the principles of foot self-examination and care. Patients should have a small mirror that they can use to examine the bottoms of their feet. Inform the patients why this is so important and instruct them to observe the nail care procedure closely so it can be repeated at home. Provide patients with the following instructions.

- The best time to trim nails is after a bath or shower when the nails are the softest.
- Keep toenails trimmed. Cuticles are not to be cut and caution patient not to use sharp objects to pry at the toenail corners which could injure the nail fold and cause infection.
- Keep feet and nails clean.
- Use moisturizing lotion to prevent dry skin from cracking.
- Never treat calluses, blisters, ingrown nails, or wounds at home because doing so can lead to serious infection. Contact the health care provider.
- Shoes should be comfortable, with support and adequate toe room. Patients should not go bare foot. Synthetic blend socks help wick foot moisture.
- Inspect feet daily. Use a mirror to inspect the soles of the feet if necessary. If neuropathy is present, caution the patient that injury or infection may occur without discomfort. Instruct patient to notify health care provider if there are signs of infection, inflammation, or foot injury, such as skin color or temperature change, increased warmth, redness, swelling, bruising, blisters, ulcers, or breaks in the skin.
- Visit the health care provider regularly and be sure the feet are examined at each visit.

COMPLICATIONS

Localized infection may develop in patients who have diabetes and poor circulation or when the procedure is not gently performed.

PRACTITIONER FOLLOW-UP

- Foot care usually must be performed about every 6 weeks.
- Monitor the feet at each visit for problems.

RED FLAGS

- Patient will need referral if patient develops ulcers or foot sores.
- If patient has arterial or venous lower extremity insufficiency, patient will need vasculature evaluation and possible surgical referral.

CPT BILLING

11720—Debridement of nail(s) by any method(s); 1 to 5 ■ **11721**—Debridement of nail(s) by any method(s); 6 or more

REFERENCES AND RELATED RESOURCES

Boulton A, Armstrong D, Albert S, et al: Comprehensive foot examination and risk assessment: a report of the Foot Care Interest group of the American Diabetes Association, with endorsement by the American Association of Clinical Endocrinologists, *Diabetes Care* 31:1679–1685, 2008.

Eddy J: Diabetic foot care: tips and tools to streamline your approach. *J Fam Practice* 58:646–653, 2009.

Edmonds M, Foster A, Sanders L: *A practical manual of diabetic foot care*, ed 2, Malden, MA, 2008, Blackwell.

McCulloch D: Evaluation of the diabetic foot. In Nathan D, editor: *UpToDate*, Waltham, MA, 2014, UpToDate. Accessed November 1, 2014.

Corn and Callus Management

Kent D. Blad and Sabrina Jarvis

DESCRIPTION

Most calluses and corns may be treated conservatively. Problems that are more extensive require minor surgical intervention by a podiatrist or surgeon. Minor, conservative treatment is discussed in this section.

ANATOMY AND PHYSIOLOGY

A *callus* represents the gradual development of a thickened stratum corneum in a localized area of tissue, resulting from continued physical trauma. Increased risk for corns often results from both biomechanics and inherited foot type. Common precipitating causes include friction from poorly fitting shoes along the inner aspects of the sole, heel, and great toe and pressure on the distal digit of the fingers from holding a pencil or pen; any area that is exposed to repeated friction and pressure may be affected.

Corns are well-demarcated, hyperkeratotic lesions that are present over bony prominences and involve the stratum corneum or "horny layer" of the skin. A corn is either soft or hard and is caused by pressure secondary to an unyielding structure.

With a *hard corn,* the phalangeal condyle under the skin and an unyielding material over the skin generates pressure and friction. A painful lesion develops over the dorsolateral aspect of the proximal interphalangeal joint of the fifth toe. The lesion is firm, dry, and tender and can have surrounding erythema and heat if acutely irritated.

A bursa may even develop. Hard corn removal often requires surgical resection, and these patients should be referred to a podiatrist.

The *soft corn* is usually interdigital; the most common place is the fourth web space. It is caused by pressure imposed by the lateral side of the base of the fourth proximal phalanx, the medial condyle of the head of the fifth proximal phalanx, or both.

INDICATIONS

Corns and calluses should be removed if there is pain, swelling, and/or redness that hinders the patient's ambulation or ability to wear shoes.

CONTRAINDICATIONS

There are none.

PRECAUTIONS

Practitioners should proceed cautiously in diabetic or immunocompromised patients.

Referral to a podiatrist is indicated for the following:

- Corns that are deeply imbedded or extensive in nature or that extend into the nail bed.
- Hard corns that may require resection of the head and neck of the proximal phalanx.

ASSESSMENT

- Take a complete history and ascertain any foot complaints of pain or injury.
- Examine and palpate all foot surfaces, examining for evidence of trauma, infection, deformity, or stress.

PATIENT PREPARATION

- Instruct the patient to wash the toes and web spaces twice a day with household soap, to dry them completely, and to apply an antifungal, antibacterial powder and a lamb's wool or self-adherent rubber web spacer ("doughnut"; found in the foot care section of a retail store).
- Instruct the patient to use over-the-counter salicylate pads, which soften the tissue continuously for 7 to 10 days.
- Patients should soak their feet in warm water for 20 minutes the night before the procedure to soften tissue. The skin may be scrubbed with a pumice stone to remove any loose tissue. The feet may be soaked again before the procedure.

EQUIPMENT

- Lamb's wool or self-adherent web spacer
- No. 15 scalpel
- Pumice stone, sanding board, or electric burr

Procedure

REMOVAL OF HARD OR SOFT CORNS

Remove any over-the-counter pads and débride with a pumice stone, rubbing deeply to remove the firm inner core. A scalpel may be used to remove this core.

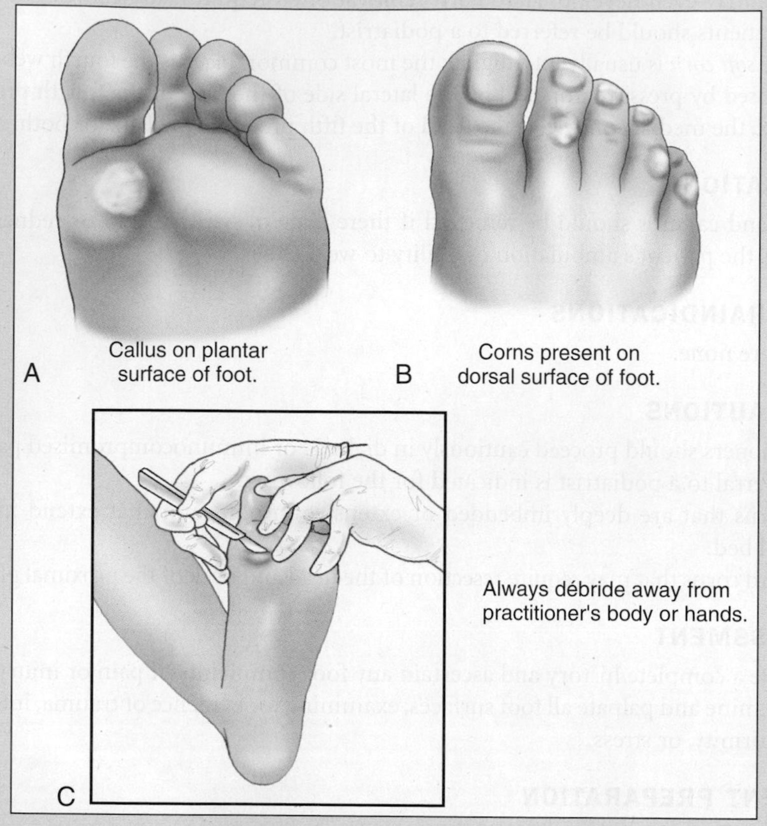
Callus on plantar surface of foot.
A
B
Corns present on dorsal surface of foot.
Always débride away from practitioner's body or hands.
C

FIGURE 2-41 Examining and removing a callus. Check plantar surface (**A**) for callus and dorsal surface (**B**) of toes for corns. **C,** Always débride away from practitioner's body or hands.

REMOVAL OF CALLUSES

1. Use a sanding board, pumice stone, or electric burr to thin and smooth any thick or rough calluses.
2. Proceed slowly so that a firm, intact layer of skin remains after sanding.
3. A scalpel can be used to slice off layers of very thick calluses (Figure 2-41).

PATIENT EDUCATION POSTPROCEDURE

Removal of Hard or Soft Corns

- Keep the toes dressed for 3 weeks, in proper position, followed by 3 weeks of taping the toes together loosely with lamb's wool between them.
- Report any signs of infection (redness, increased pain, swelling, warmth, foul-smelling discharge) at once.

Removal of Calluses

- Remove the source of irritation to prevent the recurrence of calluses.
- May rub lotions with heavy oil base or 40% urea creams into clean, dry skin to keep tissue softer.

COMPLICATIONS

- Bleeding
- Infection

PRACTITIONER FOLLOW-UP

Evaluate the patient within 1 week for signs of infection and the extent of healing.

Débridement may need to be performed every 6 to 8 weeks because the condition usually reoccurs.

Advise the patient to wear shoes that are wider, especially in the toes, and have a higher fit over the foot to prevent repetitive rubbing. Patients may wish to pad the area to take pressure off the areas of pain or use orthotics or shoe inserts. Keep skin soft with creams.

■ CPT BILLING

11055—Paring or cutting of benign hyperkeratonic lesion (corn or callus); single lesion ■ **11056**—Paring or cutting of benign hyperkeratonic lesion (corn or callus); 2-4 lesions ■ **11057**—Paring or cutting of benign hyperkeratonic lesion (corn or callus); more than 4 lesions

REFERENCES AND RELATED RESOURCES

Lyman TP, Vlahovic TC: *Foot care from A to Z.* http://www.medscape.cmo/viewarticle/735531_6. Medscape Family Medicine. Accessed December 21, 2014.

Pfenninger JL, Fowler GC: *Procedures for primary care physicians*, St Louis, 2011, Mosby.

Walsh HJ, Klenerman L: *Physical signs in orthopaedics*, London, 1999, British Medical Journal.

Ingrown Toenail and Paronychia Management

Kent D. Blad and Sabrina Jarvis

DESCRIPTION

Ingrown toenails are a common problem, and they can cause significant pain and disability. Toenail removal, either partial or total, is the procedure indicated for conditions in which a spur or splinter of nail has invaded the sulcus and subsequent subcutaneous tissue (*onychocryptosis*). As the splinter portion of the nail continues to grow within the sulcus, inflammation in the surrounding tissue occurs (*paronychia*),which may even lead to infection at times.

ANATOMY AND PHYSIOLOGY

Shoes that are too tight or toenails that are improperly cut can cause painful swelling, redness, and tenderness around the corner of the toenail on the great toe.

Three stages of ingrown toenails have been described:

- The first stage is characterized by redness, pain, and slight swelling.
- The second stage is characterized by swelling, pain, and redness with infection and suppuration. Stages 1 and 2 ingrown toenails can be successfully treated with conservative management or partial nail removal, as described in this procedure.
- The third stage is characterized by granulation tissue formation and hypertrophy of the nail wall, with all the characteristics of the second stage more pronounced. Stage 3 ingrown toenails are best treated with more aggressive, surgical procedures under local anesthesia, and the patient should be referred to the proper specialist (Figure 2-42).

2

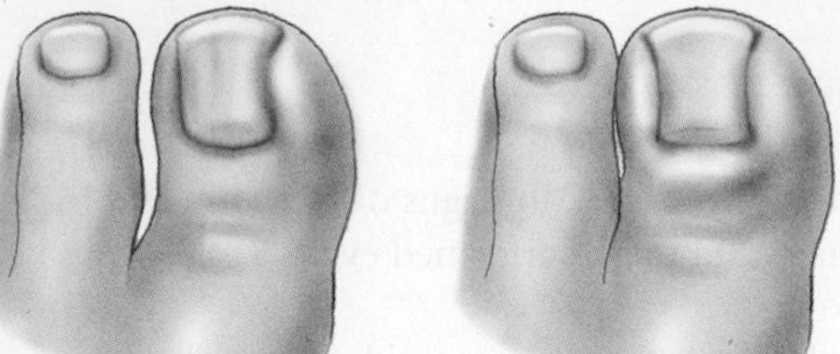

FIGURE 2-42 Stages of ingrown nails.

2

INDICATIONS

- Onychocryptosis (ingrown nail)
- Onychomycosis (fungal infection of the nail)
- Onychogryposis (deformed, curved nail)

CONTRAINDICATIONS

- History of allergy to local anesthetic agents
- Bleeding disorders
- Anticoagulant therapy
- Diabetes mellitus
- Peripheral-vascular disease
- Peripheral neuropathy
- Patients who are immunocompromised
- Pregnancy (with use of phenol)

PRECAUTIONS

Take care to not damage the soft tissue around the toes.

ASSESSMENT

- Assess which stage of nail ingrowth is present. Look for evidence of inflammation or infection of the surrounding soft tissue.
- Assess for evidence that the patient is immunocompromised or has a decreased circulation, placing him or her at higher risk for infection.
- Assess for evidence of bleeding risk or history.

PATIENT PREPARATION

- Obtain consent from patient, after discussion of risks and benefits.
- Before the procedure, the patient should be instructed to wear open-toed shoes, such as sandals, when he or she comes to the office, because of postoperative bandages.
- The practitioner should soak the patient's affected toe or toes in an antiseptic/germicidal solution for about 15 to 20 minutes. This may be performed during the patient education time or while preparing the patient for the procedure.
- Practitioners should explain the procedure sufficiently to ensure the cooperation of the patient or caregiver because home treatment for several weeks is required.

TREATMENT ALTERNATIVES

- Conservative management
- Partial nail removal
- Referral to specialist for more radical surgical treatments
- Consider antibiotics if infection present

EQUIPMENT

CONSERVATIVE MANAGEMENT

- Antiseptic/germicidal solution and a pan for soaking toe or toes
- Gloves
- Scissors to trim nail edge
- Nail elevator
- Cotton for packing and protection
- Antibiotic ointment (optional)

PARTIAL NAIL REMOVAL

- Antiseptic/germicidal solution and pan for soaking toe or toes
- Gloves
- Anesthetic agent without epinephrine (see "Anesthesia: Topical, Local, and Digital Nerve Blocks, Procedure") with syringe and needle
- Povidone-iodine or other skin preparation antimicrobial solution
- Tourniquet—penrose drain (optional)
- Nail elevator / hemostat
- Nail splitter / Mayo scissors
- Forceps
- Beaver blade
- Hemostat
- Curette
- Phenol (optional)
- Antibiotic ointment
- Sterile bandage and tape
- Silver nitrate

Procedure

Follow universal precautions.

CONSERVATIVE MANAGEMENT

1. Patient may soak foot the night before the procedure, and then wrap the foot or toe in a wet cloth and cover with plastic. This will help soften the nail.
2. Once the nail is softened and cleaned, cut off the offending nail corner.
3. Then thin the middle third of the nail (10 to 15 mm) by filing the upper surface until the nail matrix can be seen beneath.
4. Elevate the nail edge and remove any debris or infected material. Minimal amounts of granulation tissue can be reduced by the application of silver nitrate.
5. Pack a small piece of cotton firmly under the nail edge. Cotton wool soaked in 60% alcohol may also be used.
6. If the cuticle is swollen or infected, apply an antibiotic ointment before packing.
7. If the medial edge of the toenail is involved, protect it by taping cotton between the first and second toes to keep them from touching.
8. If the lateral edge is involved, protect it by taping the cotton to the outside of the ball of the toe, keeping the toenail from touching the inside of the shoe.

PARTIAL NAIL REMOVAL

1. Patient may soak foot the night before the procedure, and then wrap the foot or toe in a wet cloth and cover with plastic. This will help soften the nail.

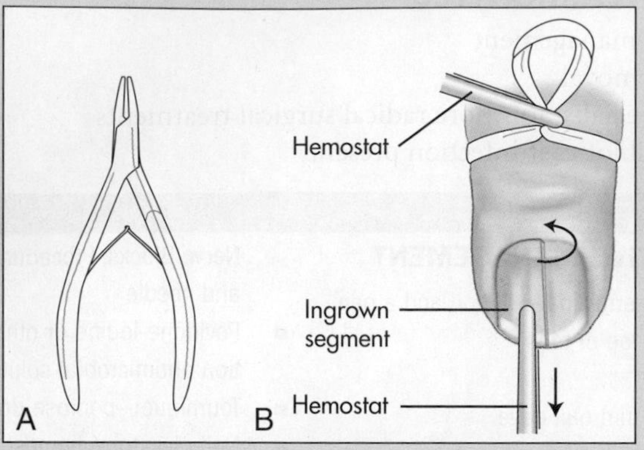

FIGURE 2-43 Equipment and technique for removing ingrown nail. **A**, Nail splitter. **B**, Technique for nail removal after nail has been split. Grasp that portion of the nail to be removed lengthwise with a straight hemostat, and remove it using a steady pulling motion with a simultaneous upward twist of the hand toward the affected side.

2

2. Position the patient comfortably in a supine or semirecumbent position.
3. Administer a bilateral digital nerve block with 2% lidocaine (without epinephrine). The purpose is to block sensory fibers of the dorsal and plantar digital nerves (see "Anesthesia: Topical, Local, and Digital Nerve Blocks, Procedure").
4. Clean the toe with an antiseptic solution, such as povidone-iodine.
5. Apply a tourniquet (optional). Use of a tourniquet is to decrease bleeding and to maintain more localized anesthesia.
6. Use the nail elevator / hemostat to free the nail sulcus and eponychium from the nail plate.
7. Split a 2- to 3-mm wedge of nail with the nail splitter / Mayo scissor.
8. Push the beaver blade under the eponychium to free the remainder of the nail.
9. Remove the wedged section using the hemostat by carefully rotating the separated portion toward the remainder of the healthy nail plate (Figure 2-43). This separates any buried portion of the nail and prevents embedding of a spicule of nail. The distal-most portion of the nail will have a feather look if it has been removed intact.
10. Curette the matrix and nail bed to remove any missed nail and additional debris.
11. Apply silver nitrate for cautery of the nail bed.
12. Apply phenol to cauterize and destroy that part of the matrix from which the wedge has been removed (optional). In the absence of phenol, the growth of new nail takes approximately 8 to 12 months in an adult.
13. Remove the tourniquet.
14. Apply an antibiotic ointment, such as bacitracin, with a piece of Owens silk or similar medium to the surgical area. Apply a sterile 2 × 2 gauze and wrap with self-adhesive tape.

PATIENT EDUCATION POSTPROCEDURE

- Rest the foot and keep it elevated for 12 to 24 hours.
- Remove the bandage the night after the surgery, and soak the foot 5 to 10 minutes in plain, warm water (never hot water). If there is difficulty removing the bandage during the initial soak, place the entire bandage into the water for 5 to 10 minutes to allow for easy removal.

- Soak the toe for 10 to 15 minutes twice a day in an antiseptic/germicidal solution or a 1:120 bleach solution (1 tablespoon of bleach per 2 quarts of water with a little liquid soap) to clean the toe and kill germs.
- During the soaks, massage the swollen part of the cuticle outward and bend the corners of the offending nail upward.
- After soaking, dry the foot, and cover the nailbed with an antibiotic ointment.
- Reapply the cotton packing, if used, after each soaking. Then cover with a bandage.
- Watch for any red streaks up the foot or leg, fever or chills, or warmth and pain. If these signs are present, call the practitioner immediately.
- Normally, there is a small amount of drainage for 1 to 2 weeks after surgery.
- If the cuticle becomes swollen or infected (oozes pus or other secretions), triple antibiotic ointment should be applied five or six times a day.
- Wearing sandals or going barefoot (where it is safe to do so) prevents continued pressure on the toenail. When closed-toed shoes are worn, be sure there is plenty of room in the toes and protect the toe or toes from further injury with cotton padding.
- Practitioners should inform the patient that ill-fitting shoes need to be replaced with properly fitting shoes.

PREVENTION

Ingrown toenails are most frequently a result of incorrect cutting of the nails. Never cut the nail so short that part of the nailbed is exposed. The free edge should be cut straight across. Direct the growth of the nail over the cuticle edge instead of into it. Excessive pressure on the nails caused by wearing tight shoes or constrictive hosiery, even for as short a period as 1 week, may also lead to ingrown or imbedded nails.

COMPLICATIONS

- Infection
- An upward-turned deformity of the distal nailbed and pulp
- Ischemia of the toe from the constricting bandage.

PRACTITIONER FOLLOW-UP

- Patient to follow-up in 2 days.
- Evaluate for regrowth of the nail and the return of symptoms.
- Recheck the nail in 1 to 2 weeks after the procedure or sooner, if there are signs and symptoms of infection.
- If incision and drainage were required, consider dicloxacillin (250 mg, four times daily) or cephalexin (500 mg, three to four times daily) for 7 to 10 days. If MRSA is suspected, then consider TMP-SMX, 2 double-strength tablets, twice daily.
- If symptoms persist despite treatment, refer the patient to a podiatrist.
- Prescribe pain medications if needed.

RED FLAGS

- Ischemia of toe
- Loss of blood flow

CPT BILLING

11730—Avulsion of nail plate, partial or complete, simple; single ■ **11732**—Each additional nail plate (List separately in addition to code for primary procedure). Must be used in conjunction with

11730. ■ **10060**–Incision and drainage of abscess (e.g., carbuncle, suppurative hidradenitis, cutaneous abscess, cyst, furuncle, or paronychia); simple or single ■ **10061**–Complicated or multiple

REFERENCES AND RELATED RESOURCES

Goldstein B, Goldstein A: Paronychia and ingrown toenails. In Dallavalle R, Levy M, editors: *UpToDate*, Waltham, MA, 2014, UpToDate. Accessed December 17, 2014.

Pfenninger J, Fowler G: *Pfenninger and Fowler's procedures for primary care*, ed 3, Philadelphia, 2011, Elsevier.

Usatine RP, Smith MA, Chumley H, Mayeaux Jr EJ: *The color atlas of family medicine*, ed 2, New York, 2013, McGraw-Hill.

2

Subungual Hematoma Evacuation

Kent D. Blad and Sabrina Jarvis

DESCRIPTION

Subungual hematoma is a common injury seen in the primary care setting. The patient usually presents with a direct trauma or squeezing injury to the fingernail or toenail, which creates bleeding between the nail bed and the fingernail. As the hematoma develops, it can cause severe pain. The procedure to drain the hematoma usually brings immediate relief from pain. It minimizes the possibility of secondary pressure effects to the digit and dystrophy of the nail bed and matrix and helps prevent unnecessary delay in regrowth of the nail plate.

ANATOMY AND PHYSIOLOGY

When there is bleeding between the nail bed and the nail, the resulting subungual hematoma slowly expands over several hours, resulting in persistent and often throbbing pain. Causes other than trauma include systemic pathology, medications, drug reactions, and aging.

INDICATIONS

This procedure is indicated for visible, painful subungual hematomas that involve less than 50% of the nail bed.

CONTRAINDICATIONS

This procedure is contraindicated when any of these conditions are present: a fracture of the nail bed or distal phalanx, a laceration of the nail bed, a subungual hematoma that involves more than 50% of the nail bed, or a wound contamination.

▶ RED FLAGS

Refer the patient to a specialist for the following situations:

- Crushed or fractured nail
- Fractured phalanx
- Presence of a subungual melanoma (a malignant, pigmented tumor beneath the nail)
- Hematomas involving more than 50% of the nail bed because these may indicate a laceration of the underlying nail bed

ASSESSMENT

- The hematoma can usually be recognized by the presence of a blue-black or blue-purple area under the nail at the site of the trauma that is exquisitely and increasingly painful.
- Examine the injured digit to determine the extent of the injury. Using your thumb and index finger, gently squeeze the lateral and medial sides of the proximal interphalangeal joint. If this area is pain free, an extensive fracture may not be present. The examiner may then proceed distally to determine whether a more extensive fracture is possible. If the examiner suspects a nondisplaced fracture, a splint should be applied in an anatomic (slightly curved) position until the swelling has decreased.
- Radiographs of the involved digits are recommended to detect associated distal phalangeal fractures (terminal tuft fracture) when there is a reasonable index of suspicion.
- A simple nail trephination procedure usually does not require an analgesic. If there is a fracture or nail matrix injury, consider a digital nerve block with lidocaine without epinephrine or with bupivacaine.

PATIENT PREPARATION

Explain the procedure to the patient. Include possible risk of pain if contact with the nail bed is made during the procedure and the risk of clotting and recurrence of the hematoma following the procedure. Inform the patient that spontaneous nail avulsion may still occur at a later date.

Subungual hematomas with uninjured nail folds are treated with a nail trephination procedure. A more extensive injury may require removal of the nail.

EQUIPMENT

- Gloves
- Povidone-iodine or other antiseptic/germicidal solution
- Electrocautery device or carbon laser (cautery trephination)
- Single bevel, 18-gauge needle or mesoscission device (boring trephination)
- A 29-gauge needle and 1-ml syringe (distal nail subungual hematoma)
- Sterile gauze
- Antibiotic ointment
- Bandage
- Splint (if necessary)

Procedure

Follow universal precautions.

1. Wash the finger with soap and water, and then rinse and dry.
2. Clean the nail with povidone-iodine swabs.
3. Over the hematoma, avoid the lunula and nail matrix and use the electrocautery or carbon laser to burn a hole through the nail to allow for drainage of the blood (Figure 2-44).
4. Alternatively, an 18-gauge needle can be rotated through the nail to the hematoma to allow the blood drain.

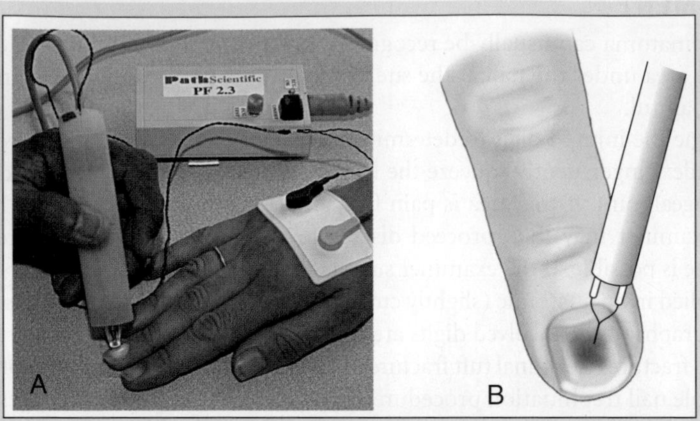

FIGURE 2-44 Procedures for subungual hematoma. **A,** The PathFinder is a mesoscission device that drills into the nail plate, but not into the nail bed, to release the pressure from a subungal hematoma. **B,** A cautery unit may be used to perforate the nail and evacuate the subungual hematoma. **(A,** Reprinted with permission from Path Scientific.)

5. Alternatively, the mesoscission device can be used to create several small holes within the nail to drain the hematoma. The device uses electrodes to determine skin electrical resistance, which aids in calculating the depth of the boring to help avoid injury to the nail bed.
6. Alternatively, if the injury is a simple distal nail subungual hematoma (effective for distal toe injuries), a 29-gauge needle can be inserted under the nail and advanced proximately until the hematoma is reached. The syringe plunger is gently pulled back and the hematoma is evacuated. Gentle pressure to the nail may be needed to help express the blood.
7. After the blood has been drained and pressure and pain have been relieved, clean the area again with alcohol.
8. Apply a light dressing to the nail.
9. The patient may use a splint for 2 or 3 days on the injured finger to protect it from further injury and pain.

PATIENT EDUCATION POSTPROCEDURE

- Soak the affected digit two or three times a day and to keep a light dressing over the area until the empty space has completely closed.
- Keep the injured extremity elevated as much as possible to reduce the swelling.
- Notify the practitioner if the pain persists, if drainage becomes purulent or foul smelling, or if there is a change in the sensation of the finger, a fever, or redness of the skin surrounding the injury.
- Nail discomfort should be alleviated as time progresses; however, if bleeding returns, pain worsens, or the injury is not getting better, call or return to the office.

COMPLICATIONS

- *Onycholysis* (slow loosening of the nail from its bed, usually beginning at the free or loosened end and progressing to the root)

- Transient or permanent nail deformity
- Infection

PRACTITIONER FOLLOW-UP

The patient's discomfort should improve within 48 to 72 hours. Follow-up is usually not needed unless there was more extensive injury.

RED FLAG

If the pain worsens or infection occurs, refer the patient to a podiatrist.

CPT BILLING

11740—Evacuation of subungual hematoma

REFERENCES AND RELATED RESOURCES

Fastle R, Bothner J: Subungual hematoma. In Stack A, editor: *UpToDate*, Waltham, MA, 2012, UpToDate. Accessed November 1, 2014.

Mayorga O: Subungual hematoma drainage, 2014. http://emedicine.medscape.com/article/82926-overview. Accessed December 21, 2014.

Salter S, Ciocon D, Gowrishankar T, Kimball A: Controlled nail trephination for subungual hematoma, *Am J Emerg Med* 24:875–877, 2006.

Tos P, Titolo P, Chirila N, et al: Surgical treatment of acute fingernail injuries, *J Orthop Trauma* 13: 57–62, 2012.

Tully A, Trayes K, Studdiford J: Evaluation of nail abnormalities, *Am Fam Physician* 85:779–787, 2012.

Nail Avulsion

Kent D. Blad and Sabrina Jarvis

DESCRIPTION

At times, a patient presents with the nail torn, or avulsed, from the nail bed, requiring treatment to reduce pain, remove sharp, torn edges, and facilitate the regrowth of a healthy nail.

ANATOMY AND PHYSIOLOGY

The eponychium overlies the base of the nail, covering the nail-forming germinal matrix. Sometimes the nail has been crushed, or the nail has been traumatically torn away by an external force (sometimes a piece of machinery), or the toenail may have caught on something and is torn loose.

INDICATIONS

This procedure is indicated for partial or complete separation of the nail from the nail bed.

CONTRAINDICATIONS

Refer the patient to an orthopedic hand surgeon or a podiatric surgeon if fractures are involved.

PRECAUTIONS

An avulsed nail is usually very painful. Care should be taken to relieve the pain and to reassure the patient.

ASSESSMENT

- Determine the degree of the avulsion. The nail may be completely avulsed, partially held in place by the nail folds, or adhered only to the distal nail bed.
- Sometimes the exposed nail bed has a pearly appearance and minimal bleeding, making it seem like the nail is still in place when actually it has been completely removed.
- Obtain radiographs to determine whether there is a fracture of the underlying bone if crushing or high-velocity shearing force was responsible for the avulsion.

PATIENT PREPARATION

- Explain the procedure to the patient, discussing risks and benefits.
- Determine the presence of any allergies to medication or anesthetic agents.

TREATMENT ALTERNATIVES

The patient should be referred to an orthopedic hand surgeon or a podiatric surgeon for treatment if a fracture is involved.

EQUIPMENT

- Sterile gloves
- Normal saline
- Anesthetic materials for digital block (see section on Anesthesia)
- Suturing materials if required
- Straight hemostat
- Nonadherent dressing, such as Telfa, petrolatum gauze, or Xeroform gauze
- Gauze and adhesive tape for fingertip dressing
- 2-Octyl cyanoacrylate (DERMABOND), if needed, to glue a loose nail
- Vaseline gauze to make a stent

Procedure

Follow universal precautions.

1. Perform a digital nerve block to completely anesthetize the digit (see "Anesthesia: Topical, Local, and Digital Nerve Block").
2. If the nail is still partially attached, remove it by separating it from the nail fold using a straight hemostat.
3. Irrigate the nail bed with normal saline solution to cleanse the area.
4. Cut away the distal free edge of the nail and remove only loose, cuticular debris. Do not débride any area of the nail bed, sterile matrix, or germinal matrix.
5. If lacerations are present, carefully reapproximate with fine (6-0 or 7-0) absorbable sutures. This is necessary to make certain that the new nail can grow in without deformity.

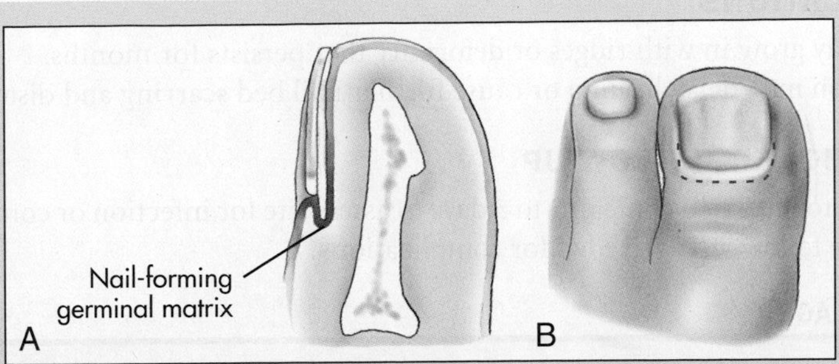

FIGURE 2-45 Replacing a nail that has been avulsed. **A,** Nail or stent in place. **B,** Nail under the eponychium.

6. In cases with very little trauma, the nail bed may be covered with a nonadherent dressing (such as Telfa). Although the dressing offers some protection to the nail bed, the nail will still be very tender and easily damaged until the new nail grows in. In addition, no dressing is truly nonadherent with this type of injury, requiring the provider to see the patient daily for a few days to prevent painful adherence. If regular gauze is used, it will stick to the nail bed and require lengthy soaks and gentle pulling to release it. This is very painful for the patient, so it should be avoided.
7. In most cases, try to reinsert the nail under the eponychium and apply a dressing (Figure 2-45). If the nail does not fit tightly under the eponychium, it may require suturing at the base. Many clinicians prefer to use 2-octyl cyanoacrylate topical skin adhesive (DERMABOND) to glue a loose-fitting nail back into place. The patient's own nail is the most comfortable dressing, so it should be used if possible. Nails that have sustained only minimal trauma can often grow normally if carefully replaced in their proper anatomic positions.
8. If the nail is badly damaged, missing, or contaminated, making it unusable, it may be replaced with a substitute. A nail substitute may be made out of a sheet of Vaseline gauze or Xeroform gauze that is cut to fit. This stent should be tucked under the eponychium where the nail would be placed before applying the dressing.
9. Apply the dressing.

PATIENT EDUCATION POSTPROCEDURE

- Keep affected hand or foot elevated as much as possible for 48 to 72 hours.
- A first-generation cephalosporin should be taken prophylactically for 3 or 4 days if the nail was crushed, wound was contaminated, or if the patient is immunocompromised. Tetanus prophylaxis may also be required.
- The stent should stay in place until the nail bed hardens. This helps prevent the development of synechiae and future nail deformities. The stent will be pushed out as the new nail grows and separates spontaneously.
- Change dressings every 3 to 5 days.
- If sutures were used, remove within 7 to 10 days.
- Complete regrowth of an avulsed nail usually takes place at a rate of about 1 mm per week. Thus the new nail will take from 6 to 12 months to be complete.

COMPLICATIONS

- Nail may grow in with ridges or deformity that persists for months.
- Infection may delay healing or cause further nail bed scarring and distortion.

PRACTITIONER FOLLOW-UP

- Patient to return to clinic in 3 to 5 days to assess site for infection or complications.
- Provide follow-up as needed for complications.

RED FLAGS

- Unresolved bleeding
- Unresolved pain
- Tissue necrosis
- Fractures in digit

CPT BILLING

11730–Avulsion of nail plate, partial or complete, simple; single ■ **11732**–Each additional nail plate. List separately in additional to code for primary procedure. This code must be used in conjunction with 11730.

REFERENCES AND RELATED RESOURCES

Pfenninger J, Fowler G: *Pfenninger and Fowler's procedures for primary care*, ed 3, Philadelphia, 2013, Elsevier.

Usatine RP, Smith MA, Chumley H, Mayeaux Jr EJ: *The color atlas of family medicine*, ed 2, New York, 2013, McGraw-Hill.

SKIN TRAUMA RESULTING FROM BITES OR FOREIGN BODIES

DESCRIPTION

The skin, in its role in protection of the body, experiences many insults from foreign objects. This section discusses bites; trauma caused by foreign bodies, such as fishhooks, rings, and splinters; and body piercings. The emphasis is on management of the problems that occur.

Animal and Human Bites

Kent D. Blad and Sabrina Jarvis

DESCRIPTION

Bite trauma results from teeth that tear, puncture, or crush the skin. People often present to medical personnel after sustaining an animal bite because of a fear of contracting rabies. Young children and teenagers experience up to 50% of all animal bites. Animal bites occur most commonly when young children are poorly supervised and they surprise or disturb an animal that is eating or sleeping, when children try to hug an unfamiliar animal, or when people try to separate fighting animals.

People with a human bite are less likely to be seen or reported; however, emergency care is also required to prevent bacterial wound infections and to promote healing of the wound.

ANATOMY AND PHYSIOLOGY

The skin trauma may involve structures in the subcutaneous and muscular layers of tissue. Irregular lacerations that cause disruption and misalignment of tissue are common because of the nature of the wound. In addition to the trauma, the saliva of cats and dogs may contain organisms that cause bacterial infections, such as gram-negative bacteria like *Pasteurella multocida,* whereas the saliva from humans may contain a high concentration of gram-positive bacteria, such as *Staphylococcus aureus,* streptococci, and gram-negative bacteria, such as *Proteus, Escherichia coli, Pseudomonas, Neisseria,* and *Klebsiella* sp. Up to 30% of all human bites may also be infected with *Eikenella corrodens,* which can be resistant to semisynthetic penicillins. Less common bites by other wild animals or pets, such as raccoons, groundhogs, or monkeys, may also contain pathogenic organisms.

INDICATIONS

Procedure is required if there is suspicion of infection or tissue necrosis.

CONTRAINDICATIONS

Patients who have facial wounds, particularly of any cartilage areas, or other areas of the body where the blood supply has been disrupted, should be referred to a plastic surgeon for emergency treatment.

PRECAUTIONS

- All animal bites should be reported to the local health department.
- Do not introduce irrigating solution deep into puncture wounds.
- The ability of a wound to heal well often correlates with how well the wound has been cleansed and debris has been removed.

ASSESSMENT

- Determine whether an animal or human made the bite and a general picture of the incident. An unprovoked attack by an animal or an animal that acts in a bizarre manner is more likely indicative of having rabies.
- Identify the time of the incident.
- Obtain a history of the current medical status of the patient, any allergies, medication use, and status of immunization.
- Determine the severity of the injury. Evaluate the location, size, depth, and structures that are involved, including the bone, muscle, nerve, and vascular system. Carefully assess for bone and joint involvement.
- Assess for general risk of infection. Young children, older individuals, or patients who are immunocompromised or have serious chronic diseases are more likely to develop infections. Bites of the lower extremities in individuals who have poor circulation also place an individual at greater risk of infection. Assess the specific risk of infection and consider the following factors:
  - Time since the bite occurred: prolonged time is associated with greater risk.
  - Amount of contamination: puncture wounds have greater risk.
  - Degree of vascularity: good circulation decreases risk of infection and poor healing.

2

PATIENT PREPARATION

- Obtain written consent for treatment after discussing risks and benefits.
- Obtain a Gram stain and anaerobic and aerobic wound cultures if infection is suspected.
- For bites on hands or feet, soak the extremity in a 50:50 solution of povidone-iodine and 0.9% sodium chloride for 15 minutes. Irrigate the wound with 500 ml of this solution if unable to soak the extremity.
- For crush wounds, elevate the bitten area above the heart and apply cold packs.

TREATMENT ALTERNATIVES

- Radiography to rule out bone injury or retained teeth (cat bite) in the wound and referral to specialist if appropriate.
- Referral of patients who have bites of the face, hands, and genitalia, or bites in close proximity to the joints or bones to the appropriate specialist.
- Referral of patients who are suspected of early wound infection to infectious disease specialist.

EQUIPMENT

- Povidone-iodine solution, 250 ml and 0.9% Sterile NaCl. Mix to a 50:50 ratio
- Sterile and nonsterile gloves
- A 50-ml syringe
- A 20-ml syringe
- An 18- to 20-gauge needle
- A 2-ml syringe, 27- to 30-gauge needle, and lidocaine 1% solution for injection
- Sterile scissors
- Sterile curved hemostats
- Sterile forceps
- Suture material if needed (see "Suturing Simple Lacerations")
- 4 × 4 gauze pads for cleaning skin and dressing
- Culture swab
- Topical antibiotic agent, such as Bactroban or Polysporin
- Iodoform gauze ¼-, ½-, or 1-inch wide

Procedure

Follow universal precautions.

1. When the wound has been soaked in the povidone-iodine or NaCl solution, position the patient comfortably with the injured area well exposed to light.
2. Provide anesthesia of the wound with buffered lidocaine 1% solution.
3. Cleanse the skin with povidone-iodine solution.
4. Using clean gloves and a syringe with an 18-gauge needle, irrigate the wound with 500 ml of sterile NaCl. Use an irrigation pressure that is fairly high.
5. Using sterile gloves and forceps, remove any devascularized tissue and debris.
6. For a large puncture wound, pack the wound with iodoform gauze, leaving a 1-inch tail protruding from the opening.
7. If the wound is clean and uninfected and open lacerations are located anywhere other than the face, hand, genitalia, joints, or close to bones, use either staples, tape, or sutures to close them. Prophylactic antibiotics should be considered if wound is not superficial or patient presents greater than 8 hours after bite.

Do not use buried absorbable suture; this may act as a foreign body and serve as a site for inflammation.

8. If the wound is already infected, delay repair until after the application of the saline dressings for 3 to 5 days or it let heal by secondary intention, and leave it open. Prescribe antibiotics for 7 to 10 days in these patients and for patients who are debilitated or immunocompromised. The current drug of choice is amoxicillin-clavulanate for 5 to 10 days or until the infection clears.
9. Apply a topical antibiotic if there is a large, denuded area or a deeply contaminated wound.
10. Apply gauze dressing.
11. Rabies prophylaxis may be required, depending on the recommendation of the county health department. If the bite is from a domestic animal that is behaving strangely or from a bat, coyote, fox, opossum, raccoon, or skunk, start rapid rabies vaccination. Rodents, rats, squirrels, hamsters, and rabbits in the United States do not usually transmit rabies. In all cases, follow health department recommendations. Bat bites may include treatment of others in a family even without a confirmed bite.
12. Consider tetanus prophylaxis (see "Wound Care").

PATIENT EDUCATION POSTPROCEDURE

- Apply an ice pack for 15 minutes every hour for the first 24 hours.
- Elevate the injured body part and immobilize for 48 hours.
- Observe for signs and symptoms of infection and report back to office if they develop.
- Take acetaminophen with codeine (Tylenol No. 3) every 4 to 6 hours for severe pain, and then acetaminophen or ibuprofen every 4 to 6 hours for mild pain.
- To reduce the risk of serious infection, take oral antibiotics for 5 to 7 days as prophylaxis. Amoxicillin plus clavulanate (Augmentin) 875/125 mg twice a day is the current Centers for Disease Control and Prevention recommendation for all bites.

COMPLICATIONS

- Systemic infection, localized abscess, cellulitis
- Septicemia
- Osteomyelitis, septic arthritis, tenosynovitis

PRACTITIONER FOLLOW-UP

- Evaluate the status of the wound within 2 days, and look for signs of infection and the extent of healing.
- All bites should be reported to local health department.

RED FLAGS

- Necrotic tissue
- Deep puncture
- Facial wounds

■ CPT BILLING

See previous section for repairs (closures)

12001 – 13160—Codes vary depending on location, size, and degree of complexity

REFERENCES AND RELATED RESOURCES

Baddour L: Soft tissue infections due to dog and cat bites. In Sexton D, editor: *UpToDate*, Waltham, MA, 2014, UpToDate. Accessed December 17, 2014.

Pfenninger J, Fowler G: *Pfenninger and Fowler's procedures for primary care*, ed 3, Philadelphia, 2011, Elsevier.

Usatine RP, Smith MA, Chumley H, Mayeaux Jr EJ: *The color atlas of family medicine*, ed 2, New York, 2013, McGraw-Hill.

2

Fishhook Removal

Kent D. Blad and Sabrina Jarvis

DESCRIPTION

A fishhook that has been accidentally caught in subcutaneous tissue may be difficult to remove without tearing the tissue. The hook must be removed without the barb damaging the tissue.

ANATOMY AND PHYSIOLOGY

Fishing is a popular sport in which the fishhook injury often occurs. Not only does the hook damage the subcutaneous tissue, but it may be difficult to remove the hook without causing further damage. The hook itself is often contaminated with gram-positive organisms, such as *Staphylococcus aureus* and *Streptococcus pyogenes*, from the skin. The hook is often contaminated from the pond, lake, river, or saltwater source and empiric antibiotics may be ordered to provide coverage for such organisms as *Aeromonas* and *Mycobacterium marinum*.

INDICATIONS

The fishhook must be removed when it is lodged in any subcutaneous tissue to relieve pain and anxiety, to reduce the risk of bacterial infection, and to promote healing.

CONTRAINDICATIONS

Primary care providers should not attempt to remove a fishhook that is embedded in or near the eyes, neck, arteries, ligaments, tendons, wrists, genitals, or other neurovascular structures. These require the special skills of a surgeon.

PRECAUTIONS

Special immobilization may be required for children who have a fishhook embedded in their skin before removal may be attempted.

ASSESSMENT

- Assess location of fishhook, depth, and any contraindications to removal by primary care provider.
- Obtain history of allergies and tetanus immunization status.

PATIENT PREPARATION

Explain the procedure to the patient.

TREATMENT ALTERNATIVES

- Pull-through technique may be used to remove multibarbed hooks. One disadvantage is it does create a second skin wound site.
- Angler's string-yank method works best on nonmobile body areas.

EQUIPMENT

ALL METHODS OF REMOVAL

- Nonsterile gloves
- Protective eye wear
- Antiseptic skin cleanser
- A 3-ml syringe with 27- to 30-gauge, ½-inch needle
- Lidocaine 1%

PULL-THROUGH TECHNIQUE

- Pliers or nonsterile hemostats
- Wire cutter

ANGLER'S STRING-YANK METHOD

- Silk suture (size 0 or larger), umbilical tape, or 2 to 3 feet of string

Procedure

ALL METHODS OF REMOVAL

Follow universal precautions.

1. Position the patient with the fishhook well visualized in the light.
2. Put on gloves.
3. Scrub the skin with antiseptic cleansing solution around the fishhook.
4. Inject 1% lidocaine at the point of the hook.
5. After hook is removed, irrigate wound with normal saline and apply antibiotic ointment and dressing.
6. Tetanus prophylaxis may be required (see "Wound Care").

PULL-THROUGH TECHNIQUE

1. Grab the fishhook shaft with the pliers or hemostat and force the fishhook tip up through the skin (Figure 2-46).
2. Cut off the eye of the fishhook close to the skin with wire cutters, and then move the pliers or hemostat to the sharp end of the hook and pull up and out.
3. Tetanus prophylaxis may be required (see "Wound Care").

ANGLER'S STRING-YANK METHOD

1. Tie suture material, umbilical tape, or string around the hook at the point at which it enters the skin (Figure 2-47).
2. With your finger, push the hook farther into the skin, and then lift the shank of the hook parallel to the skin. This should disengage the barb.
3. Using the string or suture, quickly jerk out the hook.
4. Tetanus prophylaxis may be required (see "Wound Care").

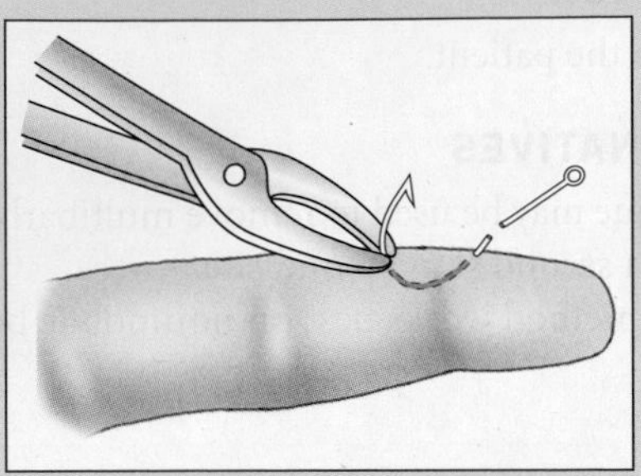

FIGURE 2-46 Pull-through method for removing a fishhook. After cutting off the eye of the fishhook close to the skin, attach pliers or hemostat to the sharp end of the hook and pull out the hook.

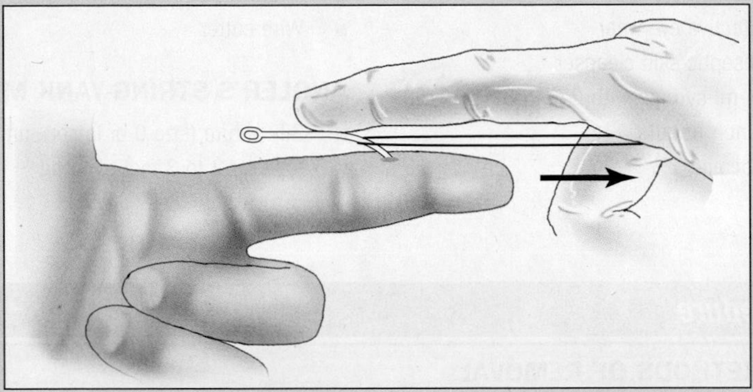

FIGURE 2-47 Angler's string-yank method. Pull the fishhook downward with your finger. Using string or suture, quickly jerk out the hook.

PATIENT EDUCATION POSTPROCEDURE

1. Soak the injured area three times daily in warm water for 2 days.
2. Watch for signs of infection. Call or see the health care provider if there is any indication of infection.
3. Consider empiric antibiotics if fishhook was deeply embedded in area sensitive to infections, such as earlobes, fingers, etc.
4. Use acetaminophen or ibuprofen every 4 to 6 hours as needed for pain.
5. Discuss methods to prevent another accident with a fishhook.

COMPLICATIONS

- Infection

PRACTITIONER FOLLOW-UP

Evaluate the patient within 48 hours for signs of infection and the extent of healing.

RED FLAG

Refer if fishhook is embedded in a body area that requires removal by specialist surgeon.

■ CPT BILLING

10120—Incision and removal of foreign body, subcutaneous tissues; simple ■ **10121**—Incision and removal of foreign body, subcutaneous tissues; complicated

REFERENCES AND RELATED RESOURCES

Bothner J: Fish-hook removal techniques. In Stack A, Wolfson A, editors: *UpToDate*, Waltham, MA, 2014, UpToDate. Accessed October 23, 2014.

Haynes III J, Hines T: Fishhook removal. In *Pfenninger and Fowler's procedures for primary care*, ed 3, Philadelphia, 2010, Elsevier, pp 121–122.

Khan A: Fish hook injury: removal by "push through and cut off" technique: a case report and brief literature review, *Trauma Monthly* 19:e17228, 2014.

Tick Removal

Kent D. Blad and Sabrina Jarvis

2

DESCRIPTION

Ticks can transmit the organisms responsible for Lyme disease (which is the most common tick-borne disease in America), Rocky Mountain spotted fever, and other related diseases. To decrease the risk of infection and potential serious sequelae, it is important for the health care provider to remove ticks intact and as quickly as possible.

ANATOMY AND PHYSIOLOGY

Ticks are arthropods and usually go through four life stages: egg, larva, nymph, and adult. Depending on the type of tick and its life stage, it can take from 10 minutes to 2 hours to prepare to feed. The tick uses its mouthparts to attach to the host. The tick inserts its feeding tube and may produce a cement-type secretion to allow better adherence with the skin surface. Feeding may continue for several days before the engorged tick detaches from its host.

Ticks can transmit several diseases. *Lyme disease* is caused by the spirochete *Borrelia burgdorferi*. Lyme disease is transmitted by the ixodid or smaller deer tick. The female deer tick is about 2 to 3 mm long and has a red body and black legs. Ticks are usually in the nymph stage when they transmit Lyme disease, so they are very tiny and easy to overlook. This nymph stage usually occurs from May through August.

Rocky Mountain spotted fever (RMSF) is caused by *Rickettsia rickettsii* and is transmitted by the American and brown dog tick and the Rocky Mountain wood tick. Ticks may also carry other tick-transmitted diseases, including Colorado tick fever, Southern tick-associated rash illness, relapsing fever, Q fever, tularemia, tick paralysis, etc.

INDICATIONS

Ticks attached to the body must be removed as soon as possible.

CONTRAINDICATIONS

Do not apply hot matches, occlusion, caustics, or noxious chemicals to the tick.

PRECAUTIONS

If a tick is removed in less than 36 hours, the chance of transmission of Lyme disease is greatly decreased.

It is important not to squeeze the body of the tick when removing it because squeezing will push fluid from the tick into the human. If fluid from the tick gets on the hands, wash them well with soap and water to prevent contamination.

ASSESSMENT

Tick-borne illnesses can develop over the course of a few weeks from the initial bite. Common symptoms include fatigue, headache, generalized muscle aches, fever, chills, and a distinctive rash depending on the type of illness. For example, the circular rash characteristic of Lyme disease is called erythema migrans and can present from 3 to 30 days. If left untreated, the patient may develop central nervous system, musculoskeletal, and cardiac symptoms. In Rocky Mountain spotted fever, the rash appears 2 to 5 days after the onset of fever. The rash is nonpruritic with pink macules that start on the wrist, forearms, and ankles and spread to the trunk.

PATIENT PREPARATION

Explain the procedure before and then again as it is carried out. Try to eliminate misconceptions about ticks, how to remove them, and sequelae.

TREATMENT ALTERNATIVES

- None

EQUIPMENT

- Clean gloves
- Fine-tipped tweezers or small forceps
- Alcohol wipe
- Povidone-iodine swab
- Bottle with alcohol for saving tick (optional)

Procedure

GENERAL METHOD OF REMOVAL

1. Clean the area with an alcohol wipe.
2. Wearing clean gloves, grab the tick with the forceps at a point of attachment (mouth), not by the body of the tick (Figure 2-48).
3. Pull straight up firmly, but with gentle traction. Do not twist or crush. Pull until tick is free. If part of the head or mouthparts remains, a punch biopsy technique may be used to remove the involved skin.

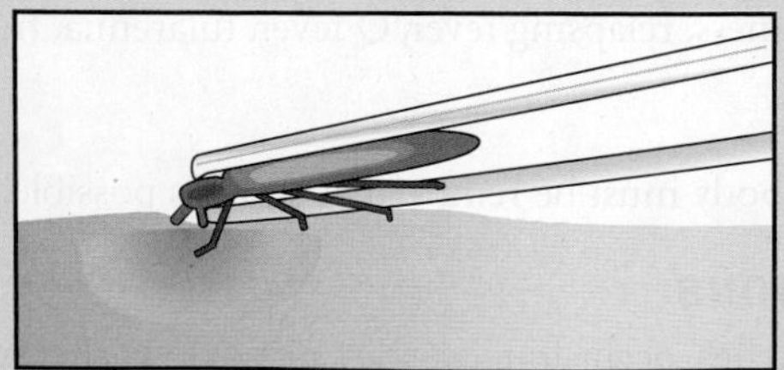

FIGURE 2-48 Procedure for tick removal. Grasp the tick as closely to the skin as possible and pull gently, allowing the tick to back out of the site.

4. A bump is often left on the skin that looks like the tick's head. Do not try to dig this out; it often is not the tick but rather is the cementum secreted by the tick, which later can be scraped off.
5. Put the tick in a bottle with alcohol if its identification is desired. If not, flush the tick down the toilet.
6. Clean the area with povidone-iodine.

PATIENT EDUCATION POSTPROCEDURE

- The patient and family should monitor for possible local or systemic infection over the next few weeks. The common symptoms include fever, fatigue, headache, generalized aches and pains, and characteristic rashes for the type of disease. These rashes include erythema migrans (Lyme disease), similar type "bulls eye" rash (Southern tick-associated rash illness), and pink macules rash (Rocky Mountain spotted fever). The patient is to immediately notify the health care provider if any of the these symptoms develop.
- Provide teaching to help in the prevention of further infestations if exposed to ticks:
  - Shower or bathe as soon as possible after being outdoors (within 2 hours) to wash off and find ticks that may be on the body.
  - Perform a total body search for ticks using a mirror. Parents should examine their children with a focus on the scalp, in and around ears, under arms, behind knees, and on legs.
  - Examine all clothing and gear for ticks. Clothing may be placed in a dryer for an hour with the heat on high.
- Instruct patients that ticks can be better avoided by wearing protective clothing, primarily long-sleeved shirts and long trousers, light-colored clothes where ticks can be seen, and pant cuffs that are tucked into boots or socks. Repellents that contain permethrin may also be applied to clothing, and DEET (diethyltoluamide)-containing products can be used on skin to reduce risk. Use care in the application of DEET, particularly to the skin of children.

COMPLICATIONS

- The most frequent complication is infection of the area, which is usually prevented by cleansing the area with povidone-iodine.
- Rarely, bites cause a delayed hypersensitivity reaction with fever, pruritus, and urticaria.
- A granuloma can develop if a tick is removed improperly, leaving tick parts in the skin. If a firm, pruritic, red papule or nodule persists at the site of tick attachment, removal by a surgeon may be necessary.

PRACTITIONER FOLLOW-UP

Usually no follow-up is necessary. Based on the clinical practice guidelines from the Infectious Diseases Society of America, a one-time dose of doxycycline may be considered for Lyme disease prophylaxis if the bite involved a deer tick or it was estimated to be embedded for 36 hours or longer (time is known or tick is partially engorged), and there is a more than 20% rate of localized infection with ticks carrying *B. burgdorferi*.

It is recommended that the prophylaxis is begun within 72 hours from the time of the initial bite.

- Uncomplicated bites can be painful and leave a red puncture wound that takes 1 to 2 weeks to heal.
- Do not obtain serologic testing in the asymptomatic patient.

RED FLAG

Refer patients to an infectious disease specialist if they develop systemic illness secondary to tick bite.

2

CPT BILLING

Use E/M code appropriate for visit. If no incision was made, you cannot use 10120, since this code is for incision and removal of foreign body.

REFERENCES AND RELATED RESOURCES

Centers for Disease Control and Prevention: *Tick removal*, 2014. http://www.cdc.gov/ticks/removing_a_tick.html. Accessed January 15, 2015.

Centers for Disease Control and Prevention: *Tickborne diseases of the U.S.*, 2014. Retrieved from Tickborne diseases of the U.S. http://www.cdc.gov/ticks/diseases/index.html. Accessed January 15, 2015.

James D: Tick removal and prevention of infection. In *Pfenninger and Fowler's procedures for primary care*, ed 3, Philadelphia, 2011, Elsevier, pp 241–243.

Wormser G, Dattwyler R, Shapiro E, et al: The clinical assessment, treatment, and prevention of Lyme disease, human granulocytic anaplasmosis, and babesiosis: clinical practice guidelines by the Infectious Diseases Society of America, *Clin Infect Dis* 43:1089–1134, 2006.

Foreign Body Removal from Skin

Kent D. Blad and Sabrina Jarvis

DESCRIPTION

Wooden, metal, or glass fragments may inadvertently become lodged into the superficial dermis or subcutaneous tissue. They must be removed completely, or their presence sets up a site for infection.

ANATOMY AND PHYSIOLOGY

Superficial splinters are commonly embedded in the skin after sliding or shoving motions against wood. Patients frequently partially remove splinters, but cannot remove deep particles that have broken off.

Organic foreign bodies create an inflammatory response in the tissues, which then serve as a site for infection if any part is left beneath the skin.

INDICATIONS

This procedure is indicated for:

- Relatively superficially located splinters or foreign bodies that patients have been unable to remove.
- Pain or inflammation from foreign body.

CONTRAINDICATIONS

The patient should be referred to a surgeon if it is unclear whether a wooden foreign body is embedded deep within the skin or when the splinter is confirmed to be very deep or on the face. If a radiograph cannot confirm the foreign body, a high-resolution ultrasound study with a linear-array transducer that focuses in the near field of view, computed tomography scan, or magnetic resonance imaging scan may be used to localize the foreign body in these cases.

PRECAUTIONS

- Wooden splinters are particularly difficult to remove because of their friability and tendency to fragment. Splintered glass can also present a challenge.
- Do not cut down deeply into the tissue to excise a splinter. Refer the patient to a surgeon if needed to cut down deeper than can be closed with superficial sutures.
- Do not make an incision across a skin line, neurovascular bundle, or tendon.
- Do not attempt to remove a splinter in a bloody field. The source of bleeding must be stopped before attempting to remove the splinter.

ASSESSMENT

- Take a good history to try to identify the source of the splinter, time of puncture, any attempts to remove the splinter by the patient, and any sequelae to date.
- A puncture wound may be seen and the splinter may be palpated over the length of the splinter. If the splinter has gone into the skin at a 90-degree angle, running the flat surface of a needle firmly over all of the skin pushes the splinter, leading to sharp pain, which may help the patient localize the spot.
- Clarify patient's tetanus immunization status.

PATIENT PREPARATION

- Explain the procedure to the patient, including risks and benefits.
- Young children may require restraints.
- Obtain written patient consent.

TREATMENT ALTERNATIVES

Very small and superficial slivers can be removed by rubbing a needle over the surface of the skin to loosen them, and then picking them out with an 18-gauge needle. The patient can then clean the skin with soap and water.

Some splinters penetrate straight into the skin and are difficult to grasp with forceps or tweezers. Soaking the area in hot saltwater several times a day may cause the splinter to swell, causing it to protrude slightly from the skin so that it can be grasped by tweezers and pulled straight out. Clear plastic tape or hair removal wax can be used as an alternative method in removing a fine splinter.

EQUIPMENT

- Povidone-iodine or equivalent antimicrobial solution
- A 3-ml syringe and needle for infiltrating tissue
- Lidocaine 1% with epinephrine solution
- Sterile gloves
- No. 15 scalpel blade
- 18-gauge needle
- Suture set (may be required to close area)

2

Procedure

Follow universal precautions.

1. Clean the skin with povidone-iodine or other antimicrobial agent.
2. Infiltrate the area locally with 1% lidocaine with epinephrine (do not use on fingertips or areas of cartilage) (Figure 2-49).
3. Ensure that the area of the splinter is well illuminated.

If the sliver is visible or can be palpated, the following is appropriate:

1. Using sterile gloves and a No. 15 scalpel blade, cut down over the entire length of the sliver, completely exposing it so it can be lifted out with the tip of a needle.
2. Irrigate the area with normal saline solution to ensure that all splinter fragments are removed best as possible.
3. Close the wound with sutures or wound closure strips if required.
4. Give tetanus prophylaxis if necessary (see "Wound Care").

If the sliver is not visible or easily palpable, but seems to be buried within subcutaneous tissue, the following is appropriate:

1. Create a bloodless field by applying a tourniquet if a digit is involved.
2. At the puncture site, make a narrow oval incision on the skin surface around the puncture.
3. Undermine the outer wound edges with the scalpel blade, and then excise the central skin plug along with the subcutaneous tissue containing the foreign body.
4. Close the wound with sutures or wound closure strips.
5. Place antibiotic ointment and dressing over the site.
6. Give tetanus prophylaxis if necessary (see "Wound Care").

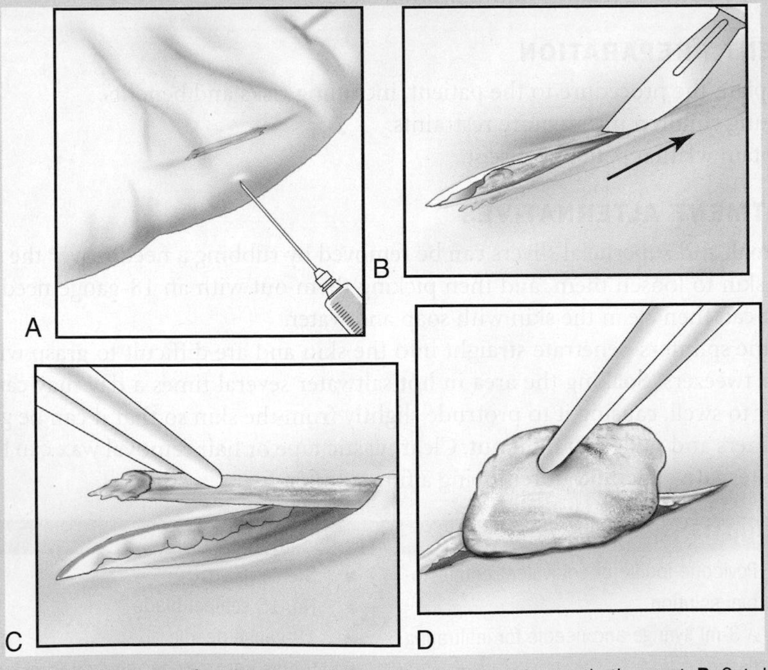

FIGURE 2-49 Procedure for removing splinter. **A,** Inject skin with anesthetic agent. **B,** Cut down to sliver with blade. **C,** Lift out splinter with forceps. **D,** Clean track with wet gauze fluff.

PATIENT EDUCATION POSTPROCEDURE

- Observe for signs/symptoms of infection.
- Take acetaminophen or ibuprofen if needed for mild pain.
- Return to clinic in 2 days for recheck of infection site.
- Return to clinic in 7 to 10 days for suture removal if suture was used.

COMPLICATIONS

- Infection
- Trauma to local structures, such as nerves or blood vessels
- Bleeding
- Scarring from wound
- Partial removal of object

▶ RED FLAG

If a patient returns because of nonhealing or recurrent evidence of inflammation, infection, or drainage, assume that the wound still contains a foreign body. The patient should then be referred to a surgeon.

2

REFERENCES AND RELATED RESOURCES

Armstrong D, Meyr A: Basic principles of wound management. In Sanfer H, Eidt J, Mils J, Billings J, editors: *UpToDate*, Waltham, MA, 2014, UpToDate. Accessed December 17, 2014.

Pfenninger J, Fowler G: *Pfenninger and Fowler's procedures for primary care*, ed 3, Philadelphia, 2011, Elsevier.

Usatine RP, Smith MA, Chumley H, Mayeaux Jr EJ: *The color atlas of family medicine*, ed 2, New York, 2013, McGraw-Hill.

Ring Removal

Kent D. Blad and Sabrina Jarvis

DESCRIPTION

Local swelling and edema that occur after a bee sting, sprain, or crushing injury to a finger may result in swelling around a ring that cuts off lymphatic draining and restricts circulation. Rings often have to be cut off, despite patient objections and personal attachment to the ring, to prevent circulatory and nerve impairment of the finger.

Young children, who create tourniquets with objects such as hair, string, or rubber bands, may not be able to communicate the degree of pain they are in until substantial swelling and ischemia has occurred. Removal of these constricting bands is generally difficult and may require local anesthetic and patient work with a magnifying mirror and large-gauge needle.

ANATOMY AND PHYSIOLOGY

Swelling around the ring serves to produce a tourniquet effect on the digit. If the swelling is extensive, obstruction in the lymphatic drainage results in greater swelling and constriction. This may lead to venous and even arterial circulation compromise. Permanent tissue damage may result if the circulation cannot be promptly restored.

INDICATIONS

Swelling of the finger around a ring often serves as a tourniquet and causes pain and loss of sensation, and must be removed as soon as possible. An additional indication would be a history of an injury, bite, or sting to a digit with a ring, with or without edema.

CONTRAINDICATIONS

Refer the patient to an orthopedic surgeon or emergency room for the following situations:

- Suspected open or closed fracture of digit
- Neurovascular compromise
- Deeply embedded ring

PRECAUTIONS

A radiograph may be required to rule out fracture of the finger if there has been a traumatic injury that caused the swelling.

If the swelling is very mild and transient and the patient is sufficiently responsible to observe for signs of vascular damage, the ring may be left in place and the patient can elevate the finger and apply ice until the swelling resolves.

ASSESSMENT

- Determine cause of swelling and time of injury.
- Perform examination to assess for neurovascular compromise of the digit assessing for color, skin temperature, capillary refill, and reduced sensation including two-point discrimination. Reassess digit after ring removal.
- Determine whether ring must be cut off or can be removed by another method.

PATIENT PREPARATION

Keep the hand elevated and apply an ice pack or cool compresses. Explain the procedure and its benefits and risks to patient.

TREATMENT ALTERNATIVES

Alternative methods for ring removal should be tried before cutting the ring. The method that is used should depend on the extent of the swelling and the degree of skin breakdown around the ring. Begin with the first method, and try successive methods as needed.

1. Apply an ice pack and elevate the extremity to limit further swelling. Often, the ring can be pulled off within a few minutes.
2. Lubricate the finger with soap, water-based lubricant, or glycerin. Provide gentle proximal traction on the skin beneath the ring. Twist the ring off of the finger (Figure 2-50).
3. Slip the end of a braided suture or umbilical tape under the ring with forceps or with a paperclip that has the string threaded through it. Wind a tight, single-layer coil of suture down the finger, compressing the swelling as you go down the finger. Pull up on the end of the suture under the ring, and then slide and wiggle the

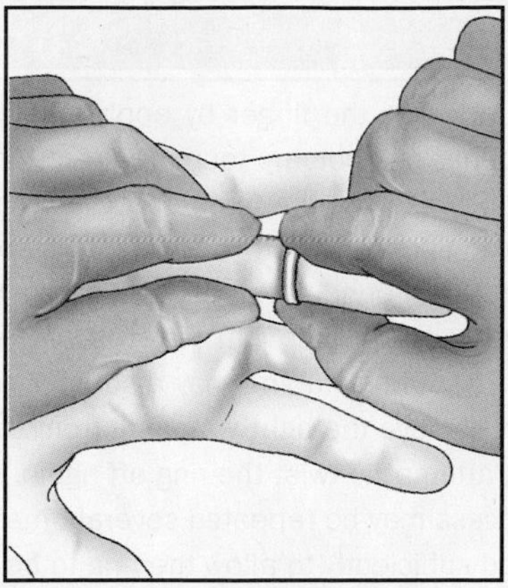

FIGURE 2-50 Pull skin taunt and twist off ring.

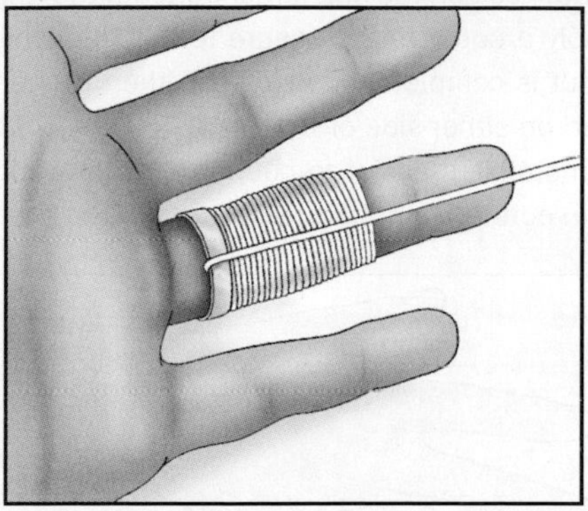

FIGURE 2-51 String technique.

ring down over the coiled suture and off the end of the finger (Figure 2-51). This technique cannot be used if there is a fracture, dislocation, or open injury to the digit.

4. If a digit is extremely swollen and there is an injury, a cut finger from a powder-free surgical glove can be placed over the digit. Using small, curved hemostats, the glove finger is gently advanced under the ring. Pull the glove finger over the ring and gently start to pull and rotate the glove material back down the finger, taking the ring with it.

EQUIPMENT

- Ice pack
- Braided suture or umbilical tape
- Soap and water
- Blood pressure cuff
- Ring cutter, carbide dental drill, Dremel cutting tool (Dremel, Racine, Wis), or orthopedic pin-cutter and cast spreader

Procedure

1. Force all of the blood from the finger by applying a tightly wrapped spiral of Penrose drain or rubber phlebotomy tourniquet around the exposed portion of the finger (Figure 2-52). Elevate the hand above the head, wait for 15 minutes, and then inflate a blood pressure cuff to 100 mm Hg above the patient's systolic pressure as a tourniquet around the upper arm above the finger. (You may have to tape the cuff together or wrap it with cotton case padding to keep the Velcro from pulling apart. The rubber tubing may also have to be clamped to avoid a slow air leak.) Then, remove the tight wrapping from the finger and, leaving the tourniquet in place, attempt to twist the ring off again, using soap and water for lubrication. This process may be repeated several times until the swelling in the finger has decreased sufficiently to allow the ring to be removed.
2. If the ring is still too tight or if there is too much pain to allow these techniques to be attempted, the clinician may use a circular-blade ring cutter to cut through a narrow ring band. Position the ring cutter beneath the ring, grip the saw handle, and begin to apply a squeezing pressure to the ring while turning the circular blade until the cut is complete. The ring can then be bent apart with pliers or hemostats placed on either side of this break (Figure 2-53). If the band is made of wide or hard metal, it is easier to cut out a 5-mm wedge from the ring using an orthopedic pin-cutter. Then, take a cast spreader, place it in the slot left by

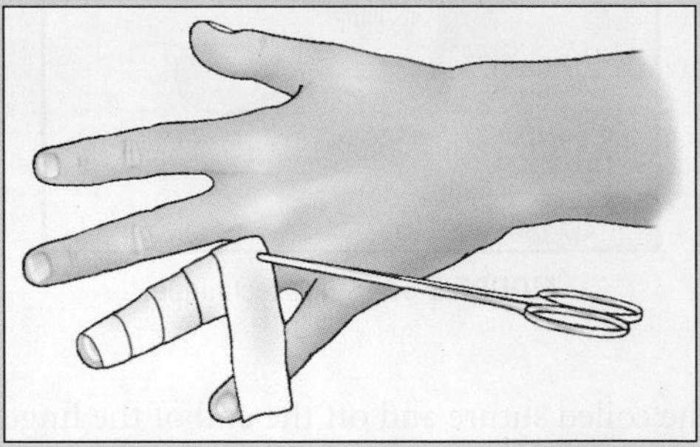

FIGURE 2-52 Tourniquet technique.

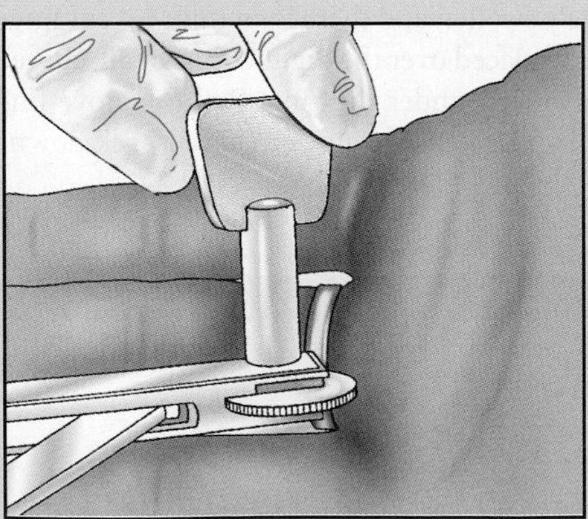

FIGURE 2-53 Ring-cutter technique.

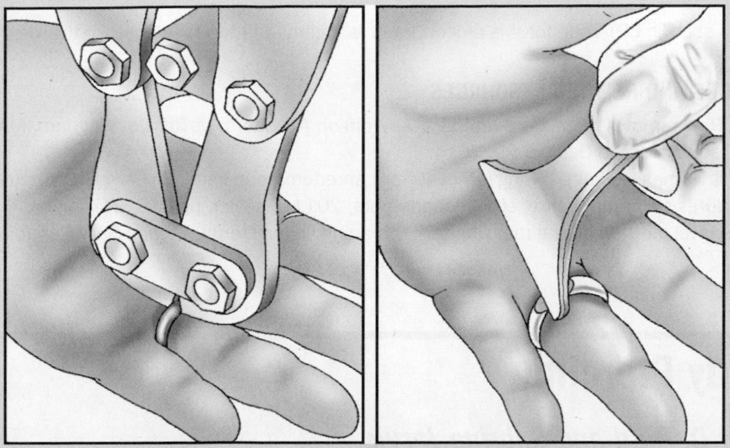

FIGURE 2-54 Orthopedic pin-cutter technique.

the wedge, and spread the ring open. The ring might also be cut with a Dremel cutting tool or a dental drill. Each of these has a sharp-edged grinder attachment that can cut steel (Figure 2-54).

3. Use a large syringe and flush the area vigorously with 50 to 100 ml of 0.9% sodium chloride to remove any metal filings from the area.
4. If finger skin is injured, apply antibiotic ointment and dressing.
5. If the digit has a contaminated wound, consider antibiotic coverage.
6. The patient may require a tetanus booster (see "Wound Care").

PATIENT EDUCATION POSTPROCEDURE

- Instruct the patient to monitor finger for swelling and signs of infection if skin has been denuded.
- Instruct patient to immediately notify health care provider if finger becomes cool, mottled, and/or dusky, or if decreased sensation develops.

COMPLICATIONS

- No complications are expected if the ring is removed in a timely manner or if the swelling is not extensive.
- If the skin is abraded, infection may develop in denuded area.
- Unable to cut or remove the ring.
- Loss of circulation to the digit.

PRACTITIONER FOLLOW-UP

Reevaluate neurovascular status of finger within 24 hours after the procedure if the skin was broken, the removal was difficult, or there was substantial swelling of the finger.

RED FLAG

Obtain emergency consult with hand surgeon if unable to remove ring or digit remains with neurovascular compromise once ring is removed.

2

CPT BILLING

There is no specific CPT code for this procedure. It is included in the E/M code for the visit.

REFERENCES AND RELATED RESOURCES

Bothner J: Ring removal techniques. In Stack A, Wolfson A, editors: *UpToDate*, Waltham, MA, 2014, UpToDate. Accessed October 29, 2014.

Haynes III J, Haynes A, Hines T: Ring removal from an edematous finger. In *Pfenninger and Fowler's procedures for primary care*, ed 3, Philadelphia, 2011, Elsevier, pp 215–217.

Kates S: A novel method of ring removal from the aging finger, *Geriatr Orthop Surg Rehabil* 1:78–79, 2010.

2

Body Piercing

Kent D. Blad and Sabrina Jarvis

DESCRIPTION

The primary care provider is most commonly asked to aseptically pierce the earlobes for cosmetic reasons. Other body parts (e.g., eyebrows, lips, tongue, nares, nipples, navel, penis, and vulva) are also pierced so that jewelry can be inserted into openings, although these piercings are usually not done by trained medical personnel. This section focuses primarily on how to perform ear piercing. Health care professionals are commonly asked to remove piercing jewelry in emergencies, a task that can be somewhat difficult.

ANATOMY AND PHYSIOLOGY

A needle may be inserted through the subcutaneous tissue or ear cartilage. When a surgical-grade wire is left in place, the skin granulates and the epithelium gradually grows down into the area, leaving a permanent opening or sinus through which an earring can be inserted and removed at will.

INDICATIONS

- The procedure is elective and performed when requested by the patient or a child (with parental permission).
- Patients may present with complications from body piercings.

CONTRAINDICATIONS

- Epidermoid cyst or local skin infection
- History of keloid formation
- Chronic steroid use and coagulation disorders
- Immunodeficiency syndromes
- Pregnancy

PRECAUTIONS

Individuals who are allergic to nickel (approximately 10% to 20% of the population) can develop a contact dermatitis to earrings after the ears have been pierced. This is manifested as a pruritic, erythematous rash on the lobes. A patch test can be performed to confirm this allergy. Individuals with a nickel allergy should be instructed to wear earrings made of high-quality surgical stainless steel, platinum, titanium, niobium, and 14- or 24-karat gold. Piercing of the helix should be discouraged. The blood supply of the helix is limited; this results in longer healing and increased susceptibility to infection.

ASSESSMENT

- Assess earlobe for injury, rash, or scar tissue.
- Assess for evidence of keloid formation at other sites of injury or surgery.
- Question patient concerning any allergy to nickel or metals commonly found in earrings.

Ear Piercing

PATIENT PREPARATION

- Explain the procedure and its benefits and risks to the patient. The patient should give written informed consent. Minors should not have ears pierced without the written permission of the parent or guardian.
- Practitioners should instruct patients that they will feel a quick pinch or pressure as the lobe is pierced.
- If the patients desire, ice cubes or topical anesthetic may be used before the procedure to anesthetize the earlobe. Practitioners may have the patients hold the earlobe between two ice cubes for 1 to 2 minutes.

TREATMENT ALTERNATIVES

There are two methods by which the earlobe can be pierced: with a disposable sterile needle or with a device or an instrument. Because of the risk to practitioners of accidentally piercing their own skin with the needle, the "gun" method is safer and is described in this procedure.

There are a variety of devices for ear piercing. The traditional model uses a spring mechanism and presterilized studs and matching friction backs. The stud has a point that pierces through the earlobe. Some of the newer ear piercing guns use a disposable cartridge.

There are also newer ear piercing devices that do not use a spring, but a handgrip. The provider manually squeezes the grip, which forces the stud through the earlobe. Some of these newer devices use earrings in capsules that permit the earring to be loaded into the device without the health care provider touching them.

EQUIPMENT

- Ear-piercing kit (gun, needles, and backing)
- Fine surgical skin-marking pencil or marker
- Cleansing solution: ethyl alcohol or povidone-iodine
- Ice cubes or topical anesthetic agent (optional)

Procedure: Ear Piercing

Follow universal precautions.

1. Position the patient on a stool or elevate the examination table so that the ears are at the practitioner's eye level.
2. Clean the earlobe, front and back, with cleansing solution.
3. Use a surgical marking pen to place a small dot on the earlobe where the ear is to be pierced (Figure 2-55). This ensures correct placement. Do not place the dot too heavy or too low because earrings may cause the hole to tear. For the first ear piercing, place the dot on the center of each earlobe. For a second ear piercing, have the patient remove existing earrings. Following the natural line of the earlobe, place the dot approximately ⅜ of an inch up from the first hole. For the third ear piercing, have the patient remove existing earrings. Following the natural line of the earlobe, place the dot approximately ⅜ of an inch up from the second hole. Have the patient check the position of the dots in a mirror. If the patient is dissatisfied, remove the dots using an alcohol swab and mark the ear again.
4. Position the earlobe between the front and rear portions of the piercing device; the nose of the device should be over the placement dot.
5. Gently squeeze the handle of the piercing device until the earring has been released from the device and has been inserted in the earring back. The earlobe is now pierced.
6. Release your hand pressure on the device and gently pull the earlobe forward to free the earring back.
7. Repeat the process for the other ear.
8. If the ear is pierced in the wrong location, remove the earring and apply pressure to the site. Do not repierce the ear for at least 24 hours.

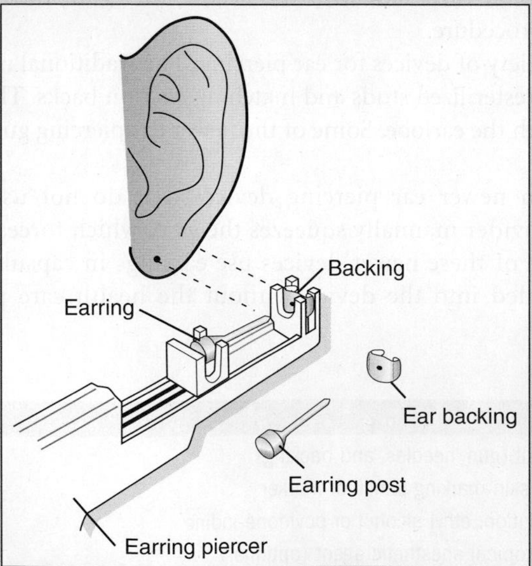

FIGURE 2-55 Ear-piercing technique.

2

PATIENT EDUCATION POSTPROCEDURE

- Avoid the use of strong soaps, cosmetics, and hair spray on the newly pierced earlobes.
- Keep hands and hair away from the newly pierced earlobe.
- Caution patient to expect a small amount of serosanguinous drainage and crust around the front and back of the earring post until healing occurs. Instruct patient to wash hands with soap and water before touching the ear. Use a cotton swab moistened with mild, fragrance-free antibacterial soap and water to clean the earlobe twice a day. (Do not use alcohol or hydrogen peroxide, which may dry the area.)
- Rotate the earrings twice a day to prevent crusting.
- If the earlobe becomes tender, red, and crusty, apply warm compresses four times a day for 24 hours. If this continues or a purulent drainage develops, notify the practitioner. The earrings may have to be removed so the area can heal.
- Do not use antibiotic ointment, such as bacitracin, neomycin, or polymyxin B sulfate because they are petroleum-based ointments that may increase the risk of infection and delay healing.
- The studs or earrings must remain in place for 6 weeks before being removed or replaced with different earrings.

Other Types of Piercings

- The health care provider should offer proactive education for adolescents and young adults on positive body image and self-esteem. Body piercing discussion should include objective information on the piercing procedures, loosely regulated studios, and potential health risks.
- The eyebrows, cheeks, and nares may heal after piercing within 6 to 8 weeks because they are in vascular areas, open to the air.
- The tongue usually has a large amount of swelling, particularly at the beginning. This may require a larger device to be inserted, and it is replaced with a smaller one when the swelling subsides. Swelling may resolve faster if the patient sucks gently on ice for 2 to 3 days. The tongue is a very vascular structure and usually heals in 4 to 6 weeks.
- Any piercings of the mouth, lips, or uvula may interfere with breathing and be associated with aspiration of jewelry, chipped teeth, gingival injury, and infection. Antiseptic, alcohol-free mouthwash should be used with oral piercings, especially after eating or smoking, to decrease the risk of infection.
- Navel piercings are the slowest to heal and the most likely to become infected because of the moist environment or constrictive clothing. Some navel piercings take up to 9 months to heal. The scars from navel piercings may not stretch uniformly in a patient who becomes obese or pregnant, causing pain or discomfort.
- Nipple piercings may take 8 to 16 weeks to heal. Healing is delayed by the wearing of a brasserie and other constrictive clothing. The piercing may also burrow through into the lactation ducts.
- Genital piercings may heal rapidly over 6 to 8 weeks because they are in vascular areas; however, the infection rate is high. Condoms should be used while genital

piercings are healing and to cut down irritation from certain types of lubricants and spermicides. Condoms are often torn by jewelry, particularly the Prince Albert, the ring that goes through the male urethra and out through the glans, which may be worn to increase the sexual sensitivity for the wearer and partner. Double condoms or condoms with extra room at the tip may be used. Men who are uncircumcised are at risk for the development of paraphimosis and genital injury and for potential impotence.

■ CPT BILLING

69090—Ear piercing

Jewelry Removal

Kent D. Blad and Sabrina Jarvis

DESCRIPTION

In an emergency, piercing jewelry should be removed if swelling or bleeding is present in a pierced area or if the patient is undergoing a radiography or surgery. Jewelry parts can present a choking hazard if they are inadvertently swallowed by a patient who is unconscious.

There are several types of body jewelry. These include barbells, capture ball rings, tubes, labrets, flared eyelet flesh tunnels, studs, and safety pins. If the patient is unable to remove the jewelry, the health care provider may need to assist. The provider should be sensitive to the patient's cultural background with the goal to remove the jewelry without damaging it and preventing injury to the patient.

Nose studs, eyebrow rings, and barbell studs on the lip, tongue, or genitalia can usually be unscrewed. For barbells and studs, ring closing pliers or forceps can be used to grasp the ball and turn it counterclockwise as the stud or bar is held stable. Care must be taken not to lose the ball. A ring opening pliers or forceps can be inserted into the center of a capture ball ring and the ring spread open. The ball is held in place by tension and should drop out, allowing the ring to then be removed.

For other jewelry, the screwing mechanisms are often quite different and not always immediately obvious. If the patient is not able to tell the clinician how to remove them, valuable time may be wasted.

If the piercing has been in place and the site well established, the jewelry may be removed without concern that the hole will immediately close off. If there is concern that the hole may seal off, temporary, radiolucent, polypropylethylene jewelry is available commercially.

Patients who have multiple piercings may also need to be tested for human immunodeficiency virus and hepatitis because the risk for contamination of piercing needles and exposure to the virus increases with multiple piercings.

COMPLICATIONS

- Delayed healing and infection, often by *Staphylococcus aureus, Pseudomonas* spp., and group A β-hemolytic *Streptococcus*
- Cyst formation or sepsis

- Keloid formation
- Earlobe deformity with earring tearing through the skin
- Embedded earring stud or backing if the patient has the backing on too tightly
- Pain, allergic reactions, damage to the vasculature, bleeding, and neuroma
- Risk of human immunodeficiency or hepatitis B virus transmission and tetanus
- Delayed treatment for infection, leading to systemic infections that require hospitalization and/or surgical debridement and drainage

PRACTITIONER FOLLOW-UP

- With localized infection, removing or keeping the jewelry is controversial and should be decided on a case-by-case basis. Consider antibiotics if appropriate.
- Instruct patient to return to clinic or emergency room if swelling, infection, and/or bleeding develop at piercing sites.

RED FLAG

Refer patient to appropriate specialist if piercing has caused anatomic injury or systemic infection.

REFERENCES AND RELATED RESOURCES

Holbrook J, Minocha J, Laumann A: Body piercing: complications and prevention of health risks, *Am J Clin Dermatol* 13:1–17, 2012.

Larkin B: The ins and outs of body piercing, *AORN J* 79:330, 333–335, 337–342, 2004.

Schmidt R, Armstrong M: Body piercing in adolescents and young adults. In Blake D, editor: *UpToDate*, Waltham, MA, UpToDate. Accessed December 17, 2014.

Valenzuela P: Body piercing. In *Pfenninger and Fowler's procedures for primary care*, ed 3, Philadelphia, 2011, Elsevier, pp 1597–1604.

Zipper Injuries

Kent D. Blad and Sabrina Jarvis

DESCRIPTION

Skin may become entrapped and crushed between the metal teeth and the slide of the zipper, thereby painfully attaching the article of clothing to the body part involved. This is common with the tissue of the penis, chin, or abdomen.

INDICATIONS

Skin that is caught in the teeth of the zipper.

CONTRAINDICATIONS

There are none.

PRECAUTIONS

Do not cut away or excise the skin. This is unnecessary and very upsetting to the patient.

2

ASSESSMENT

- Identify clearly the amount of skin that is entrapped.
- Assess the degree of discomfort and anxiety in the patient. Provide sedating medication or distraction as needed.

PATIENT PREPARATION

- Discuss risks and benefits.
- Some offices require informed written consent for this procedure.
- Explain clearly to the patient in advance what will be done. Make certain the patient knows that the clinician will not cut or tear his or her skin. This is particularly anxiety provoking if the skin that is entrapped is from the penis.
- Have the patient lie down, and position the patient carefully with good illumination of the affected area. Optional: Drape the patient's face or create a visual barrier to restrict patient from observing the procedure.

TREATMENT ALTERNATIVES

- First try using mineral oil lubricant.
- If mineral oil is not effective, try cutting away the zipper slide.

EQUIPMENT

- Povidone-iodine solution
- Sterile 4 × 4 sponges to scrub area
- 1% Buffered lidocaine (plain), 5 ml
- A 5-ml syringe and ⅝-inch, 15-gauge needle
- Mineral oil (30 ml) or other lubricant
- Scissors
- Metal snips or orthopedic pin cutter
- Two heavy-duty surgical towel clamps

Procedure

Follow universal precautions.

1. For most patients, but especially for children, the face may have to be draped to decrease anxiety. Parents may have to hold the arms of children to prevent movement.
2. To allow comfortable manipulation of the zipper and the article of clothing, paint the trapped skin area with a small amount of povidone-iodine and infiltrate the skin with 1% buffered lidocaine (plain).
3. Apply mineral oil to the skin area and zipper. The oil will lubricate the moving parts of the zipper, and with some traction, the skin is often freed without having to cut the zipper.
4. If the zipper has not pulled away, cut the zipper away from the article of clothing to decrease weight and tension on the entrapped area. This may sometimes be done in such a manner that the article of clothing is not destroyed.

5. Using metal snips or an orthopedic pin cutter, cut the zipper slide in half. If the two halves of the slide do not comc apart, then take two heavy-duty surgical towel clamps and place their tongs into the side grooves at both ends of the slide. Gripping the clamps firmly in each hand, pull your wrists firmly in opposite directions. The two halves of the slide will usually pop apart, releasing the entrapped skin (Figure 2-56).
6. Pull the exposed zipper teeth apart.
7. Cleanse the crushed skin.
8. Apply an ointment, such as povidone-iodine or bacitracin, to the affected area.
9. Tetanus prophylaxis should be provided as needed.

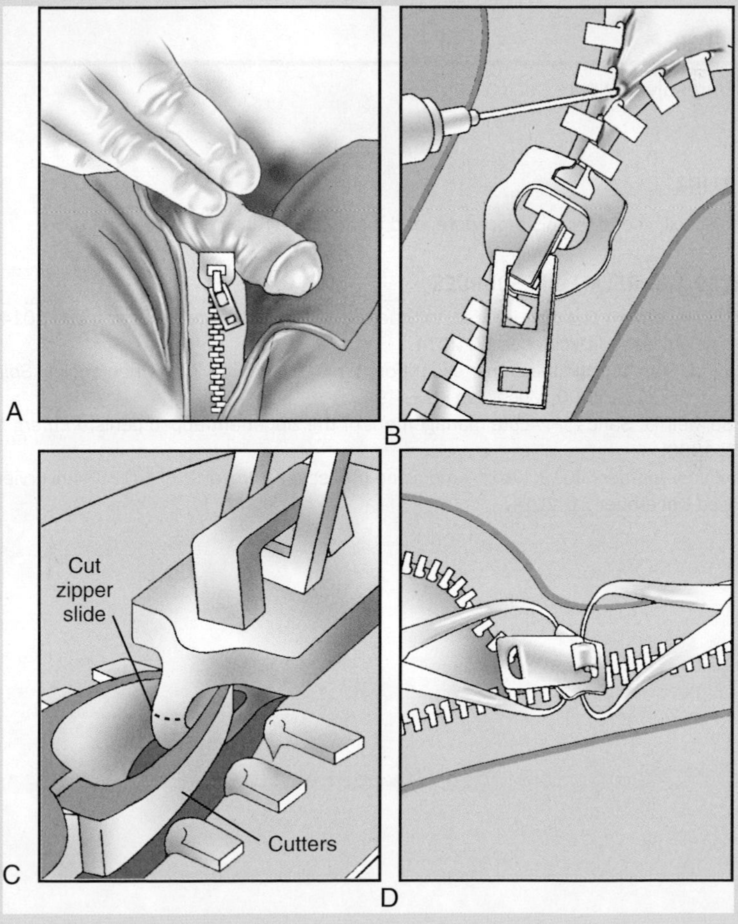

FIGURE 2-56 Removing zipper caught on skin. **A**, Penis caught in zipper. **B**, Injection of lidocaine. Cut zipper slide with a metal snip or an orthopedic pin cutter (**C**), or use two heavy-duty surgical towel clamps (**D**).

2

PATIENT EDUCATION POSTPROCEDURE

- The patient should keep the area clean and without dressing if possible.
- The area should be covered with antibiotic ointment for several days.
- The patient may take acetaminophen to reduce soft tissue pain.
- There should be no long-term consequences to this problem.
- The patient may be encouraged to discard clothes with metal zippers and to buy plastic zipper closures in preference.

COMPLICATIONS

- Potential bleeding
- Skin tear or laceration

PRACTITIONER FOLLOW-UP

Usually not needed.

RED FLAG

- Unresolved zipper stick

CPT BILLING

There is no specific code for this procedure, and it should be reflected in the E/M code.

REFERENCES AND RELATED RESOURCES

Bothner J: Management of zipper injuries. In Stack A, editor: *UpToDate*, Waltham, MA, 2014, UpToDate. Accessed December 17, 2014.

Buttaravoli PM, Stair TO, editors: Zipper caught on penis or chin. In *Minor emergencies: Splinters to fractures*, St Louis, 2000, Mosby, pp 492–494.

Nolan JF, Stillwell TJ, Sands JP: Acute management of the zipper-entrapped penis, *J Emerg Med* 8:305, 1990.

Saxena A: *Zipper injuries*, 2013. http://emedicine.medscape.com/article/1413584-overview. Accessed December 21, 2014.

3

Eye, Ear, Nose, and Mouth Procedures

Joanne Rolls

EYE PROCEDURES

Most procedures involve evaluating and treating injuries to the cornea. After a careful examination to diagnose the problem, the primary care provider is often required to refer the patient to an ophthalmologist. If in doubt about the course of action, referral is always the best course.

ANATOMY AND PHYSIOLOGY

Primary care procedures that involve the eye require a good understanding of the external and internal structures. A review of the internal structures helps the health care provider remember the short distance between the outside body and the brain (Figure 3-1).

ASSESSMENT

The most important thing to assess with any eye injury is whether the patient can see. Do not forget to perform basic visual acuity testing with all patients who have an eye injury. Remember to find out about previous visual history, especially related to trauma, and to measure visual acuity in both eyes, corrected and uncorrected if applicable. The physical assessment should also include extraocular movements (EOM) testing, pupillary direct and consensual reaction to light testing, inversion of the upper lids and fluorescein staining if necessary. Assess for tearing, photophobia, drainage, blurred or double vision, and redness. Loupe glasses may also help with your assessment. Box 3-1 lists ophthalmology problems requiring same-day care.

▶ RED FLAG

Situations requiring immediate emergency evaluation or ophthalmic referral:

- Acute angle-closure glaucoma
- Central retinal artery occlusion
- Trauma to the eye or injury in which intraocular damage is suspected because of the mechanism of injury (e.g., small object propelled toward the eye, hammering metal, etc.)
- Temporal arteritis
- Vitreous hemorrhage
- Retinal tear or detachment

- Blood in the anterior chamber of the eye
- Fixed, distorted, or dilated pupils
- Change in visual acuity
- Visible flecks of steel or iron surrounded by a rust ring
- Foreign body embedded inside the eyeball or deeply lodged in the sclera or cornea
- Painless loss of vision
- Chemical burns or chemical or liquids in the eye *(immediate management is eye irrigation with normal saline)* or iron or steel foreign bodies frequently form ring-shaped orange stains that cause a low-grade inflammation and impair vision
- Patients who are uncooperative

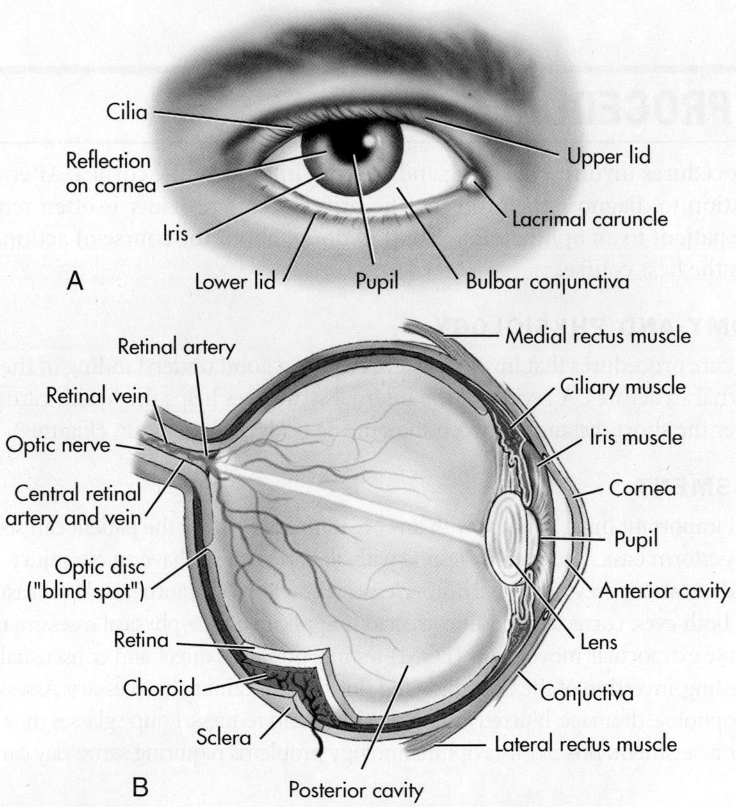

FIGURE 3-1 Structures of the eye. **A**, External. **B**, Internal.

BOX 3-1 Ophthalmology Problems Requiring Same-Day Care

- Acute and/or severe pain
- Blurred vision that is not helped by repeated blinking or putting on glasses
- Double vision
- Pain involving contact lenses, especially extended-wear lenses
- Seeing halos around objects (symptom of acute angle-closure glaucoma)
- Seeing light flashes, black dots, or a curtain effect (symptom of retinal detachment)
- Sensitivity to light; photophobia
- Sudden loss of vision, with or without pain

Removal of a Foreign Body From the Eye

DESCRIPTION

The most common ocular injury is caused by a simple foreign body. Corneal abrasions, erosion, or lacerations may produce similar symptoms depending on the severity of the injury. Not all foreign body injuries are associated with pain. Glass embedded in the cornea may be particularly difficult to detect because it is clear.

ANATOMY AND PHYSIOLOGY

Common sites of foreign bodies in the eye are the conjunctival fornix of the upper lid, within the lid fissure, sunk into an angle of the anterior chamber inferiorly, within the posterior wall, or within the vitreous cavity.

INDICATIONS

- Unilateral foreign body sensation
- Red eye
- Eye trauma
- Unilateral eye irritation in contact lens wearers

A primary care provider can remove foreign bodies embedded in the conjunctival sac or in the corneal epithelium that are easily seen without magnification. Fluorescein staining outlines the area.

CONTRAINDICATIONS

- Do not use corticosteroids in the eye without consultation with an ophthalmologist. Steroids can cause rapid activation of herpes, promote the growth of fungi, potentiate the collagenolytic effect of enzymes of organisms, such as *Pseudomonas,* and impair wound healing.
- Patient should not be discharged with anesthetic eye drops.
- A patient who is uncooperative (patient has a mental deficiency or dementia, or a young child).

A list of emergency conditions that require immediate treatment is found in Box 3-1.

PRECAUTIONS

- The eye globe should not be pressed against at any time.
- Foreign bodies may serve as a source of infection.

ASSESSMENT

- Obtain a history (full description of the current episode, relevant past history, allergies, whether the injury was employment related, status of tetanus booster, etc.).
- Check visual acuity.
- Perform a complete focused examination of the eyes including EOMs, pupillary examination.

PATIENT PREPARATION

During an eye examination, the patient may be frightened, upset, and apprehensive. If the patient has pain, he or she will keep the eye shut tightly as a defense mechanism.

The patient will need reassurance, so explain each step of the procedure. A topical local anesthetic agent is required to permit adequate inspection of the eye. Explain that the anesthetic usually takes effect immediately, but will not completely block sensation.

TREATMENT ALTERNATIVES

Some foreign bodies are fairly superficial and may be removed with eye irrigation.

- Holding the eye open with one hand, flush the eye with normal saline irrigating solution squirted under gentle pressure from a bulb syringe. Alternatively, use a 1-L bag of normal saline with or without a Morgan lens.
- Do not use extreme pressure.
- Continue flushing eye until particle floats away.

EQUIPMENT

- Bright light
- Snellen eye chart
- Sterile normal saline
- Topical anesthetic drops (proparacaine HCl 0.5%)
- Topical antimicrobial drops or ointment
- Eye spud or small-gauge needle (25 gauge)
- Fluorescein-impregnated strips
- Penlight or cobalt blue light or Wood's lamp or slit lamp if available
- Sterile cotton-tipped applicator
- Ophthalmoscope
- Loupe glasses (optional)

3

Procedure

1. Instill 1 to 2 drops of 0.5% topical anesthetic and wait about 1 minute.
2. Inspect the cornea and sclera using a light source. Open the lids wide, using your thumb and index finger. If a foreign body is detected, use the removal technique for a particle before proceeding (see "Removal Techniques").
3. Apply fluorescein dye.
   a. Moisten the tip of a dye strip with sterile saline.
   b. Touch the strip to the conjunctiva. (If you are staining both eyes, use separate strips to prevent cross-contamination.)
   c. Instruct the patient to blink the eye gently and to look straight ahead.
   d. Shine a penlight or cobalt blue light at an oblique angle across the cornea. Bright green areas indicate a true corneal abrasion. A minute corneal foreign body can be seen in the concentration of fluorescein in the area surrounding it.
   e. Irrigate eyes to prevent chemical conjunctivitis from the fluorescein.
4. Evert the upper eyelid to examine the upper conjunctiva (Figure 3-2).
   a. Instruct the patient to look down with both eyes.
   b. Grasp the eyelashes of the upper lid and gently pull the lid down and slightly outward away from the eye.

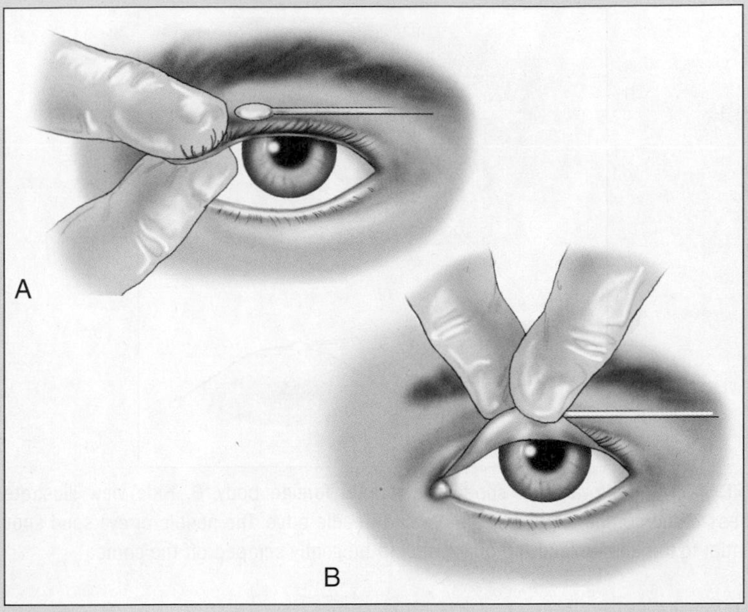

FIGURE 3-2 Evert the upper eyelid to examine the upper conjunctiva. **A,** Grasp the upper eyelashes between the thumb and index finger and, with the tip of the other index finger or a cotton-tipped applicator, press gently on the skin at the upper lateral border of the tarsal plate. **B,** Pull outward on the lashes and rotate the tarsal plate upward until it forms a right angle with the eyeball. A gentle tug upward should flip the plate into eversion, clearly exposing the conjunctival surface of the upper lid.

c. Apply a gentle pressure directly on the lid (on the upper edge of the tarsus on the skin side, about 10 mm above the upper lid margin) using a small cotton-tipped applicator.
d. Simultaneously pull the lashes upward.
e. Examine the upper conjunctiva.
f. Remove the foreign body if present (see "Removal Techniques").
g. When the foreign body is removed, release the upper lid and ask the patient to look up. The eyelid will readily flip back to its normal position.

5. Examine the lower eyelid.
a. Have the patient fix his or her gaze upward; grasp the lower eyelashes, and pull the lid away from the eyeball.
b. Place the tip of your free index finger on the cheek over the inferior orbital margin and push the skin upward to expose the lower lid conjunctiva.

6. Removal techniques.
a. Instruct the patient to gaze on a distant object.
b. Hold the eyelid apart with the thumb and index finger.
c. Gently wipe the cornea or upper tarsal conjunctiva once with a sterile cotton swab moistened with sterile normal saline or ocular irrigating solution. If the particle does not dislodge with this gentle brushing maneuver, stop. The corneal epithelium could be damaged by continued swabbing.

3

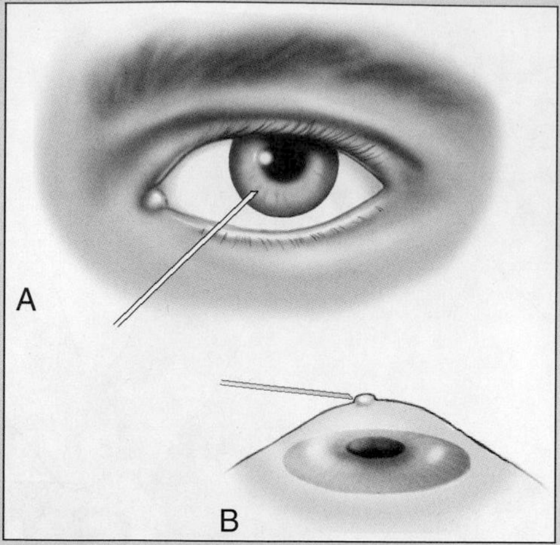

FIGURE 3-3 **A,** Removal of a superficial corneal foreign body. **B,** Side view illustrates the thickness of the cornea relative to the beveled needle edge. The needle or eye spud should be tangential to the cornea, and the object should be gently scraped off the cornea.

d. If the particle remains embedded, slip an eye spud or the beveled edge up of a 25-gauge needle attached to a syringe (some recommend an 18-gauge needle) under the particle and lift it off the cornea. Several attempts may be necessary (Figure 3-3).
e. Keep the instrument parallel to the surface of the cornea to prevent pressure, which could lead to perforation.
f. After the foreign body is removed, retest visual acuity and apply an antibiotic ointment.

3

PATIENT EDUCATION POSTPROCEDURE

- Instruct the patient to return within 24 hours for reevaluation if he or she has any problems, especially if there is any blurred vision. The majority of superficial injuries heal without difficulty.
- Warn the patient always to wash the hands with soap before applying an eye ointment, manipulating an eyelid, or touching any part of the eye.
- Teach the patient how to instill an eye ointment: Without touching the tip to the eye, pull down the lower lid and place a line of ointment just inside. Close the eye and look all around. Advise the patient that vision will be blurry after instillation; the patient should not attempt to drive or perform tasks that require hand-eye coordination.
- Instruct the patient to avoid rubbing the eyes.
- Warn the patient that the foreign body sensation may return temporarily when the anesthetic agent has worn off.
- Tell the patient who wears contact lenses not to wear them until he or she is seen by an ophthalmologist.
- Advise the patient to wear protective glasses when working around flying particles, such as dust, sawdust, glass, metal, or sand.

COMPLICATIONS

- Continued pain (do not prescribe numbing drops for home use)
- Infection

PRACTITIONER FOLLOW-UP

- The anesthesia lasts about 15 minutes.
- Corneal injuries usually heal within 24 hours after the foreign body is removed.
- A follow-up examination by an ophthalmologist 1 to 2 days after the injury is recommended.
- The patient should return to the ophthalmologist if symptoms are persistent or recurrent.

CPT BILLING

If a patient comes in for a procedure only, there is no E/M code charge. The charge for the office visit is the procedure itself.

65205—Removal of foreign body, external eye; conjunctival, superficial

REFERENCES AND RELATED RESOURCES

Pokhrel P, Loftus S: Ocular emergencies, *Am Fam Physician* 76(6):829–836, 2007.
Turner A, Rabiu M: Patching for corneal abrasion, *Cochrane Database Syst Rev* (2):CD004764, 2006.

Treatment of Corneal Abrasion

DESCRIPTION

Simple, minor corneal abrasions can be treated by the primary care provider. See Box 3-1 for triage priority.

ANATOMY AND PHYSIOLOGY

Because the inner eyelid so frequently rubs across the cornea, the surface must be kept smooth and lubricated. When foreign bodies invade the cornea or a corneal abrasion destroys the integrity of the corneal epithelium, significant pain results.

INDICATIONS

- A history of the eye being scratched
- Foreign body sensation and pain in eye
- Complaints of irritation in contact lens wearers (remove contact lens, evaluate, and then refer to ophthalmologist)
- Photophobia (especially in children)

RED FLAGS

- Evidence of penetrating eye injury
- Hypopyon or hyphema
- Corneal infiltrate or ulcer
- Significant vision loss, with or without pain

3

CONTRAINDICATIONS

- Practitioners should NEVER prescribe topical anesthetic agents. These products retard corneal healing and may allow for corneal abrasion to progress to corneal ulcers.
- Practitioners should avoid prescribing steroids for the eye unless advised by an ophthalmologist. These products retard healing and promote overgrowth of virus and fungus.

PRECAUTIONS

Contact lens wearers who have corneal abrasions require special precautions. Help the patient remove and discard disposable contact lenses. Evaluate if the corneal abrasion is due to the contact lens or other cause. Treat with an antibiotic ointment that provides coverage for pseudomonas. See patient daily for follow-up until resolution.

Contact lens wearers who have severe abrasions may require referral to an ophthalmologist.

ASSESSMENT

- Obtain a history (full description of the current episode and the mechanism of injury, past relevant history, allergies, status of tetanus booster, etc.).
- Check visual acuity, perform a focused examination.

PATIENT PREPARATION

Tell the patient that he or she will not feel pain if anesthetic drops are used, but that he or she will feel pressure.

TREATMENT ALTERNATIVES

3

If corneal abrasion is due to the wearing of contact lens, the lens should be immediately removed. Removal of this irritation often allows for a mildly irritated eye to heal without other forms of intervention. An ophthalmologist should confirm the status of the eye and when or if contact lenses can be used again.

EQUIPMENT

- Snellen eye chart
- Sterile normal saline or ophthalmic irrigating solution
- Topical anesthetic drops (proparacaine HCl 0.5%)
- Topical antimicrobial ointment (sulfacetamide 10%)
- Fluorescein-impregnated strips
- Penlight or cobalt blue light
- Ophthalmoscope
- Eye patch and paper tape
- Loupe glasses (optional)

Procedure

1. Instill 1 or 2 drops of topical anesthetic and wait about 1 minute.
2. Inspect the cornea and sclera using a light source. Open the lids wide using your thumb and index finger.

3. Apply fluorescein dye.
    a. Moisten the tip of a dye strip with sterile saline.
    b. Touch the strip to the conjunctiva. (If you are staining both eyes, use separate strips to prevent cross-contamination.)
    c. Instruct the patient to blink the eye gently and to look straight ahead.
    d. Shine the penlight or cobalt blue light at an oblique angle across the cornea. Bright green areas indicate a true corneal abrasion. A minute corneal foreign body can be seen in the concentration of fluorescein in the area surrounding it. A linear corneal abrasion suggests a foreign body beneath the lid (Figure 3-4). If you suspect a foreign body beneath the lid, the lid must be everted and swept, and the foreign body removed.
4. Irrigate the eyes to prevent chemical conjunctivitis from the fluorescein.
5. If an abrasion is seen:
    a. Instill 1 or 2 drops of additional anesthetic agent.
    b. Instill a cycloplegic agent if the patient has significant spasm and pain (contraindicated in children).
6. Apply an antibiotic ointment.
7. Reexamine in 24 hours using fluorescein.
    a. If the abrasion has healed, give antibiotic drops for 3 days.
    b. If the abrasion is smaller, instill a cycloplegic and an antibiotic ointment and examine again in 24 hours.
8. Refer to an ophthalmologist if the eye is not healing well or if cloudiness or drainage appear. Maintain a low-threshold for referral in contact lens wearers.
9. Recheck visual acuity before discharging the patient.

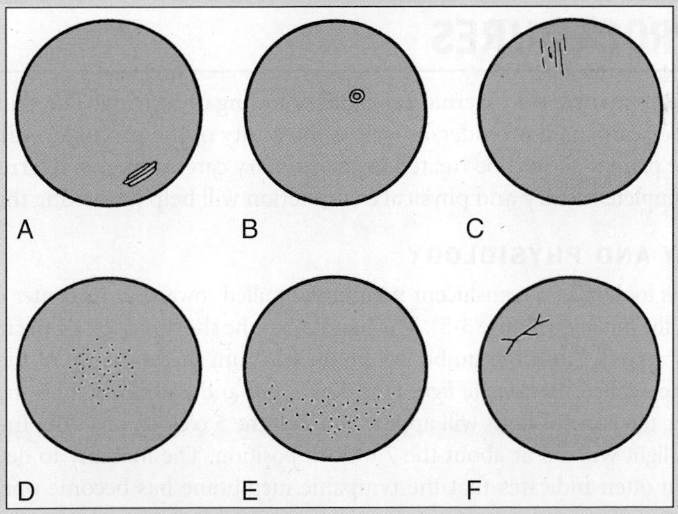

FIGURE 3-4 Corneal defect staining patterns for specific injuries. **A,** Typical abrasion. **B,** Abrasion around a corneal foreign body. **C,** Abrasion from a conjunctival foreign body under the upper lid. **D,** Abrasion from excessive wearing of a contact lens. **E,** Ultraviolet exposure (resulting from sunlamp exposure, welding, or snow blindness). **F,** Herpetic dendritic keratitis. (From Pfenninger JL, Fowler GC: *Pfenninger and Fowler's procedures for primary care physicians,* ed 3, Philadelphia, 2011, Saunders.)

3

PATIENT EDUCATION POSTPROCEDURE

- Instruct the patient to return in 24 hours for reevaluation if symptoms are not resolving.
- The patient will need reevaluation every day until the abrasion is healed.
- It is best that the patient not drive, watch television, or read until eye has healed.

COMPLICATIONS

Some significant abrasions promote adhesions that cause the cornea to stick to the lid. This situation should be followed by a specialist.

PRACTITIONER FOLLOW-UP

- Reevaluate the eye daily until the abrasion is healed.
- Refer to an ophthalmologist if the abrasion is not healing properly or signs and symptoms of infection occur.
- Refer contact lens wearers to their ophthalmologist.

REFERENCES AND RELATED RESOURCES

Shields SR: Managing eye disease in primary care, part 2: how to recognize and treat common eye problems, *Post Grad Med* 108:83, 91, 2000.

Tingley DH: Consultation with the specialist: eye trauma: corneal abrasions, *Pediatr Rev* 20:320, 1999.

Turner A, Rabiu M: Patching for corneal abrasion, *Cochrane Database Syst Rev* (2):CD004764, 2006.

Vorvick L, Reinhardt R: 5 Common eye complaints, *J Fam Practic* 62(7):345–355, 2013.

Wipperman J, Dorsch J: Evaluation and management of corneal abrasions, *Am Fam Physician* 87(2):114–120, 2013.

EAR PROCEDURES

Ear procedures involve the external ear canal or testing of hearing. The skill and experience of the health care provider, as well as the acuity of the problem, will determine whether the patient should be treated in the primary care setting or referred to a specialist. A complete history and physical examination will help in making that decision.

ANATOMY AND PHYSIOLOGY

The *eardrum* looks like a translucent membrane pulled inward at its center over one of the ossicles, the *malleus* (Figure 3-5). The handle and the short process of the malleus may also been observed. From the umbo, where the eardrum meets the tip of the malleus, a light reflection called the *cone of light* fans downward and anteriorly. This means that in the right ear, the cone of light will appear at about the 5 o'clock position. In the left ear, the cone of light will fall at about the 7 o'clock position. The inability to determine the cone of light often indicates that the tympanic membrane has become opaque due to infection.

On the tympanic membrane, but above the short process, lies a small portion of the eardrum called the *pars flaccida.* The remainder of the tympanic membrane is called the *pars tensa.* Anterior and posterior malleolar folds extend obliquely upward from the short process and separate the pars flaccida from the pars tensa. These folds are usually visible only if the eardrum is retracted. A second ossicle, the *incus,* can sometimes be seen through the drum if it is very clear (Figure 3-6).

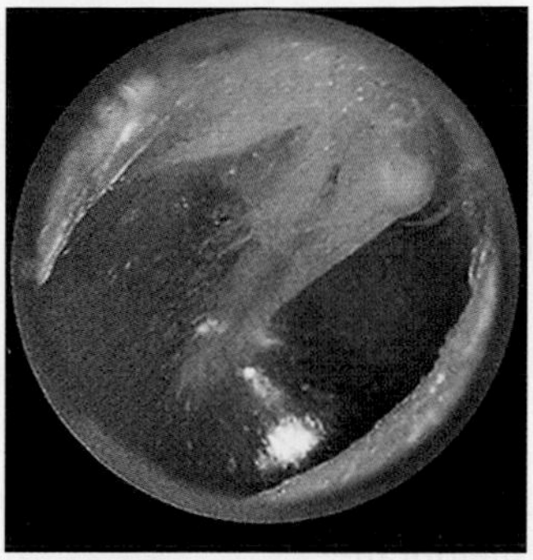

FIGURE 3-5 Normal tympanic membrane. (From Ball JW, Dains JE, Flynn FA, et al: *Seidel's guide to physical examination*, ed 8, St Louis, 2015, Elsevier.)

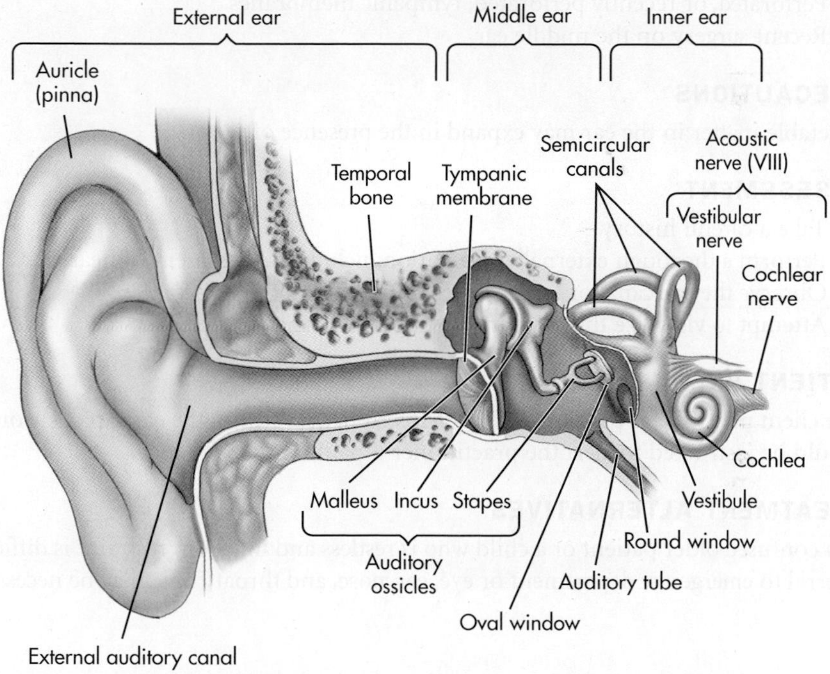

FIGURE 3-6 The structures of the ear.

Removal of a Foreign Body From the Ear

DESCRIPTION

It is not uncommon for a foreign object to become stuck in an ear canal. It is quite common for children, particularly toddlers, to put objects into their ear canals. Such objects as pebbles, beads, beans, folded paper, and button batteries are commonly found in children's ears. After the age of 9 months, once the pincer grasp is fully developed, any number of foreign body types can be inserted into the pediatric patient's ear. In adults the most common foreign bodies are insects that accidentally enter the ear canal. Objects such as matchsticks or cotton-tipped swabs that have been used to relieve itching or soreness in the ear are also common in adults. The main symptoms of a foreign body in the ear canal are sudden pain, a feeling of fullness, and noise in the ear (usually buzzing or roaring). Sometimes irritation of the nerves in the ear canal may cause hiccups. Children often do not complain of these symptoms, but may have a discharge from the ear, especially if the object has been in the ear for some time.

INDICATIONS

Any foreign object lodged in the ear canal should be removed to prevent infection or disruption of the tympanic membrane.

CONTRAINDICATIONS

- Tympanostomy tubes
- Perforated, or recently perforated, tympanic membranes
- Recent surgery on the middle ear

PRECAUTIONS

Vegetable matter in the ear may expand in the presence of water.

ASSESSMENT

- Take a careful history.
- Perform a thorough external examination including assessment of hearing.
- Observe the ear canal of the unaffected ear with an otoscope.
- Attempt to visualize the tympanic membrane of the affected ear.

PATIENT PREPARATION

The client may feel ear pressure while the instrument is within the ear canal. He or she should be instructed to alert the practitioner if pain occurs.

TREATMENT ALTERNATIVES

In a confused older patient or a child who is restless and in whom restraint is difficult, referral to emergency department or eye, ear, nose, and throat clinic may be necessary.

EQUIPMENT

The tools that are necessary will vary depending on the foreign object and its location.

- Blunt ear curette or ear spoon
- Ear or 60-ml syringe
- Basin of warm water
- Emesis basin
- Towel
- Otoscope
- One of the following agents to immobilize an insect for removal from the ear: microscope oil, 2% lidocaine, 4% lidocaine, or 2% viscous lidocaine

Procedure

1. Visualize the foreign object; if it is not immediately visible, place the tip only of the otoscope outside the ear canal and retract the pinna superiorly and posteriorly to aid in visualization (Figure 3-7).
2. If the object CANNOT be visualized, pour warm water into the clean basin; fill the irrigating syringe with warm water, expelling air; place the syringe tip into the canal; and direct a stream of water upward, not toward, the tympanic membrane. After irrigating the canal with 60 ml of water, examine the canal and the returned solution for the presence of the foreign object.
3. If the object CAN be visualized, retract the pinna superiorly and posteriorly with your nondominant hand, gently insert the curette or spoon along the canal until the object is grasped, and remove the object.
4. If a live insect is visualized, you should kill or immobilize it before you attempt to remove it. Place a chemical agent in the ear and wait for the insect to stop wiggling. Microscope oil kills the insects in about 45 seconds; lidocaine takes a bit longer.
5. Prescribe antibiotic ear drops if any injury has occurred to the canal.

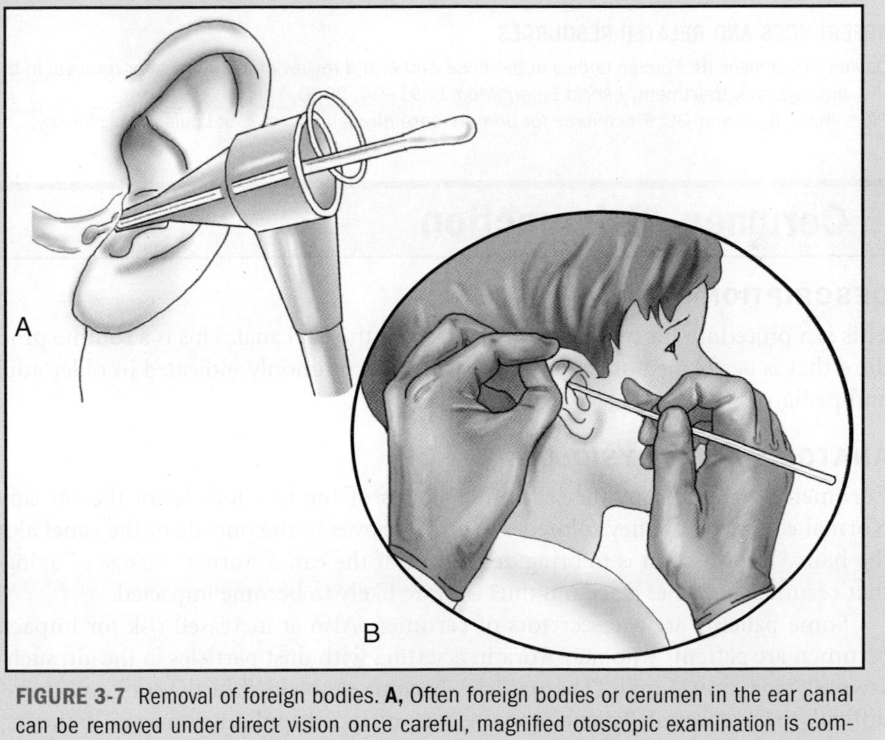

FIGURE 3-7 Removal of foreign bodies. **A,** Often foreign bodies or cerumen in the ear canal can be removed under direct vision once careful, magnified otoscopic examination is completed. **B,** Notice how the patient's head is supported and the practitioner's hand rests on the face.

PATIENT EDUCATION POSTPROCEDURE

- Keep small objects out of reach of young children.
- Educate children to not put objects into their ear, but that, if it happens again, to tell you or another adult immediately.
- Notify the practitioner if there is any hearing loss or bleeding, continued pain, or discharge from the ear.

COMPLICATIONS

- Local pain

PRACTITIONER FOLLOW-UP

The patient should be seen for follow-up if one of the following should occur:

- Bleeding
- Discharge
- Continuous ear pain
- Loss of hearing

CPT BILLING

If a patient comes in for a procedure only, there is no E/M code charge. The charge for the office visit is the procedure itself.

69200—Removal foreign body from external auditory canal; without general anesthesia

REFERENCES AND RELATED RESOURCES

Davies PH, Benger JR: Foreign bodies in the nose and ear: a review of techniques for removal in the emergency department, *J Accid Emerg Med* 17:91–94, 2000.

Pfenninger JL, Fowler GC: *Procedures for primary care physicians*, ed 3, St Louis, 2011, Mosby.

Cerumen Disimpaction

DESCRIPTION

This is a procedure for removing cerumen from the ear canal. This is a routine procedure that is performed on an elective basis. It is commonly indicated in older adults and pediatric patients.

ANATOMY AND PHYSIOLOGY

Cerumen is produced by the sebaceous glands of the hair follicles of the ear canal. Normal cerumen is honey colored. Cerumen moves to the outside of the canal along the hairs. The function is to bring debris out of the ear. A normal change of aging is that cerumen becomes drier and thus is more likely to become impacted.

Some patients are oversecretors of cerumen. Also at increased risk for impacted cerumen are patients who may work in a setting with dust particles in the air, such as sawmills and cotton mills. The particles become embedded in the wax and make it difficult to be removed. Patients who use cotton-tipped applicators may push the cerumen back into the canal and up against the tympanic membrane.

INDICATIONS

- If an ear canal is obstructed by cerumen and infection is not suspected, irrigation is warranted.

- Removal is frequently required to allow visualization of the tympanic membrane in a child.
- Dizziness, pressure sensation, pain, or tinnitus is present.
- Auditory acuity can be enhanced.
- Frequently both ears are involved, although the patient may have more symptoms involved with one ear.

CONTRAINDICATIONS

- Integrity of the tympanic membrane is in doubt
- Suspected tympanic membrane perforation
- History of recent middle ear surgery
- Myringotomy
- Drainage from ear
- History of recurrent middle ear infections

PRECAUTIONS

- Use gentle pressure to avoid accidental tympanic membrane perforation.
- Discontinue the procedure if the patient complains of discomfort, as a precaution against an unrecognized perforation.
- Have irrigation solution at room temperature to prevent caloric stimulation.
- Aim irrigating stream at the superior wall of the ear canal to avoid compaction of the plug against the tympanic membrane.
- Use an otoscope, cerumen spoon, or curette with caution in a child or older adult who has dementia because they may resist the procedure, to avoid damage to the ear canal or tympanic membrane if the patient struggles.
- Use of a soft immobilization device fashioned from sheets is less labor intensive and often safer than complete manual restraint.
- In the older child, restraint may require one person assigned to each limb and a fifth to control the head.
- Refer to specialist in the following situations:
  - Integrity of tympanic membrane is in doubt.
  - Wax cannot be removed after two separate attempts.

ASSESSMENT

- Assess patient for history of inserting objects in ear canal, stuffed-up ears, foreign body sensation, pain, itching, decreased hearing, tinnitus, dizziness, and/or pressure sensation.
- Physical examination of the ear canal with an otoscope may show thick, dry, dark-brown cerumen that obstructs the view of the tympanic membrane. The cerumen may be visible at the entrance of the ear canal without use of the otoscope.

PATIENT PREPARATION

- An informed consent form is not necessary.
- Warn the patient that the tympanic membrane may sometimes be injured.
- The patient should alert the practitioner during the procedure if pain or discomfort occurs.
- The patient will have to assist in the procedure by holding the basin under the ear.
- Advise the patient that he or she may feel pressure, dizziness, or vertigo during the procedure.

- If possible, the patient should use wax-softening ear drops for 3 to 5 days before the procedure OR
- Place wax-softening ear drops in ears and wait 10 to 15 minutes before starting the procedure. Alternatively, use a few drops (0.25 ml) of docusate sodium (Colace) syrup in the affected ear. This stool softener will soften the cerumen enough for irrigation in about 15 minutes. (It is also bright red, so remember to warn the patient that any postprocedure fluid that drains out may be red.)

TREATMENT ALTERNATIVES

- *Cerumen spoon:* May be effective for small amounts of cerumen; there is a greater risk of injury. This is commonly used when there is a need to visualize the tympanic membrane to evaluate for infection.
- Ear candles are ineffective and are not recommended.

EQUIPMENT

SYRINGE IRRIGATION

- Otoscope
- Irrigating apparatus
  - Ear syringe *OR*
  - A 20- to 60-ml syringe with a piece of 1-cm rubber tubing; the tubing from a butterfly needle (with needle cut off) is effective
- Irrigation solution: 1:1 mixture of warm water/hydrogen peroxide
- Emesis or ear basin
- Container for irrigating solution (an emesis basin or a specimen cup)
- Protective drapes or towels

CERUMEN SPOON

- Otoscope
- Cerumen spoon
- Debrox or Cerumenex, olive oil, mineral oil, or hydrogen peroxide (optional)

3

Procedure

SYRINGE IRRIGATION

1. Position and drape the patient, preferably sitting upright. Have the patient hold the emesis basin under the ear. Put drapes on the patient's shoulder and neck (Figure 3-8).
2. Fill the syringe with body-temperature solution.
3. Retract the pinna posteriorly and superiorly with your nondominant hand. For children, retract the pinna anteriorly and superiorly.
4. Place the syringe tip at the canal opening without occluding the canal.
5. Direct a gentle flow of solution toward the superior wall of the ear canal (see Figure 3-7, *A*).

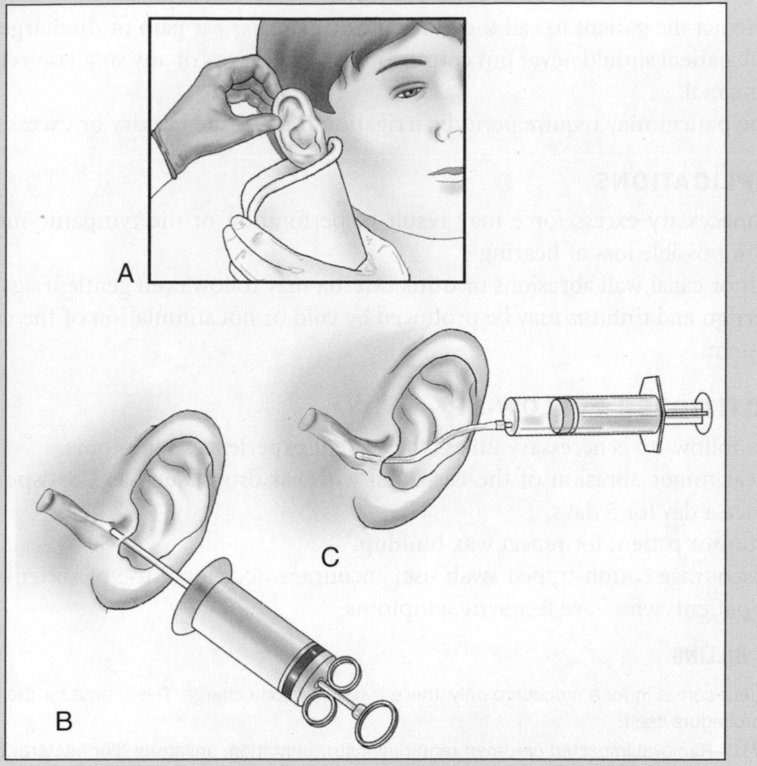

FIGURE 3-8 Procedure for removing cerumen. **A,** Basin cup that fits under ear. **B,** Typical commercial ear canal irrigation setup. The initial stream should be directed toward the superior canal. Cover the upper torso with a splash bib. **C,** Alternative irrigation setup, with butterfly tubing, with needle and butterfly removed.

6. Irrigate each ear two or three times with full syringes, observing the draining liquid for cerumen.
7. Inspect the ears with the otoscope. If wax remains, repeat step 6.
8. If the cerumen is not removed, send the patient home to use liquid earwax softener (such as Cerumenex drops or olive oil) twice a day for 4 or 5 days, and then return for repeat irrigation.
9. Inspect the canal after the procedure to ensure that there is no remaining wax and the ear canal is not abraded.

CERUMEN SPOON

1. Position the patient, preferably sitting upright.
2. Retract the pinna posteriorly and superiorly with your nondominant hand. For children, retract the pinna anteriorly and superiorly.
3. Visualize the cerumen with the otoscope.
4. Either work through the otoscope or by direct vision (see Figures 3-6 and 3-7). Remove the cerumen carefully, avoiding injury to the wall of the canal.
5. If the wax is hard, install Debrox or Cerumenex, mineral oil, or half-strength hydrogen peroxide and wait 10 to 15 minutes before repeating the procedure.
6. Inspect the canal after the procedure to assess for injury to the canal.

3

PATIENT EDUCATION POSTPROCEDURE

- Instruct the patient to call the office if he or she has ear pain or discharge.
- The patient should never put cotton-tipped applicators or any small object into the ear canal.
- The patient may require periodic irrigation if he or she has dry or excess wax.

COMPLICATIONS

- Unnecessary excess force may result in perforation of the tympanic membrane with possible loss of hearing.
- Minor canal wall abrasions or otitis externa may follow even gentle irrigation.
- Vertigo and tinnitus may be produced by cold or hot stimulation of the vestibular system.

PRACTITIONER FOLLOW-UP

- No follow-up is necessary unless the patient experiences symptoms.
- Treat minor abrasion of the ear canal with ear drops, such as Cortisporin Otic, twice a day for 5 days.
- Monitor patient for repeat wax buildup.
- Discourage cotton-tipped swab use; encourage occasional use of softening drops in patients who have frequent symptoms.

3

■ CPT BILLING

If a patient comes in for a procedure only, there is no E/M code charge. The charge for the office visit is the procedure itself.

- **69210**—Removal impacted cerumen requiring instrumentation, unilateral (For bilateral procedure, report 69210 with modifier 50).
- Removing wax that is not impacted does not warrant the reporting of CPT code 69210. Rather, that work would appropriately be captured by an E/M code regardless of how it is removed. If, however, the wax is truly impacted, then its removal should be reported with 69210 if performed by a clinician using at minimum an otoscope and an instrument such as a cerumen spoon.
- If any one or more of the following are present, cerumen should be considered impacted clinically:
    - Cerumen impairs examination of clinically significant portions of the external auditory canal, tympanic membrane, or middle ear condition.
    - Extremely hard, dry, irritative cerumen causing symptoms such as pain, itching, hearing loss, etc.
    - Associated with foul odor, infection, or dermatitis.
    - Obstructive, copious cerumen that cannot be removed without magnification and multiple instrumentations requiring clinician skills.

REFERENCES AND RELATED RESOURCES

Clegg AJ, Loveman E, Gospodarevskaya E, et al: The safety and effectiveness of different methods of ear wax removal: a systematic review and economic evaluation, *Health Technol Assess* 14(28):1–192, 2010.

New England Journal of Medicine video on removal of cerumen: [Video]. http://www.nejm.org/doi/full/10.1056/NEJMvcm0904397. May 20, 2010. Accessed May 28, 2015.

Tympanometry

DESCRIPTION

Testing of the mobility of the tympanic membrane is an indirect measure of the pressure within the middle ear.

ANATOMY AND PHYSIOLOGY

Increased pressure may represent infection or fluid associated with otitis media or serous otitis media. Tympanometry may also indicate the degree of pressure in the middle ear, eustachian tube dysfunction, or the cause of a developmental delay in hearing or speaking.

INDICATIONS

- Determine the degree of mobility of the tympanic membrane.
- Evaluate hearing loss and middle ear function.
- Evaluate the cause of ear pain.
- Make a diagnosis of or monitor recovery in middle ear infections and effusions or tympanic membrane perforations.
- Determine the effectiveness of pressure-equalization tubes in children.
- Evaluate the cause of developmental delays in hearing or speaking in children.

CONTRAINDICATIONS

- Children younger than 5 months
- Otitis externa
- Obstruction of the ear canal with cerumen or foreign body

PRECAUTIONS

Younger children may require restraints during the procedure.

ASSESSMENT

- Perform focused head, eyes, ears, nose, and throat (HEENT) examination.
- Evaluate for subauricular, postauricular, and occipital lymphadenopathy.
- Assess sinuses, nose, mouth, and throat for evidence of infection.
- Palpate tragus and pinna of ear to evaluate for otitis externa.
- Evaluate ear canal to rule out infection, effusions, or obstruction by cerumen.

PATIENT PREPARATION

- Infants and younger children may require restraints for tympanometry to be accurate.
- Provide clear instructions about what will and will not happen during the procedure. Reassure children in particular that this procedure should not hurt.

TREATMENT ALTERNATIVES

Refer patient to ear, nose, and throat specialist.

EQUIPMENT

- The tympanometry tool should have ear tips of various sizes that provide a tight seal over the external canal opening, with an air pressure range of −400 decapascals (dPa) to +200 dPa (1.02 mm H_2O = 1.0 dPa). The probe should have a 226-Hz probe tone. The best equipment has large buttons and an easy-to-read numbering system. Some systems also have a portable printer that records the scores as documentation of the results.

3

Procedure

1. Adjust and calibrate the tympanometer according to the manufacturer's instructions. Machine settings may need to be modified if altitude is above 1280 ft. Each instruction manual has a table that provides the adjustments that are required for higher elevations (Figure 3-9).
2. Have the patient sit in a comfortable position, with the ear at a comfortable height for the examiner.
3. Give directions to the patient about how to respond when he or she hears the tone.
4. Experiment until you find the ear tip that provides the best seal of the external canal and then activate the machine.
5. Grasp the pinna carefully and pull up and back (for adults) or back (for children) to make a tighter seal. Then apply the probe to the external canal. The machine reading will indicate when there is a good seal and the test switch can be turned on.
6. Follow the instructions in the instrument manual for full testing of each ear.
7. Record the readings (as directed in the instruction manual) and print out the readings if the machine includes a printer, or directly input into the electronic medical record.
8. A normal tympanogram provides a symmetric increase and decrease in tracing: recording to about 1.0 Ya-mm h (Figure 3-10).

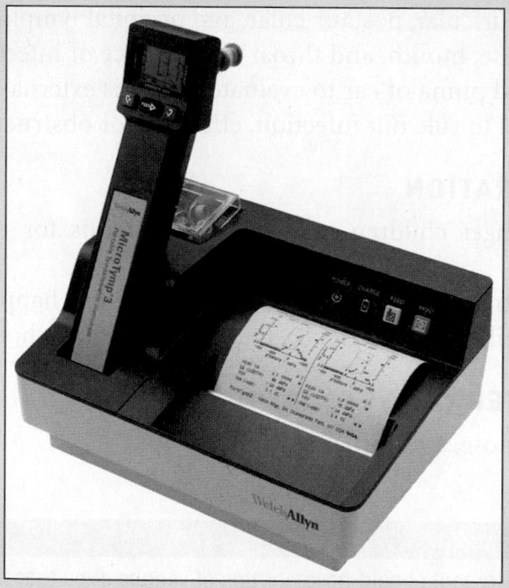

FIGURE 3-9 Portable tympanometric instrument. (Courtesy of Welch Allyn, Inc.)

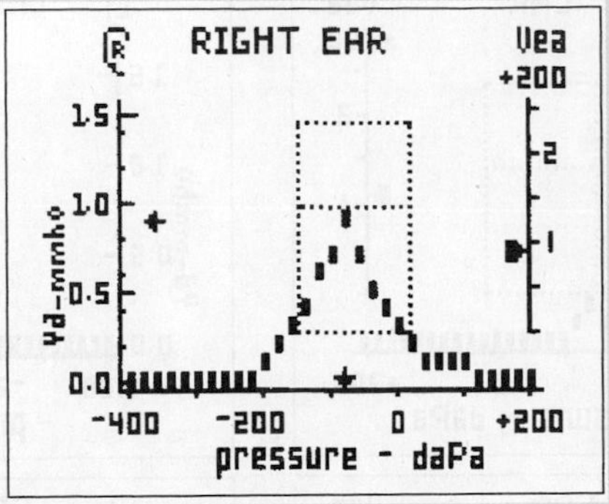

A

Tympanometric Measurement	Child's Ear (Under Age 10) 90% Range	Adult's Ear (Over Age 10) 90% Range
Peak Ya	0.2 to 0.9 mmho	0.3 to 1.4 mmho
Gradient (GR) (Tympanometric Width)	60 to 150 daPa	50 to 110 daPa
Tympanometric Peak Pressure (TPP)	-139 to +11 daPa	-83 to 0 daPa
Equivalent Ear Canal Volume (Vea)	0.4 to 1.0 cc	0.6 to 1.5 cc

B

FIGURE 3-10 Common tympanometric patterns. **A,** Tympanogram for a normal ear. **B,** Normative tympanometric data. (Courtesy of Welch Allyn, Inc.)

3

PATIENT EDUCATION POSTPROCEDURE

- Discuss the findings with the patient or family (Figures 3-10 and 3-11).
- Provide relevant follow-up, referral, or advice.
- Consider genetics referral for children who have suspected congenital hearing loss.

COMPLICATIONS

There are none.

PRACTITIONER FOLLOW-UP

Repeat testing may be required in a patient who is unable to cooperate if results are inconclusive or if the condition is expected to change.

Abnormal results require a formal referral for a formal audiology assessment.

Many children who have hearing loss do not receive follow-up care and suffer complications of hearing loss; maintain close follow-up of children who have abnormal results.

■ CPT BILLING

If a patient comes in for a procedure only, there is no E/M code charge. The charge for the office visit is the procedure itself.

92567—Tympanometry (impedance testing); both ears. Use modifier 52 if test is applied to one ear instead of two ears.

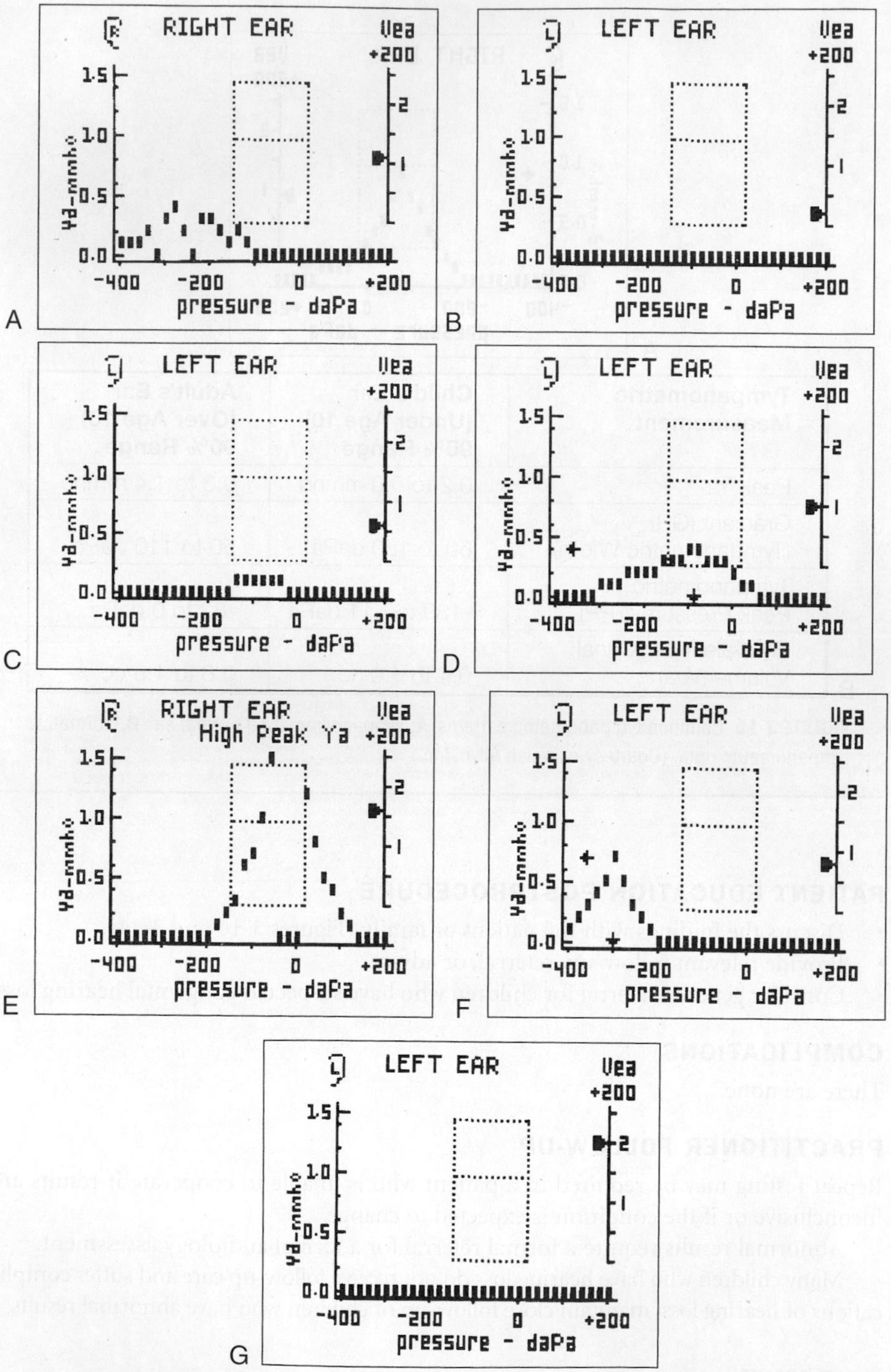

FIGURE 3-11 Common abnormal ear tympanometric patterns. **A,** Too much artifact. **B,** Ear canal occlusion. **C,** Otitis media with effusion (low peak Ya). **D,** Otitis media with effusion (tympanogram too wide). **E,** Tympanic membrane abnormalities or ossicular disruption (high static admittance). **F,** Negative middle ear pressure. **G,** Patent tympanotomy tube or perforated tympanic membrane (flat tympanogram with volume that is too high). (Courtesy of Welch Allyn, Inc.)

REFERENCES AND RELATED RESOURCES

Engel J, et al: Otoscopic findings in relation to tympanometry during infancy, *Eur Arch Otorhinolaryngol* 257:3366, 2000.

Green LA, et al: Tympanometry interpretation by primary care physicians: a report from the International Primary Care Network (IPCN) and the Ambulatory Sentinel Practice Network (ASPN), *J Fam Pract* 49:932, 2000.

Johansen EC, et al: Tympanometry for diagnosis and treatment of otitis media in general practice, *J Fam Pract* 17:317, 2000.

Joint Committee on Infant Hearing: Year 2007 Position Statement: principles and guidelines for early hearing detection and intervention programs, *Pediatrics* 120(4):898–921, 2007.

Audiometry

DESCRIPTION

Primary care providers may obtain baseline audiometry readings, which provide an objective method for the diagnosis of hearing loss. This test may be used to confirm suspicions that a hearing loss exists before referral to a specialist.

ANATOMY AND PHYSIOLOGY

Approximately 1 in 15 Americans has some degree of hearing loss, with the incidence increasing with age. Although some infants are born with hearing loss, most people do not experience deficits in hearing until after age 55. Exposure to sustained loud noises or explosions contributes to acoustic nerve damage. Some drugs have ototoxic adverse effects that damage hearing. Smoking and allergies also may exacerbate the problems of hearing loss.

Hearing loss is more likely to develop in children after prenatal infections of the mother with organisms that cause cytomegalovirus, human immunodeficiency virus, herpes, rubella, or syphilis. Maternal drug or alcohol use also may be correlated with infant hearing loss. Newborn jaundice, meningitis, head trauma, and low birth weight are additional factors associated with infant hearing loss.

INDICATIONS

- Evaluation of suspected hearing loss
- Complaints of tinnitus or exposure to loud noises
- Evaluation for pathology in children who have speech and language development delays, behavior problems, poor academic progress, and/or difficulties in interpersonal skills
- Unexplained behavior changes in the older adult that are suggestive of dementia.

CONTRAINDICATIONS

- Children younger than 6 months (inaccurate readings)
- Active otitis external infection
- Cerumen impaction

PRECAUTIONS

- Explain the procedure clearly to the patient and family.
- The test must take place in a room isolated from other loud or disturbing noises.

ASSESSMENT

- Perform a thorough ear assessment examination by palpating the external ear, and then viewing the ear canal and tympanic membrane with an otoscope with a good light.
- Make certain that there is no infection, evidence of recent trauma, or cerumen present in either ear canal. If cerumen is present, it should be removed before the testing.

PATIENT PREPARATION

- Patient should be in a comfortable position.
- Explain clearly how you wish the patient to respond to the sound that he or she will hear. For example, "Raise your hand when you hear the sound."
- Reassure the patient that this is an important and painless procedure.

TREATMENT ALTERNATIVES

If a quiet environment cannot be provided or if the patient seems confused or restless or is unable to cooperate, evaluation and testing by a trained audiologist may be necessary.

EQUIPMENT

- Choose one of a variety of hand-held models, earphone, or earplug models of audiometry tools, complete with external canal probe and ear pieces in a variety of sizes, to ensure a good seal over the external canal opening. The tool should be capable of producing frequencies between 500 and 4000 Hz.
- Use a special soundproof room, if possible.

Procedure

For use with hand-held model (Figure 3-12):

1. Select the appropriate-size ear probe, insert and check for good seal of external canal.
2. Activate the probe.
3. Grasp the pinna and pull up and back (for adults) or back (for children) to help obtain a good seal.

For use with earphone or earplug model:

1. Cover the entire concha with the equipment so that there is a good seal.
2. Follow the directions carefully in the instrument instruction manual for the testing protocol as to time, sequence, and process.
3. Record the results carefully as they are obtained.
4. Using the instruction manual, interpret results to determine whether hearing is within the normal hearing screening range.
5. If the results are not within the normal range, the test is usually repeated before referral is made to an audiologist for further testing.

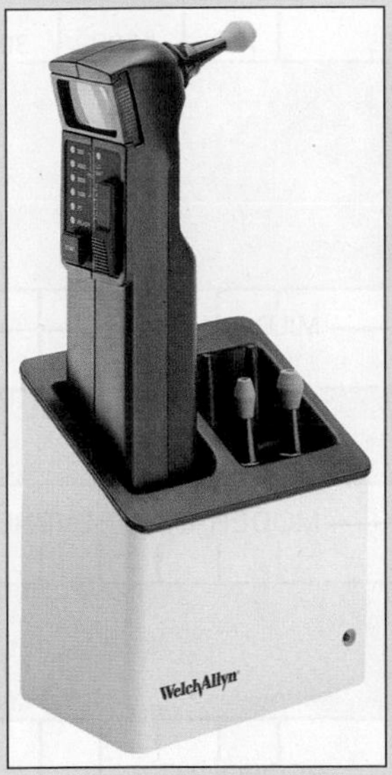

FIGURE 3-12 Sample audiometry equipment–the AudioScope 3. (Courtesy of Welch Allyn, Inc.)

PATIENT EDUCATION POSTPROCEDURE

- The results should be reviewed with the patient or family (Figure 3-13).
- Items to discuss may include possible causes of hearing loss, use of protective ear plugs when around loud noises, elimination of exposure to cigarette smoke, and treatment of allergies.
- It is important to explain the importance of following up with a certified audiologist for more extensive testing and treatment.

COMPLICATIONS

There are none.

PRACTITIONER FOLLOW-UP

Audiometric testing may be performed several times to determine a consistent hearing loss.

Referral for formal audiology evaluation is warranted for patients who have abnormal results.

■ CPT BILLING

If a patient comes in for a procedure only, there is no E/M code charge. The charge for the office visit is the procedure itself. The audiometric tests require the use of calibrated electronic equipment, recording of results, and a report with interpretation. Hearing tests, such as whispered voice or tuning fork, are considered part of E/M services and are not reported separately.

92551–Screening test, pure tone, air only ■ **92552**–Pure tone audiometry (threshold, air only) ■ **92553**–Pure tone audiometry (threshold, air and bone)

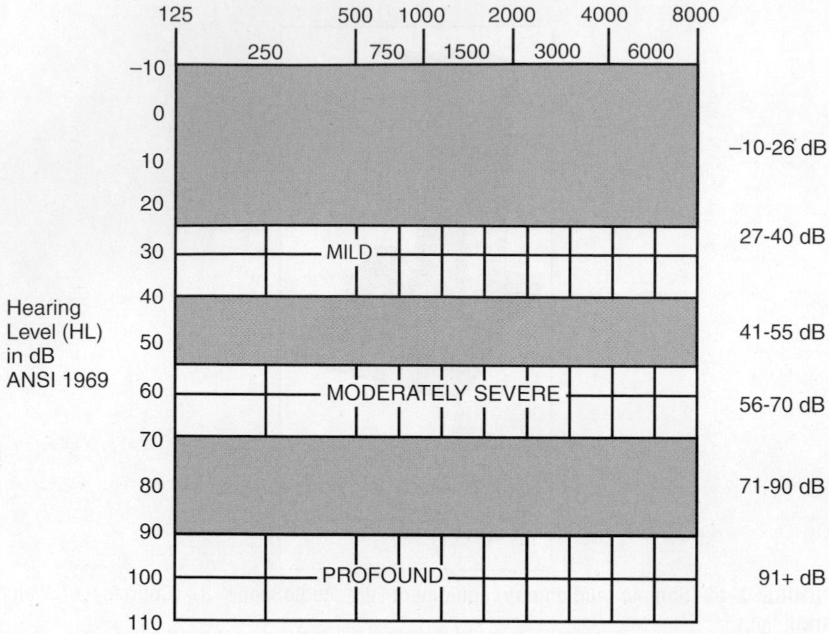

FIGURE 3-13 Normal hearing screening range. (Courtesy of Welch Allyn, Inc.)

REFERENCES AND RELATED RESOURCES

Bagai A, Thavendiranathan P, Detsky AS: Does this patient have hearing impairment? *JAMA* 295(4):416–428, 2006.

Chou R, et al: Screening adults aged 50 years or older for hearing loss: a review of the evidence for the U.S. Preventive Services Task Force, *Ann Intern Med* 154(5):347–355, 2007.

Stone KA, et al: Universal newborn hearing screening, *J Fam Pract* 49:1012, 2000.

Uy J, Forciea MA: Hearing loss, *Ann Intern Med* 158:ITC4-1, 2013.

Video of Normal anatomy of the Middle ear: [Video.] http://www.nlm.nih.gov/medlineplus/ency/anatomyvideos/000063.htm. November 11, 2010. Accessed May 28, 2015.

NOSE PROCEDURES

DESCRIPTION

Epistaxis and removal of a foreign body in the nose are procedures that often begin as primary care problems. Both of these problems may require the intervention of an ear, nose, and throat specialist if the situation is not corrected after an initial attempt at resolution.

ANATOMY AND PHYSIOLOGY

The upper third of the nose is supported by bone, and the lower two thirds is supported by cartilage. Air is channeled through the nasal cavity and anterior nares, then into the vestibule, and on through the nasal passage to the nasopharynx. The nasal septum is the medial wall of each nasal cavity; it is supported by both bone and cartilage and is covered by a mucous membrane with a rich blood supply. The vestibule is unique in that it is covered with hair-bearing skin, but not mucosa.

Laterally, the turbinates are visualized as curving bony structures covered by a highly vascular mucous membrane. A groove, or meatus, lies just beneath each of the turbinates, into which the nasolacrimal duct or paranasal sinuses empty (Figure 3-14).

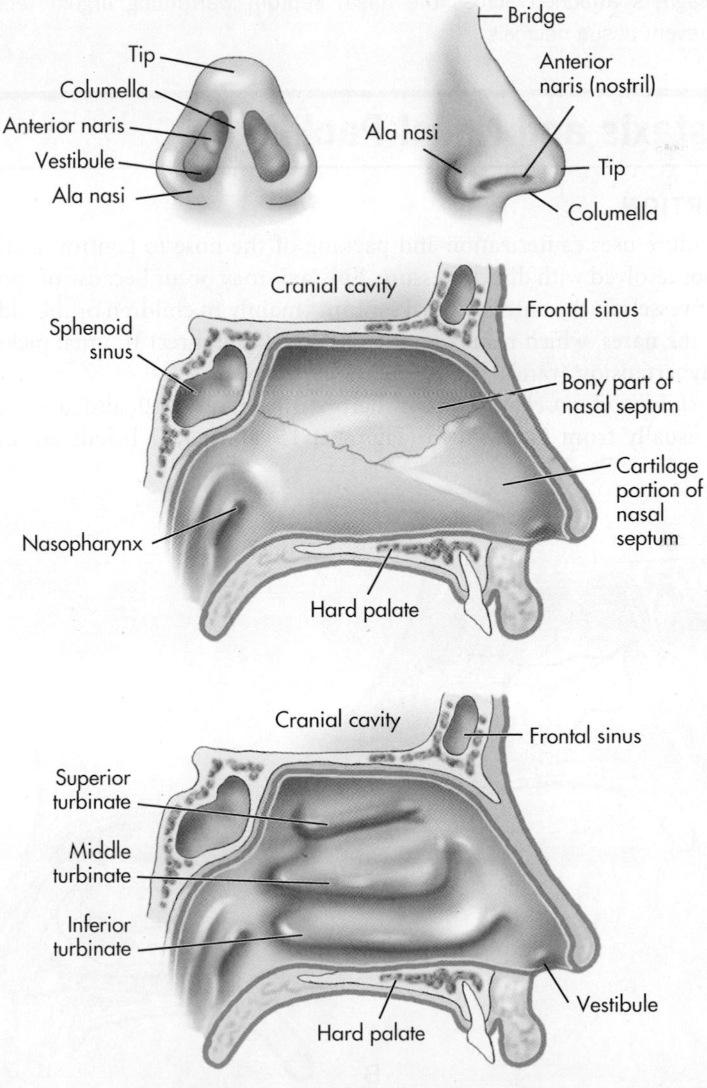

FIGURE 3-14 Anatomy of the nose and nasal cavity.

3

RED FLAGS

Nasal procedure concerns that warrant emergency evaluation or emergent ear, nose, and throat (ENT) consult:

- Epistaxis in any patient who has hemodynamic instability
- Posterior epistaxis, especially in adults managed with antiplatelet therapy
- Recurrent bleeding, which has been difficult to control
- Epistaxis lasting more than 1 hour
- Epistaxis that continues after packing has been placed
- Patients who require bilateral nasal packing
- Children who have button batteries inserted in their nose because significant tissue damage can occur in a short time period
- Magnets attached across the nasal septum warranting urgent removal to prevent tissue necrosis

Epistaxis and Nasal Packing

DESCRIPTION

This procedure uses cauterization and packing of the nose to control nasal bleeding that has not resolved with direct pressure. Epistaxis may occur because of spontaneous rupture of vessels in the anterior nasal septum (mainly in children or the older adult); drying of the nares, which results in mucosal cracking; direct trauma; picking of the nostrils; hypertension (rarely); and hematologic causes.

Most *childhood nosebleeds* occur before the age of 10 and are anterior in location, usually from Little's area (Figure 3-15). Posterior bleeds are unusual in

3

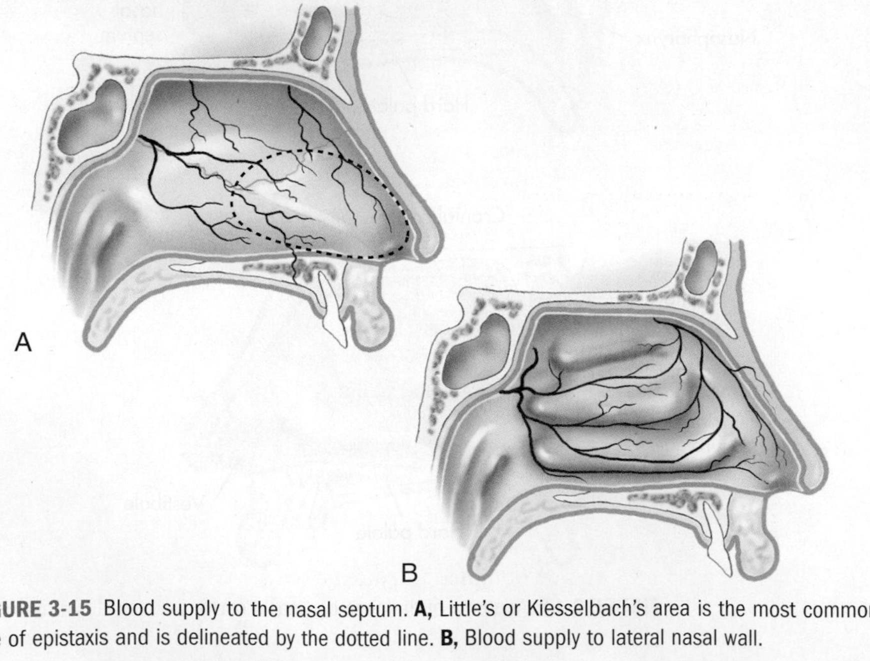

FIGURE 3-15 Blood supply to the nasal septum. **A,** Little's or Kiesselbach's area is the most common site of epistaxis and is delineated by the dotted line. **B,** Blood supply to lateral nasal wall.

children. They are more common in adults and are signaled by an inability to identify the bleeding site and the continued oozing of blood into the pharynx, despite treatment.

Trauma is the most frequent cause of nosebleeds in children. Digital trauma from the patient's finger is the most common source. Repeated local trauma causes an inflammatory response, and subsequent granulation tissue can be "picked off," causing the bleeding to occur. Nasal *foreign bodies* can also traumatize the nasal mucosa.

Breathing *dry air* is a major predisposing factor to nosebleeds. In addition, a *deviated nasal septum* may cause the nasal cavity on one side to be relatively narrowed; air passes through the narrowed side at a greater velocity, predisposing that side to nosebleeds.

Repeated *infection* and *allergic rhinitis* in childhood are also associated with nosebleeds. Repeated forceful *nose blowing* can rupture the septal venous vessels. Viral or bacterial *rhinitis* is also associated with increased vascularity of the inflamed nasal septum.

ANATOMY AND PHYSIOLOGY

In up to 90% of cases, epistaxis originates in the anterior septum in the rich vascular plexus known as Kiesselbach's plexus or Little's area. Kiesselbach's plexus is composed of the terminal septal branches of the anterior and posterior ethmoid arteries, the superior labial artery (via the external facial artery), and the sphenopalatine artery (see Figure 3-15).

INDICATIONS

This procedure is performed to control nasal hemorrhage that has not been alleviated with firm pressure, in the correct location, immediately distal to the bony portion of the septum for at least 10 to 15 minutes continuously.

CONTRAINDICATIONS

- Practitioners should use these procedures carefully if granulocytopenia is present. The relative severity of the hemorrhage needs to be weighed against the risk of a life-threatening infection.
- Practitioners should not attempt these procedures in the presence of known or suspected cribriform fracture or necrosis of the septum.
- Severe epistaxis is not a simple event. The practitioner should have the proper equipment readily available in case the patient has syncope or goes into shock, cardiac arrest, or pulmonary distress. Epinephrine and ephedrine should be used with caution or not at all in patients who have severe hypertension. Unless shock is present, epistaxis should not be treated with the patient in a supine position.
- The partial pressure of oxygen in the blood often decreases 10 mm Hg with packing in the nose because of nasopulmonary reflexes. This decrease, in conjunction with hypovolemia, hypertension, and preexisting pulmonary disease, can precipitate a stroke or a myocardial infarction in susceptible individuals. Therefore an electrocardiogram should be obtained in patients older than 40 years, and referral for workup should be made in patients who have pulmonary, renal, or cardiac disease.

PRECAUTIONS

- Posterior bleeding is unusual in children, but should be suspected when a bleeding site cannot be visualized and an anterior pack fails to control the bleeding. Posterior bleeding should be managed by an otolaryngologist in the hospital, where ligation or embolization of the vessel may be performed.
- If bilateral anterior packs are indicated, the patient will have to be referred to an otolaryngologist for possible hospital admission.

ASSESSMENT

- Obtain a complete history of current medications (especially antiplatelets and anticoagulants); circumstance leading to epistaxis, specifically if event occurred spontaneously or by any injury or trauma; and vital signs, especially blood pressure and heart rate.
- Perform an external examination of the nose and assess adequacy of patient airway.
- Attempt to visualize the turbinates and septum of both nares.
- Identify the source of the bleeding.

PATIENT PREPARATION

- The patient or the practitioner should maintain constant pressure on the nose by pinching it between the thumb and first finger as close to the facial bones as possible (Figure 3-16).
- The practitioners must provide reassurance to the patient throughout the entire procedure, making sure to explain each step to the patient before carrying out the packing.
- Also, the patient must be made aware that nosebleeds, although messy and upsetting, are rarely life-threatening.

3

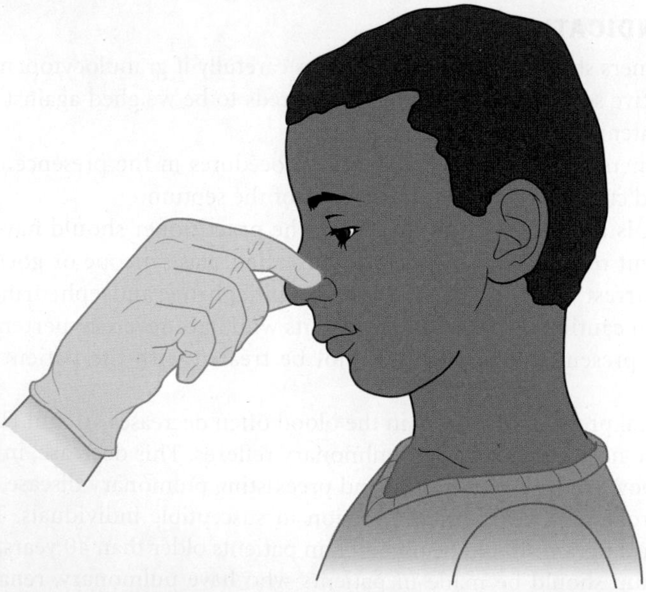

FIGURE 3-16 Direct pressure to control epistaxis. Pinch the nose to stop the bleeding.

- Practitioners should make sure the patient knows that bleeding will be controlled at the end of the procedure.
- It is important to explain that the nostril will feel full and that it will not be easy to breathe through it.
- It is also important to explain that some pressure may be felt during cauterization, but that pain should not be felt if the mucosa is properly anesthetized.

While applying direct pressure to stop bleeding, practitioners might use the time to obtain additional and important information, such as:

- The patient's general physical condition, the amount of blood lost, and the possibility of a coagulopathy. Previous bleeding episodes and methods of control should be explored. A history of trauma, surgery, allergy, recent upper respiratory infection, or a foreign body should be elicited.
- Note the patient's vital signs. Orthostatic hypotension is an important clue to moderate to severe volume loss. In children, an increase in heart rate of 10% to 15% is indicative of significant volume loss.
- Inspect the patient for signs of hemorrhagic disease (e.g., ecchymoses, petechiae, organomegaly, and telangiectasia).

TREATMENT ALTERNATIVES

- Some forms of mild repetitive bleeding can be handled with direct pressure, electrical or silver nitrate stick cautery, application of vasoconstrictors, packing with thrombin, or nasal packing.
- More significant bleeding that does not respond to packing should be referred to an ear, nose, and throat specialist.

3

EQUIPMENT

- Light source, preferably a head lamp
- Nasal speculum (Figure 3-17)
- Suction apparatus, including Fraser tips No. 5 to No. 8, 8 to 10 French suction catheter
- Cautery unit or silver nitrate sticks (optional)
- Topical thrombin or other topical coagulant (optional)
- Topical vasoconstrictor, such as epinephrine 1:1000 or phenylephrine 0.125% to 0.5%
- Expandable nasal sponges or petrolatum gauze packing
- Bayonet forceps
- Kidney basin

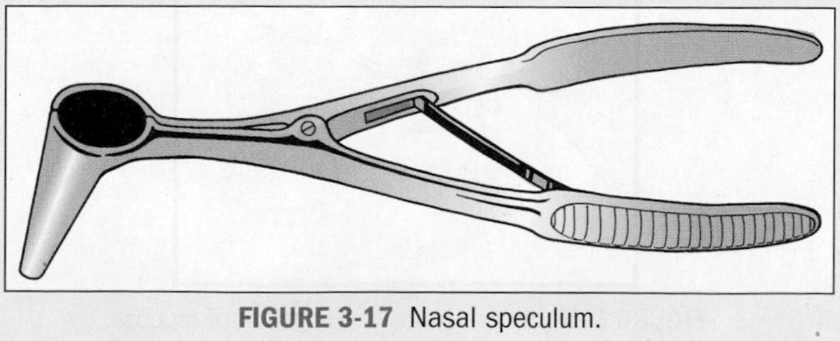

FIGURE 3-17 Nasal speculum.

Procedure

1. Attempt cauterization of the bleeding site, if visualized, first. If the site is unsuitable for cauterization or if cauterization fails to control the bleeding, perform tamponade of the bleeding area with gauze.
2. Identify the specific site of bleeding. *This is the key to success.*
3. The patient should be seated, leaning forward slightly; he or she should not tip his or her head back.
4. Before the examination, have the patient blow his or her nose to clear the nasal passages of blood clots. Suction will serve the same purpose in an uncooperative child.
5. After the removal of clots and blood, place the nasal speculum into the nares and inspect the nasal cavity for a bleeding source. Begin with the nares from which the blood first originated. Inspect the nasal cavity from anterior to posterior. Use the headlamp for better visualization.
6. To control bleeding, if pressure is not successful, try packing the nose with topical thrombin, followed by 10 minutes of firm and constant pressure, by squeezing the anterior cartilage of the nose between the thumb and index finger. This technique is safer and technically simpler than using silver nitrate sticks. Ice applied to the bridge of the nose may also help with vasoconstriction.
7. If the bleeding is still not controlled, topical application of a vasoconstrictor, such as Neo-Synephrine (phenylephrine) or epinephrine with a cotton pledget for 5 to 10 minutes is often effective. *Caution:* Although only minimal volumes of these drugs are necessary, care should be taken to anticipate and treat any untoward effects from systemic absorption.
8. Cauterization is most appropriate for visualized, anterior, oozing epistaxis that continues after conservative management. If you decide to cauterize, use silver nitrate sticks to touch the area around the bleeding site for 5 to 10 minutes. Work in concentric circles, starting away from the bleeding site. The mucosa may turn gray to black. *Note:* You cannot cauterize an actively bleeding site with silver nitrate. More vasoconstricting agents may be required to stop the bleeding (Figure 3-18).
9. If bleeding persists, proceed with nasal packing. Nasal sponges are now available for this purpose. They are inserted dry and expand when wet. They can be cut to fit the nares in any child. Also, petroleum gauze packing may be used.

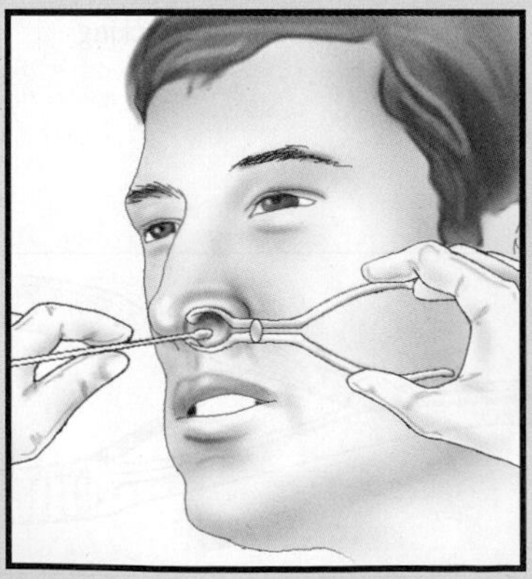

FIGURE 3-18 Silver nitrate cauterization of mucosa.

3

10. Insert the packing into the nose:
    a. Hold the nasal speculum in your nondominant hand and use your dominant hand to manipulate the bayonet forceps.
    b. Grasp the gauze strip with the bayonet forceps, forming a loop that leaves the end of the packing outside the nose (Figure 3-19, *A*). Pack the anterior nasal cavity from top to bottom by inserting successive loops of packing into the nose. Each loop should be placed under the previous loops in an accordion fashion and as far posteriorly as possible (Figure 3-19, *B*).
    c. Fill the nostril, but not too tightly, because excessive pressure may cause ischemic necrosis.
    d. When the nostril is fully packed, secure both ends of the nasal pack to the external cheek to prevent the ends from falling into the nasopharynx.
11. After packing is placed, the posterior oropharynx should be inspected for posterior bleeding. If present, consult ENT or the emergency department.
12. Packing can be removed in 2 to 4 days.

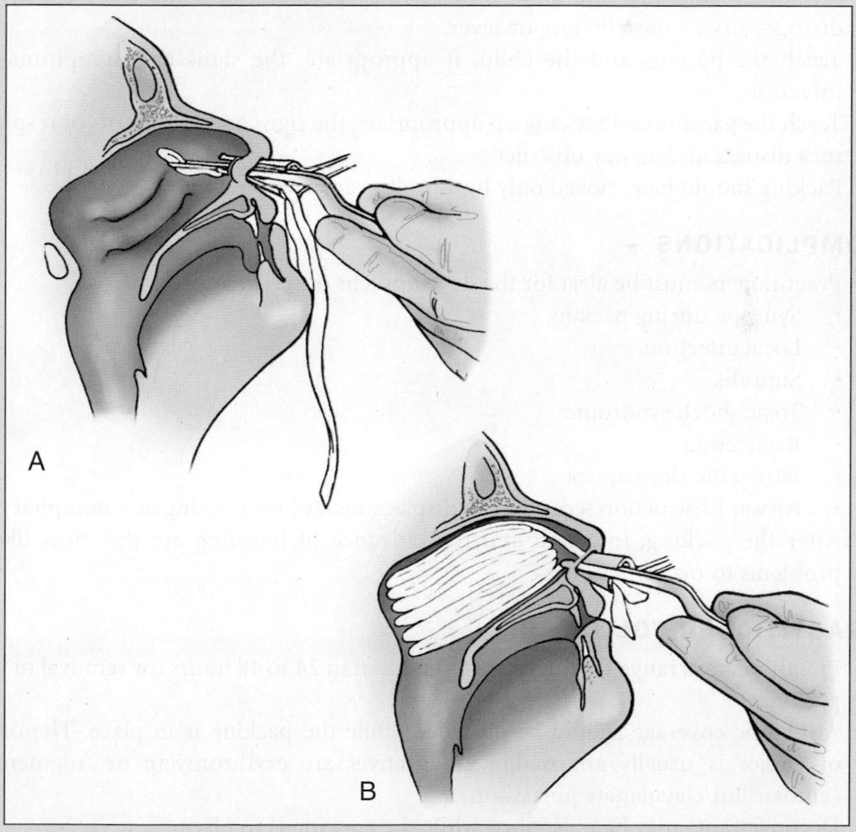

FIGURE 3-19 Nasal packing to control epistaxis. **A,** Insert anterior pack with folded end inserted first. **B,** Fold gauze pack in layers.

PATIENT EDUCATION POSTPROCEDURE

- The patient should not take aspirin or nonsteroidal antiinflammatory drugs for the next 3 to 4 days.
- The patient may take a decongestant or antihistamine for excessive mucus production.
- Instruct the patient to not blow his or her nose with the packing in the nostrils.
- Petroleum jelly should be applied to the nares daily for 4 to 5 days.
- Strenuous physical activity, bending, and sneezing should be avoided, if possible.
- Instruct the patient to follow-up with the health care provider if nosebleeds persist.
- Instruct the patient to place nothing in the nostrils.
- The patient should run a humidifier in the house during the winter months, especially at night.
- Instruct the patient to avoid the use of alcohol, which can increase the risk of rebleeding.
- If bleeding recurs, instruct the patient to apply pressure for 10 minutes while compressing the soft and bony parts of the nose.
- Instruct the patient to call the practitioner if unexplained bruises appear, if bleeding recurs and cannot be controlled by pressure, or if there is respiratory distress, airway obstruction, or fever.
- Teach the parents and the child, if appropriate, the signs and symptoms of infection.
- Teach the parents and the child, if appropriate, the signs and symptoms of respiratory distress and airway obstruction.
- Packing should be removed only by a health care provider.

COMPLICATIONS

- Practitioners must be alert for the development of the following:
  - Syncope during packing
  - Local infection
  - Sinusitis
  - Toxic shock syndrome
  - Bacteremia
  - Iatrogenic sleep apnea
  - Airway obstruction secondary to displacement of the packing into nasopharynx
- After the packing, infection and reoccurrence of bleeding are the most likely problems to occur.

PRACTITIONER FOLLOW-UP

- Practitioners arrange for the patient to be seen in 24 to 48 hours for removal of the packing.
- Antibiotic coverage should be provided while the packing is in place. The drug of choice is usually amoxicillin; alternatives are erythromycin or Augmentin (amoxicillin/clavulanate potassium).
- Decongestants may be prescribed while the packing is in place.
- Tylenol (acetaminophen) should be prescribed for discomfort.

■ CPT BILING

If a patient comes in for a procedure only, there is no E/M code charge. The charge for the office visit is the procedure itself.

30901–Control nasal hemorrhage, anterior, simple (limited cautery and/or packing any method)

■ **30902**–Control nasal hemorrhage, anterior, complex (extensive cautery and/or packing any method)

To report bilateral procedure, add modifier 50 to either procedure.

REFERENCES AND RELATED RESOURCES

Diamond L: Managing epistaxis, *J Am Acad Physician Assist* 27:35–39, 2014.

Pond F, Sizeland A: Epistaxis: strategies for management, *Aust Fam Physician* 29:933, 2000.

Schlosser R: Epistaxis, *N Engl J Med* 360:784–789, 2009.

Removal of a Foreign Body From the Nose

DESCRIPTION

This procedure describes the use of appropriate instrumentation and methods to extricate a foreign body that is positioned forward of the pharynx and can be visualized with a speculum. The extent of tissue reaction and bleeding that ensues are largely functions of the size, position, movement, and antigenicity of the foreign body. The only limits on the size and shape of nasal foreign bodies are the physical limits of the cavities into which they intrude.

Foreign bodies can remain unnoticed for long periods of time. A rhinolith is a nasal foreign body that has become mineralized. A rhinolith will continue to increase in size as mineral salts are deposited onto its surface. It is usually an incidental finding on a plain radiography.

Retained foreign bodies can be classified as animal, vegetable, or mineral. The primary reason for making these distinctions is the somewhat different approaches to their removal. Insects and other animate objects should be killed before removal is attempted. Vegetable matter tends to swell if moistened and should be removed in a dry environment if possible. Foreign objects that are round and plastic can be difficult to grasp. Vasoconstriction enlarges the nostril slightly, thereby easing the movement of the foreign body and minimizing bleeding. In patients who are very young or uncooperative, sedation may be appropriate to minimize trauma and prevent aspiration.

Foreign bodies that are most commonly found in children's noses include such objects as buttons, beads, cotton, beans, and other objects of appropriate size. Vegetable foreign bodies will absorb water from the nasal mucosa and swell with time, making removal much more difficult than insertion.

INDICATIONS

A child or adult who has a retained nasal foreign body often presents with a foul odor from the nostrils, unilateral purulent rhinorrhea, or persistent epistaxis. More commonly, the patient presents with the request for object removal.

3

CONTRAINDICATIONS/PRECAUTIONS

- The practitioner should not attempt to remove foreign bodies not easily visualized or requiring general anesthesia to remove.
- If a foreign body is large and initial attempts to remove it are unsuccessful, the procedure is likely to cause trauma or aspiration and referral to an otolaryngologist is indicated.
- Practitioners should not push the object farther into the nasopharynx, hoping that the object will be swallowed, because aspiration may occur.
- Practitioners do not irrigate, because the nasal cavity is open posteriorly and aspiration may occur.
- If it appears that prolonged attempts at removal are required, refer the patient to a specialist.
- The patient who is very young or uncooperative may require sedation to prevent trauma during an extraction.
- It is important to examine both nares and ears carefully even when only a single foreign body is suspected. It is not uncommon for children to place objects in both their nose and their ears.

PATIENT PREPARATION

- Provide reassurance throughout the entire procedure, explaining each step as it is performed.
- It is important for the patient to remain still, so as to minimize trauma to the nasal passage during the procedure.
- Advise the patient that the nostril may feel full or numb from the topical anesthesia.

3

EQUIPMENT

- Headlight or head mirror
- Nasal speculum (see Figure 3-18)
- Topical anesthetic (4% lidocaine) and vasoconstrictor (0.25% phenylephrine HCl)
- Immobilization device (optional)
- One of the following, depending on the foreign body:
  - Suction and several suction tips (8 to 10 French catheter)
  - Alligator or Hartmann forceps
  - Wire loop or curette
  - Bayonet forceps (Figure 3-20)
  - Right-angle hooks
  - No. 4 Fogarty catheter

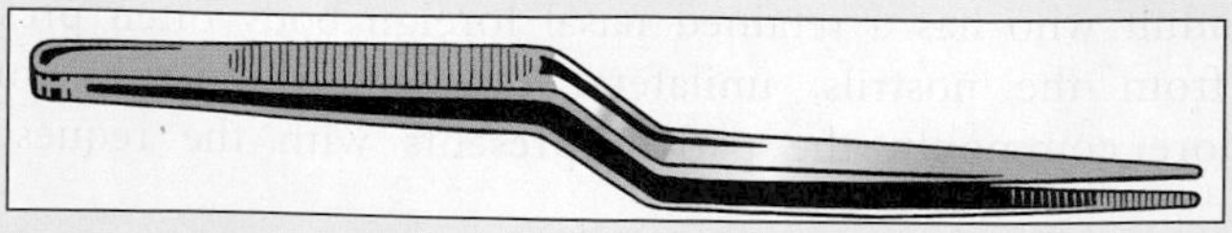

FIGURE 3-20 Bayonet forceps.

Procedure

1. Try to determine the type of object in the nostril by history from the patient or the parent to determine the best approach to removal.
2. Position the patient erect, sitting and with the head tilted forward (more of the nasal cavity is visible in this position than with the head tilted back).
3. Use the nasal speculum to visualize the nostril.
4. Apply a topical anesthetic or vasoconstrictor as spray or drops. If tissue edema is present in the nares, the practitioner can ease the removal of the foreign body by applying a topical vasoconstrictor.
5. In a cooperative child, occlude the unobstructed nostril, keep the mouth closed, and have the child forcefully blow his or her nose. This may be attempted several times.
6. Determine which instrument provides the best chance for removing the foreign body. The choice of instrument for removal of a foreign body is largely related to its exact location, shape, and composition, and the practitioner's preference.
   a. Smooth, round objects can be removed with suction or with right-angle hooks.
   b. A bayonet forceps can be used to grasp an object with a small leading edge.
   c. Objects that may break when grasped may be more easily removed with a curette or wire loop.
   d. A No. 4 Fogarty vascular catheter may be used to remove blunt nasal foreign bodies in children. Pass the catheter beyond the foreign body and inflate the balloon. Maintain slow, gentle traction on the catheter while carefully extricating the object. This technique may be less traumatic than removal with a forceps.
   e. In some cases, a lubricated No. 8 Foley catheter may be passed beneath and beyond the object, inflated with 2 to 3 ml of water, and slowly withdrawn.
   f. The Fogarty catheter may also be used to stabilize the foreign body from behind while it is removed with forceps because attempts to remove a foreign body may otherwise result in the object being forced into the oral pharynx.

PATIENT EDUCATION POSTPROCEDURE

- After extraction, any intranasal bleeding can be tamponaded with a small pack of gauze moistened with 0.5% phenylephrine.
- Residual inflammation of the nasal membranes should clear spontaneously in a few days.
- Instruct the patient to follow up with the provider if prolonged bleeding occurs.
- Teach patients or their parents the signs and symptoms of sinus infection and otitis media.
- Talk to parents of young children about how to do the following:
  - Childproof their house
  - Remove small objects within children's reach
  - Provide careful supervision of young children
  - Understand normal growth and development: hand-to-mouth activity; children's natural curiosity to stick objects in orifices (nose, mouth, ears)

COMPLICATIONS

- Complications can occur as a result of the foreign body itself, the examination, or the removal.
- Infection can closely follow the presence of a foreign body. The sinus ostia in the anterior section of the nose and eustachian tube in the posterior section of the nose can become blocked, predisposing the patient to sinusitis or otitis media. Signs of infection should be treated.
- If an object is not removed in a timely manner, a rhinolith may form. Its size gradually increases and may complicate removal or predispose the patient to serious infection.

PRACTITIONER FOLLOW-UP

- Use care during this procedure to prevent posterior dislodging of the object because the patient may swallow or aspirate it.
- Aspiration of the object into the tracheobronchial tree may precipitate bronchospasm, which is manifested by shortness of breath and wheezing. This requires referral to an emergency department for bronchoscopic removal under anesthesia.
- Instruct the patient or parents in the management of epistaxis, which may occur if nasal tissue has been irritated during foreign body removal.

■ CPT BILLING

If a patient comes in for a procedure only, there is no E/M code charge. The charge for the office visit is the procedure itself.

30300—Removal foreign body, intranasal; office type procedure

3

REFERENCES AND RELATED RESOURCES

Dane S, Smally AJ, Peredy TR: A truly emergent problem: button battery in the nose, *Acad Emerg Med* 7:204, 2000.

MOUTH PROCEDURES

Many primary care mouth procedures are performed by dentists. However, some offices may see a patient with tooth avulsion and can provide some care before they are referred to a dentist. Other procedures, like applying fluoride varnish or performing a frenulectomy, are appropriately performed in primary care and may provide an especially valuable service to those patients who have limited dental access.

ANATOMY AND PHYSIOLOGY

Above and behind the tongue is the arch, which comprises the anterior and posterior pillars, the soft palate, and the uvula. The tonsils are present in the fossae, or cavities, between the anterior and posterior pillars. The underside of the tongue is smooth, with the submaxillary gland (Wharton's duct) opening near the midline. Stensen's duct opens from each parotid gland onto the buccal mucosa near the upper second molar. In adults there are 32 teeth (12 in each jaw) (Figure 3-21).

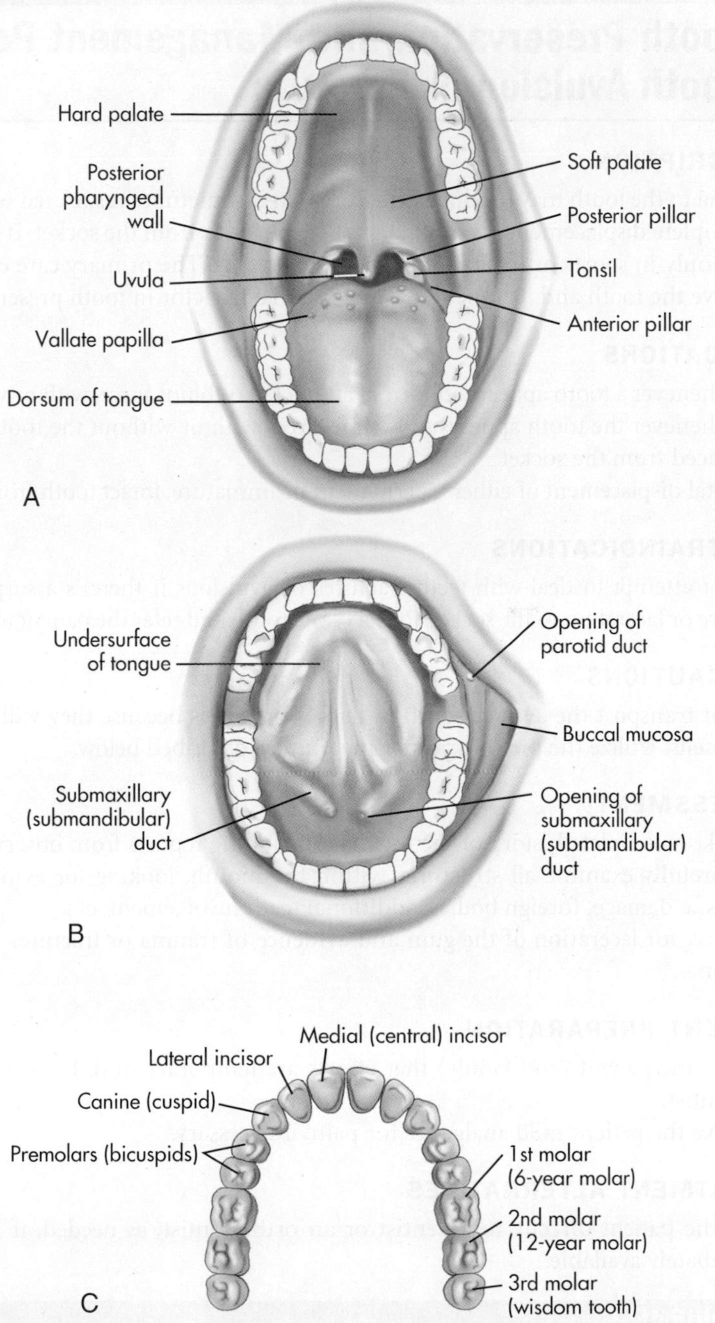

FIGURE 3-21 Anatomy of the mouth. **A,** Anatomy with tongue resting. **B,** Anatomy with tongue raised to roof of mouth. **C,** Teeth.

Tooth Preservation and Management Post Tooth Avulsion or Fracture

DESCRIPTION

Trauma to the tooth may produce a fracture that is sometimes associated with avulsion or complete displacement (exarticulation) of the tooth from the socket. It is seen most commonly in sports or in children experiencing falls. The primary care efforts are to preserve the tooth and its function. Time is a major factor in tooth preservation.

INDICATIONS

- Whenever a tooth appears abnormal after a fall or blunt force, with or without pain
- Whenever the tooth appears to be fractured, with or without the tooth being displaced from the socket
- Total displacement of either a permanent or immature, intact tooth from the socket

CONTRAINDICATIONS

Do not attempt to deal with teeth fractures or avulsions if there is a suspected facial fracture or laceration to the socket. Preserve the tooth and refer the patient to a specialist.

PRECAUTIONS

Do not transport the avulsed tooth in tissues or towels because they will dry out the tooth cells. Utilize the proper transfer medium as described below.

ASSESSMENT

- Take a complete history of the incident, including reports from observers.
- Carefully examine all structures within the mouth, looking for evidence of soft tissue damage, foreign bodies, additional teeth involvement, etc.
- Look for laceration of the gum and evidence of trauma or fractures of the facial bones.

PATIENT PREPARATION

- Tell the patient (and family) that efforts are temporary until he or she can see a dentist.
- Give the patient mild analgesics for pain, if necessary.

TREATMENT ALTERNATIVES

Send the patient directly to a dentist or an orthodontist, as needed, if he or she is immediately available.

EQUIPMENT

Transfer medium (listed in order of desirability)

- Hanks' balanced salt solution (should be available from a pharmacy)
- Milk
- Sterile 0.9% sodium chloride
- Saliva

Procedure

For a fractured tooth with total avulsion that has been out of the mouth for less than 1 hour:

1. Inspect the tooth and all tooth fragments.
2. If the tooth and root appear totally intact and not contaminated:
   a. Irrigate the tooth socket with water or saline.
   b. Hold the tooth at the distal tip, avoid touching the root and gently rinse with at least 10 ml of 0.9% sterile sodium chloride or water.
   c. Gently set the tooth back into the socket.
   d. Seek dental care.
3. If the tooth root has been contaminated:
   a. Irrigate the tooth socket with 0.9% sterile sodium chloride or water to remove any clot.
   b. Hold the tooth at the distal tip and gently rinse with a copious amount of 0.9% sterile sodium chloride or water.
   c. Gently set the tooth back into the socket.
   d. Consult with a dentist.

For a fractured tooth with total avulsion that has been out of the mouth for longer than 1 hour:

1. Locate and inspect the tooth and all tooth fragments.
2. Use gauze to gently remove debris, including attached necrotic tissue.
3. Follow the instructions for reimplanting the tooth that has been out for less than 1 hour (see step 3 above).
4. If unable to reimplant the tooth, place the fractured tooth into the transport medium.
5. Contact a dentist or an endodontist as soon as possible for treatment.

3

PATIENT EDUCATION POSTPROCEDURE

- If the tooth can be reimplanted, do not dislodge it from the socket.
- Clenching the tooth gently may allow for support of the tooth.
- Avoid talking, drinking, or chewing.
- Seek dental attention as soon as possible.

COMPLICATIONS

Delay in seeking dental assistance may result in complete loss of the tooth.

PRACTITIONER FOLLOW-UP

A dentist usually takes over the evaluation of tooth avulsion.

REFERENCES AND RELATED RESOURCES

The Dental Trauma Guide 2010: *Your interactive tool to evidence based trauma treatment*. July 1, 2014. Resource Centre for Rare Oral Diseases and Department of Oral and Maxillo-Facial Surgery at the University Hospital of Copenhagen. http://www.dentaltraumaguide.org/permanent_avulsion_treatment.aspx. Accessed December 21, 2014.

Emerich K, Wyszkowski J: Clinical practice: dental trauma. *Eur J Pediatr* 169(9):1045-1050, 2010.

Fluoride Varnish Application

DESCRIPTION

Dental caries is both a common and significant health issue for children that is often not self-limiting and can lead to persistent pain and eventual tooth loss. This disease is preventable and can be addressed in a primary care setting, especially for those patients who have little access to proper dental care. Professional fluoride varnish application likely minimizes the risk of fluorosis.

INDICATIONS

There are conflicting recommendations currently regarding the application of fluoride varnish. The United States Preventive Services Task Force recommends that all children from birth to 5 years of age receive applied fluoride varnish from their primary care providers beginning with primary tooth eruption. Both the American Academy of Pediatric Dentistry and American Dental Association recommend a risk-stratified approach. Children younger than 6, with elevated risk for dental caries, should have a 2.26% fluoride varnish (5% sodium fluoride) professionally applied every 3 to 6 months. See Table 3-1 to help determine risk for dental caries.

CONTRAINDICATIONS

There are none.

PRECAUTIONS

Sensitivity to any product ingredients.

3

TABLE 3-1 Caries-Risk Assessment Form for 0- to 3-Year-Olds (for Nondental Health Care Providers)

FACTORS	HIGH RISK	MODERATE RISK	PROTECTIVE
BIOLOGICAL			
Mother/primary caregiver has active cavities	Yes		
Parent/caregiver has low socioeconomic status	Yes		
Child has >3 between meal, sugar-containing snacks or beverages per day	Yes		
Child is put to bed with a bottle containing natural or added sugar	Yes		
Child has special health care needs		Yes	
Child is a recent immigrant		Yes	
PROTECTIVE			
Child receives optimally fluoridated drinking water or fluoride supplements			Yes
Child has teeth brushed daily with fluoridated toothpaste			Yes
Child receives topical fluoride from health care professional			Yes
Child receives regular dental care			Yes

TABLE 3-1 Caries-Risk Assessment Form for 0- to 3-Year-Olds (for Nondental Health Care Providers)—cont'd

FACTORS	HIGH RISK	MODERATE RISK	PROTECTIVE
CLINICAL FINDINGS			
Child has white spot lesions or enamel defects	Yes		
Child has visible cavities or fillings	Yes		
Child has plaque on teeth		Yes	
Circling those conditions that apply to a specific patient helps the health care worker and parent understand the factors that contribute to or protect from caries. Risk assessment categorization of low, moderate, or high is based on preponderance of factors for the individual. However, clinical judgment may justify the use of one factor (e.g., frequent exposure to sugar-containing snacks or beverages; visible cavities) in determining the overall risk.			
Overall assessment of the child's risk for dental caries: ☐ High ☐ Moderate ☐ Low			

With data from Ramos-Gomez FJ, Crall J, Gansky SA, et al. Caries risk assessment appropriate for the age 1 visit (infants and toddlers). J Calif Dent Assoc 35:687, 2007. American Dental Association Councils on Scientific Affairs and Dental Practice. Caries risk assessment form (ages 0-6). American Dental Association: Chicago, 2008.

ASSESSMENT

- A complete oral examination should be performed on pediatric patients in preparation for this procedure.

PATIENT PREPARATION

- Provide reassurance that this is a pain-free procedure
- Explain that the patient will be able to feel the varnish on the teeth until the next day

TREATMENT ALTERNATIVES

Send the patient directly to a dentist.

EQUIPMENT

- Fluoride varnish
- Gauze
- Gloves

Procedure

Applying fluoride varnish:

Follow universal precautions.

1. Position patient.
   a. Young children may be placed in a knee-to-knee position.
   b. Older children may sit on examination table.
2. Dry teeth using gauze squares.
3. Using the supplied paintbrush, apply the varnish to all surfaces of the teeth beginning with the outer upper teeth and working in. Repeat on the lower teeth.

3

PATIENT EDUCATION POSTPROCEDURE

- No brushing or flossing for 4 to 6 hours; ideally wait until next day
- Eat soft foods for the rest of today
- If colored varnish was used, this will go away in about 6 to 8 hours
- Avoid products with alcohol, like mouthwash, or hot drinks for the remainder of day

COMPLICATIONS

There are none.

PRACTITIONER FOLLOW-UP

Follow up in 3 to 6 months for repeat varnish application

CPT BILLING

If a patient comes in for a procedure only, there is no E/M code charge. The charge for the office visit is the procedure itself.

D1206—Topical fluoride varnish; therapeutic application for moderate to high caries risk patients

REFERENCES AND RELATED RESOURCES

Children's Oral Health, American Academy of Pediatrics: *Online oral health practice tools.* http://www2.aap.org/oralhealth/PracticeTools.html. Accessed December 29, 2014.

Douglass JM: *Applying fluoride varnish.* [Video.] YouTube. April 10, 2009. https://www.youtube.com/watch?v=cV5OmL7C8K4. Accessed February 5, 2015.

Selwitz R, Ismail A, Pitts N: Dental caries, *Lancet* 369:51–59, 2007.

U.S. Department of Health and Human Services: *Fluoride varnish.* 2009. http://www.ihs.gov/doh/documents/ecc/HowToApplyFluorideVarnish.ppt. Accessed December 29, 2014.

U.S. Preventive Services Task Force: *Recommendation summary,* September 2014. http://www.uspreventiveservicestaskforce.org/Page/Topic/recommendation-summary/dental-caries-in-children-from-birth-through-age-5-years-screening.

Weyant R, et al: Topical fluoride for caries prevention: executive summary of the updated clinical recommendations and supporting systematic review, *J Am Dent Assoc* 144(11): 1279–1291, 2013.

Frenulectomy

DESCRIPTION

Tongue tie is a congenital condition in which the frenulum is abnormally tight, thickened, or short. This condition affects 1.7% to 4.7% of the population and can affect feeding. Approximately 25% of infants with a shortened frenulum will experience feeding difficulty, characterized by a poor latch, clicking noise with breastfeeding, nipple pain in the mother, long feeds, or appearing unsatisfied. Division of the frenulum has been shown to significantly improve feeding in these infants within 24 hours of the procedure. It is simple and safely performed in the outpatient setting.

INDICATIONS

- Frenulectomy is indicated when a newborn infant has tongue tie, difficulty latching or breastfeeding, or who has already been evaluated by a lactation specialist. Ideally the infant is less than 2 weeks old.

CONTRAINDICATIONS

- Absence of feeding disorder
- Known bleeding or clotting disorder in the newborn
- Significant comorbidity
- Unclear diagnosis
- Posterior tongue-tie (refer to surgery)

PRECAUTIONS

Infant is older than 2 weeks.
Infant who has jaundice.

ASSESSMENT

- A complete examination and history of the newborn should be performed.
- Consultation with a lactation specialist should take place to maximize current feeding techniques.
- The degree of tongue-tie should be approximated and documented, up to 100% in which the frenulum reaches the tip of the tongue (Figure 3-22).

PATIENT PREPARATION

Informed consent should be reviewed and completed, including risks, benefits, and alternatives. This should include the risk that the procedure may not improve feeding. Give the parents time to think about the risks involved before the procedure is started.

TREATMENT ALTERNATIVES

- Consult a pediatric surgeon or HEENT specialist.
- Consult a lactation specialist.

EQUIPMENT

- Blunt-edged sterile scissors
- Sterile gauze
- Gloves
- An assistant to help secure the patient

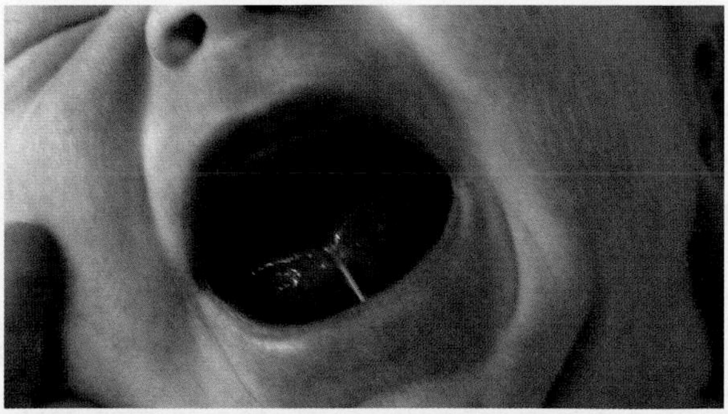

FIGURE 3-22 Tongue-tie, in which the lingual frenulum is attached near the tip of the tongue. (From Zitelli BJ, McIntire SC, Norwalk AJ: *Zitelli and Davis' atlas of pediatric physical diagnosis*, ed 6, Philadelphia, 2012, Saunders.)

Procedure

In order to perform a frenulectomy:

1. A "time-out" for parents to consider risk should be completed before the procedure.
2. There is no need for analgesia or anesthesia.
3. Infant should be swaddled securely by the assistant, who can secure the infant's shoulders using his or her wrists and using his or her hands to secure the infant's head.
4. Sugar water may be given to the infant (optional).
5. The provider should stretch the tongue-tie by pushing the tongue up with the nondominant index finger while using the thumb to keep the lower lip clear. Alternatively, the provider may use the thumb and index finger to extend the tongue on both sides of the tongue tie. The goal is to stretch the tongue-tie and avoid the submandibular ducts and lower lip.
6. The tongue-tie should be completely divided in a smooth snip with the blunt-tipped scissors.
7. Use the gauze to immediately compress the floor of the mouth.
8. Comfort the infant and immediately hand the child to the mother to feed, either by breast or bottle.

3

PATIENT EDUCATION POSTPROCEDURE

- Caregiver should monitor for effectiveness of feeding, nipple pain, and other signs of feeding difficulty.
- Infant should be fed and cared for as normal.

COMPLICATIONS

- Infection
- Sublingual hematoma
- Pain
- Bleeding

PRACTITIONER FOLLOW-UP

Follow up by phone at 24 hours for effectiveness of feeding and to assess parental concerns.

CPT BILLING

If a patient comes in for a procedure only, there is no E/M code charge. The charge for the office visit is the procedure itself.

41010—Incision of lingual frenum (frenotomy)

REFERENCES AND RELATED RESOURCES

Bowley DM, et al: Fifteen-minute consultation: the infant with a tongue tie, *Arch Dis Child Educ Pract Ed* 99:127–129, 2014.

Columbia University Medical Center Department of Otolaryngology: *Frenulectomy (tongue-tie surgery)* 2007. http://www.entcolumbia.org/frenul.html. Accessed December 29, 2014.

Emond A, et al: Randomized controlled trial of early frenotomy in breastfed infants with mild-moderate tongue-tie, *Arch Dis Child Fetal Neonatal Ed* 99:F189–F195, 2014.

Hogan M, et al: Randomized, controlled trial of division of tongue-tie in infants with feeding problems, *J Paediatr Chil Health* 41:246–250, 2005.

Wallace H, Clarke S: Tongue tie division in infants with breast feeding difficulties, *Int J Pediatr Otorhi* 70:1257–1261, 2006.

4

Respiratory Procedures

Kent D. Blad and Sabrina Jarvis

DESCRIPTION

Primary care providers often care for patients who have respiratory disorders such as asthma, chronic obstructive pulmonary disease (COPD), and pneumonia. The spirometry and peak flowmeter procedures assess lung function and assist in the diagnosis and management of pulmonary disorders. The nebulizer treatment procedure provides inhaled aerosol medication administration that can be used in both acute and chronic pulmonary conditions. The following is information relevant to all three procedures.

ANATOMY AND PHYSIOLOGY

The respiratory system is composed of increasingly smaller bronchial airways leading to alveolar sacs by which air moves in and out of the body. The alveolar sacs are sites for the interchange of oxygen and carbon dioxide. Blood capillaries surround the alveoli (Figure 4-1).

Asthma and COPD share the same physiologic abnormality of airflow limitation secondary to airway inflammation and bronchospasm, but generally involve a different clinical course and response to pharmacotherapy.

ASSESSMENT

Patients who have pulmonary disorders often present with complaints of shortness of breath, cough, chest tightness and discomfort, and wheezing. Physical findings may include adventitious lung sounds, such as crackles, wheezes, and rhonchi. Other findings may include tachypnea, use of accessory muscles, low oxygenation saturation, and cyanosis.

REFERENCES AND RELATED RESOURCES

Ball J, Dains J, Flynn J, et al: *Seidel's guide to physical examination*, ed 8, St Louis, 2014, Mosby.

Bickley L, Szilagyi P: *Bate's guide to physical examination*, ed 11, Philadelphia, 2013, Wolters Kluwer Health/Lippincott Williams & Wilkins.

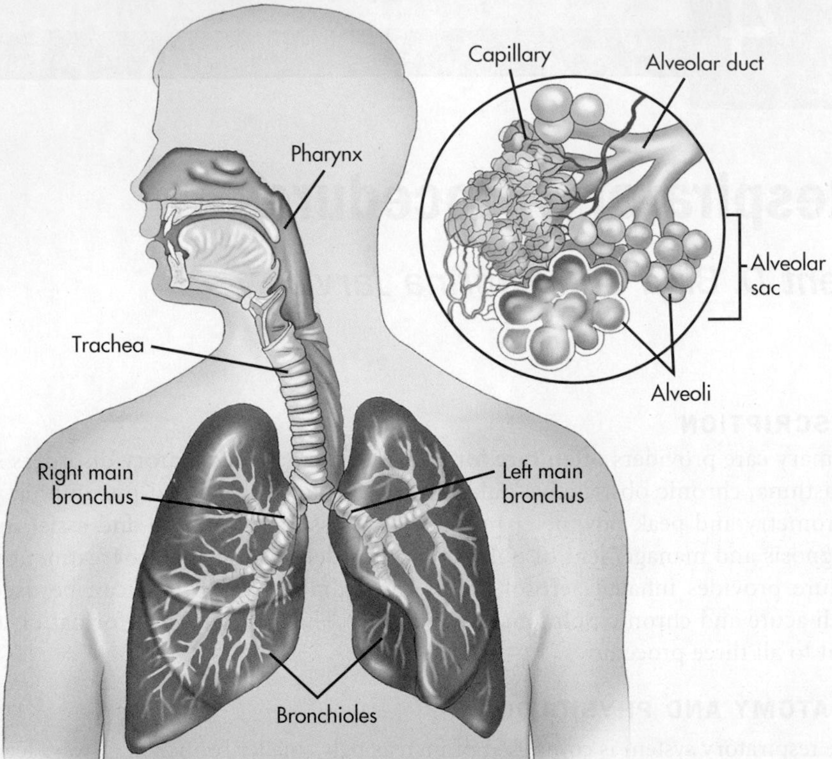

FIGURE 4-1 Anatomy of the respiratory system.

4

Nebulizer Treatment

DESCRIPTION

Inhaled medications are the mainstay of treatment in patients who have acute bronchospasm. To be effective, inhaled medications must be properly used. One method of medication administration is through the use of a metered dose inhaler (MDI). The MDI comprises a pressured canister, metering valve and stem, and a mouthpiece. Using a spacer with an MDI can help deliver more medications to the lungs. An MDI with a spacer is a very effective way of administering inhaled medications, particularly for young children.

However, anyone who has difficulty using an inhaler correctly may benefit from a nebulizer. Nebulizers are used in situations in which patients are too ill or too young or old to manage a handheld device. In addition, nebulizers may be used when larger amounts of medication are required over a longer period of administration time.

The nebulizer is a medication delivery system that generates a mist, which is inhaled by the patient. Medications delivered by this system may commonly include drugs, such as short- and long-acting beta-2 agonists and steroids.

INDICATIONS

- To deliver medications directly to the respiratory tract for the treatment of acute bronchospasm, excessive mucous accumulation, croup, and epiglottitis.

CONTRAINDICATIONS

- Hypersensitivity to medication/class/components
- Inhaled corticosteroids in patients who have a severe hypersensitivity to a milk protein allergy

PRECAUTIONS

- Short- and long-term beta-2 agonists should be used with caution in patients who have hypertension, cardiovascular disease, congestive heart failure, hyperthyroidism, diabetes, seizure disorder, hypokalemia, or hyperglycemia. Adverse effects include tachycardia, headache, nervousness, dizziness, tremor, gastrointestinal upset, hypertension or hypotension, paradoxical bronchospasm, asthma, and cough.
- Inhaled glucocorticoid steroids should be used with precaution in patients who are immunocompromised. Adverse effects include dysphonia, oral candidiasis, glaucoma, cataracts, hyperglycemia, and osteoporosis.

ASSESSMENT

- Monitor and document vital signs including pulse oximetry before, during, and after the procedure. If a peak flowmeter is used to assess dynamic lung function and therapeutic response to medical pretreatment and posttreatment, document results.
- Assess breath sounds premedication and postmedication administration, and monitor for treatment effectiveness and possible side effects.

PATIENT PREPARATION

Position patient in an upright, comfortable position to allow for maximum, deep ventilation.

EQUIPMENT

- Air compressor unit nebulizer (three nebulizer types include mesh, ultrasonic, and jet)
- Mouthpiece or mask
- Flex tube
- Nebulizer medication cup
- Compressor tubing
- Prescribed medication

Procedure

1. Set up equipment according to manufacturer instructions.
2. Place the prescribed medication in the nebulizer cup. Observe for mist with compressed air or oxygen, depending on patient condition, pulse oximetry, and/or arterial blood gas results.
3. Instruct the patient on the procedure.

4. With the patient sitting, have the patient hold the nebulizer in an upright position and close lips to form a seal around the mouthpiece. If the patient is unable to use the mouthpiece, then apply a mask attachment over the nose and mouth.
5. Instruct the patient to take slow, deep breaths until all the medication is used (average of 10 minutes).
6. In many cases, the equipment will be disposable; therefore, discard after use. If the equipment is reusable, then disassemble the equipment, rinse with manufacturer-recommended antimicrobial solution, and dry completely.

PATIENT EDUCATION POSTPROCEDURE

- If the patient is sent home with a nebulizer, instruct the patient on equipment care, medication dosing, and side effects.
- Instruct the patient to seek emergency medical care for any of the following:
  - Worsening shortness of breath that is unresolved with nebulizer treatment
  - Nasal flaring; use of accessory breathing muscles
  - Cyanosis of fingertips and/or lips

COMPLICATIONS

Adverse effects of the medications as noted above.

PRACTITIONER FOLLOW-UP

The practitioner should observe for complications of the particular medication that was used.

Schedule the patient to return to the clinic if symptoms do not change or improve.

RED FLAGS

- Inhalation injury
- Adverse reactions to medication requiring the discontinuance of the drug
- Patient is unresponsive to therapy
- Hemodynamic instability: systolic blood pressure <90 mm Hg, O_2 sat $<90\%$, heart rate <60 or >100 bpm, respiratory rate >20 bpm

CPT BILLING

94640—Pressurized or nonpressurized inhalation treatment for acute airway obstruction or for sputum induction for diagnostic purposes (e.g., with an aerosol generator, nebulizer, metered dose inhaler or intermittent positive pressure breathing [IPPB] device)

For more than one inhalation treatment performed on the same date, append modifier 76 to the nebulizer code.

J7613—Albuterol ■ **J7644**—Ipratropium bromide

Many insurance carriers consider the medication a bundled service.

REFERENCES AND RELATED RESOURCES

Buddiga P: *Use of metered dose inhalers, spacers, and nebulizers*. http://emedicine.medscape.com/article/1413366-overview. Updated June 3, 2013, Accessed May 29, 2015.

Kacmarek R, Stoller J, Heuer A: *Egan's fundamentals of respiratory care*, ed 10, St Louis, 2013, Elsevier.

4

Tashkin D, Klein G, Colman S, et al: Comparing COPD treatment: nebulizer, metered dose inhaler, and concomitant therapy, *Am J Med* 120:435–441, 2007.
Urden L, Stacy K, Lough M: *Critical care nursing diagnosis and management*, ed 7, St Louis, 2014, Elsevier.

Spirometry

DESCRIPTION

This procedure measures the amount (volume) and/or speed (flow) of air with inhalation and exhalation for the purpose of diagnosing and monitoring pulmonary disease.

ANATOMY AND PHYSIOLOGY

The rate of airflow from the lungs is determined by the elastic recoil of the lungs, the patency of the pulmonary airways, and the condition of the respiratory muscles and/or the muscular effort of the patient. Lungs have a tendency to collapse because they are elastic and under pressure from the thoracic cage. Opposed to this tendency to collapse is the airway resistance.

If airway resistance is high, which occurs with bronchospasm, edema, mucous plugs, and inflammation, airflow from the lungs is limited and air trapping results. This happens in obstructive diseases such as COPD and asthma. In restrictive diseases, the lungs lose their elastic capabilities because of fibrosis. They are not able to inflate adequately, so lung volumes are low. The rate of airflow, however, does not drop until restriction is severe or if obstructive defects coexist. This commonly occurs in sarcoidosis and asbestosis.

INDICATIONS

- Part of a standard workup of respiratory symptoms such as dyspnea, chronic cough, sputum, or wheezing
- Establish baseline lung function
- Diagnose and differentiate between restrictive and obstructive pulmonary diseases
- Assess as part of preoperative risk evaluation before anesthesia is administered or cardiothoracic surgery is performed
- Evaluate reversibility of airway obstruction and bronchial responsiveness to bronchodilators
- Monitor progression of pulmonary diseases

CONTRAINDICATIONS

- Current, painful ear infection
- Eye surgery within the past 3 months
- Chest or abdominal surgery within the past 3 months
- Myocardial infarction or stroke within the past 3 months
- History of aneurysm or collapsed lung
- History of coughing up blood within the past month

- History of syncope with forced exhalation
- Patient who is uncooperative

PRECAUTIONS

- Obtain accurate results; proper instructions must be given to ensure the test is performed correctly.
- Ensure the equipment is properly cleaned as per manufacturer recommendations because it may become a source of infection for patients who are immunocompromised.

ASSESSMENT

Gather patient information (name, age, sex, height without shoes, weight, race, and a short respiratory history).

PATIENT PREPARATION

- Explain the procedure to the patient. Explain to the patient that the machine measures how much and how fast air leaves the lungs.
- Patient should be sitting upright in chair with legs uncrossed and feet on floor.
- Use of nose clips is recommended.
- Patient should remove any dentures and restrictive clothing.
- The practitioner should explain and demonstrate the maneuvers even if the patient has performed the test before. There are three distinct test maneuver phases:
  1. **Maximal inspiration phase.** Say, "You need to take as deep a breath as you possibly can, until you can't hold any more air. Like this." The practitioner demonstrates how the mouthpiece is placed in the mouth, with the teeth around the outside and lips closed tightly around it. There should be less than 1 second between the end of inhalation and the beginning of exhalation.
  2. **"Blast" of exhalation phase.** Then instruct the patient to "Blow out as hard and as fast as possible; try to force all the air you can from your lungs, like blowing out a birthday candle." Show how to blow through the mouthpiece, using body language to emphasize the importance of maximal inhalation and maximal exhalation.
  3. **Continued complete exhalation to end of test phase.** Emphasize the need for the prolonged effort to squeeze the last little bit of air out of the lungs for at least 6 seconds for the most accurate test result.
- Ask if the patient has any questions.

TREATMENT ALTERNATIVES

Peak flowmeters are useful for monitoring the progress of the disease, but are not as sensitive as spirometry in detecting mild disease and do not provide as reliable results.

EQUIPMENT

- Spirometer (there are diagnostic and office spirometers; simple office spirometers cost less than half as much as diagnostic spirometers and are effective for most uses)

Procedure

1. Calibrate the machine following manufacturer instructions.
2. Put a new mouthpiece on the spirometer and have the patient try it. Encourage the patient to relax.
3. *Maximal inspiration:* Prompt inhalation in patient by saying, "Now take a deep breath." Coach the patient with, "MORE, MORE, ALL YOU CAN HOLD." Make sure there is a tight seal on the mouthpiece.
4. *Rapid and hard exhalation.* Prompt exhalation in patient by saying, "NOW BLAST IT OUT HARD AND FAST!!"
5. *Continue exhalation for 6 seconds:* You must coach for at least 6 seconds and no more than 10 seconds. "ALL YOU CAN. MORE. MORE. KEEP ON GOING!"
6. Repeat the procedure. There should be at least three acceptable maneuvers. The American Thoracic Society defines an acceptable and reproducible spirogram as one in which the two largest forced vital capacity (FVC) measurements are within 5% of each other and the two largest 1-second forced expiratory volumes (FEV_1) match within 5%.
7. To evaluate for bronchial responsiveness, administer the bronchodilator via a handheld inhaler.
8. Wait about 20 minutes, and then repeat this procedure.

INTERPRETATION OF RESULTS

The four values commonly used in office spirometry in assessing a patient are:

1. *Peak expiratory flow (PEF):* Measurement of how fast a patient can blow out during exhalation following a maximal inhalation; reported in liters per minute.
2. *Forced vital capacity (FVC):* Sum of TV, ERV, and IRV, or the total amount one can exhale after taking the deepest breath; normal value is 3.88 to 5.0 L.
3. *Forced expiratory volume in 1 second (FEV_1):* The volume of the FVC is exhaled in 1 second; normal volume is 3.12 to 3.96 L.
4. *Ratio of FEV_1/FVC:* Expressed in percentages with a normal range of 65% to 85%.

Interpretation of Spirometry

- Typical spirograms are shown in Figure 4-2.
  - Degree of obstruction = reduced maximal expiratory flow = reduced FEV_1 compared with the FVC (FEV_1/FVC ratio).
  - Degree of restriction = reduced volume = reduced FVC in the presence of normal or elevated FEV_1/FVC ratio.
- Reduction of the FVC and percentage of FEV_1 may be caused by obstructive and/or restrictive disease.
- The FVC is low because of chronic airway obstruction. If the FVC improves after bronchodilator use, the patient has chronic obstruction.
- A positive response to bronchodilators is defined as an increase in FVC of 15% or more and an increase in FEV_1 of 12% or more.

4

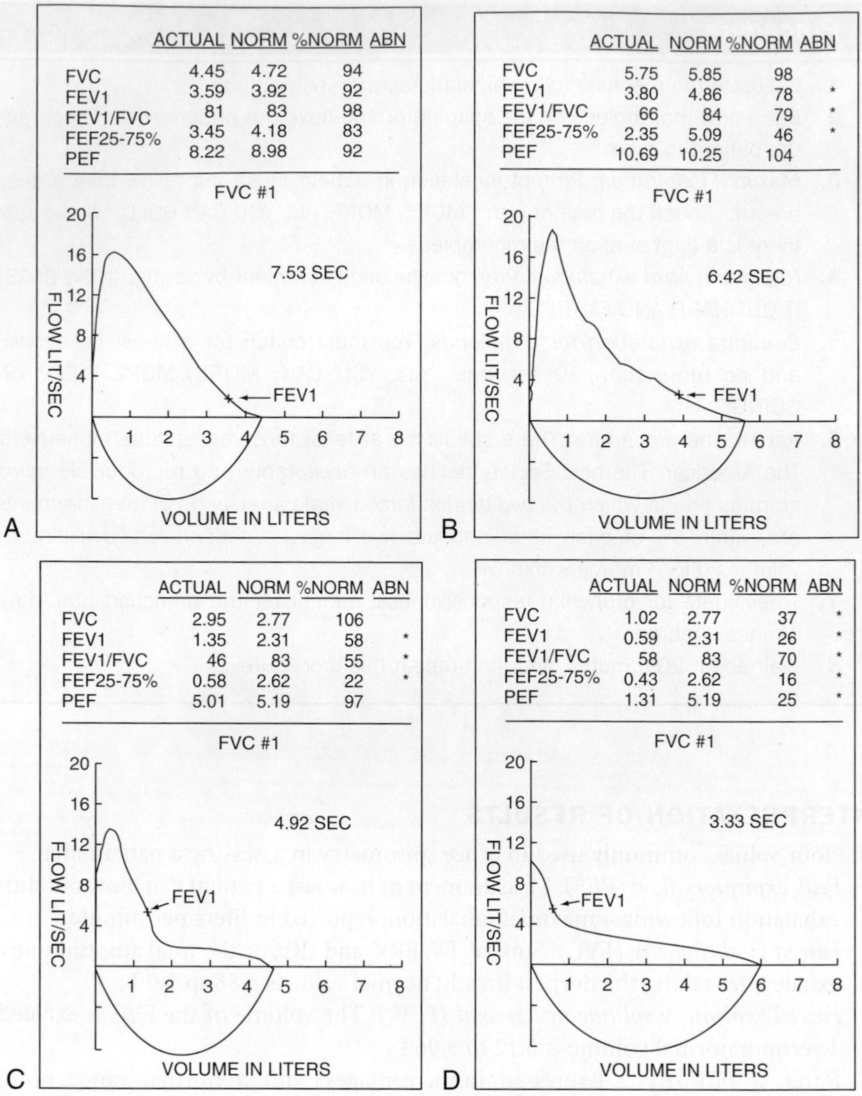

	ACTUAL	NORM	%NORM	ABN
FVC	4.45	4.72	94	
FEV1	3.59	3.92	92	
FEV1/FVC	81	83	98	
FEF25-75%	3.45	4.18	83	
PEF	8.22	8.98	92	

FVC #1

7.53 SEC

←FEV1

A VOLUME IN LITERS

	ACTUAL	NORM	%NORM	ABN
FVC	5.75	5.85	98	
FEV1	3.80	4.86	78	*
FEV1/FVC	66	84	79	*
FEF25-75%	2.35	5.09	46	*
PEF	10.69	10.25	104	

FVC #1

6.42 SEC

←FEV1

B VOLUME IN LITERS

	ACTUAL	NORM	%NORM	ABN
FVC	2.95	2.77	106	
FEV1	1.35	2.31	58	*
FEV1/FVC	46	83	55	*
FEF25-75%	0.58	2.62	22	*
PEF	5.01	5.19	97	

FVC #1

4.92 SEC

←FEV1

C VOLUME IN LITERS

	ACTUAL	NORM	%NORM	ABN
FVC	1.02	2.77	37	*
FEV1	0.59	2.31	26	*
FEV1/FVC	58	83	70	*
FEF25-75%	0.43	2.62	16	*
PEF	1.31	5.19	25	*

FVC #1

3.33 SEC

←FEV1

D VOLUME IN LITERS

FIGURE 4-2 A, Normal spirometry, showing a sharp initial peak flow, and then a relatively straight descent at about 45 degrees to the baseline. There are no stars in the ABN column, indicating that all parameters are within the normal limits. **B,** Mild obstruction, which may be difficult to detect from this spirogram alone. The FEV$_1$/FVC flags this as an obstruction. The severity of the obstruction is mild as judged by the FEV$_1$, which is 78% of the predicted value. Mild obstruction occurs gradually over many years. **C,** Moderate obstruction. The FEV$_1$/FVC is abnormal, indicating obstruction. The FEV$_1$ is 58% of normal, indicating that the obstruction is moderate in severity. Note the concave shape of the flow-volume curve, with low flows after the initially sharp peak flow. **D,** Severe obstruction with a low vital capacity. All of the parameters are abnormally low. The low FEV$_1$/FVC indicates obstruction; FEV$_1$ is only 26% of normal, showing that the obstruction is severe. A superimposed restriction may also be present because the FVC is abnormally low, but the patient tried to exhale for only about 3 seconds, so the FVC is probably underestimated. This patient had emphysema.

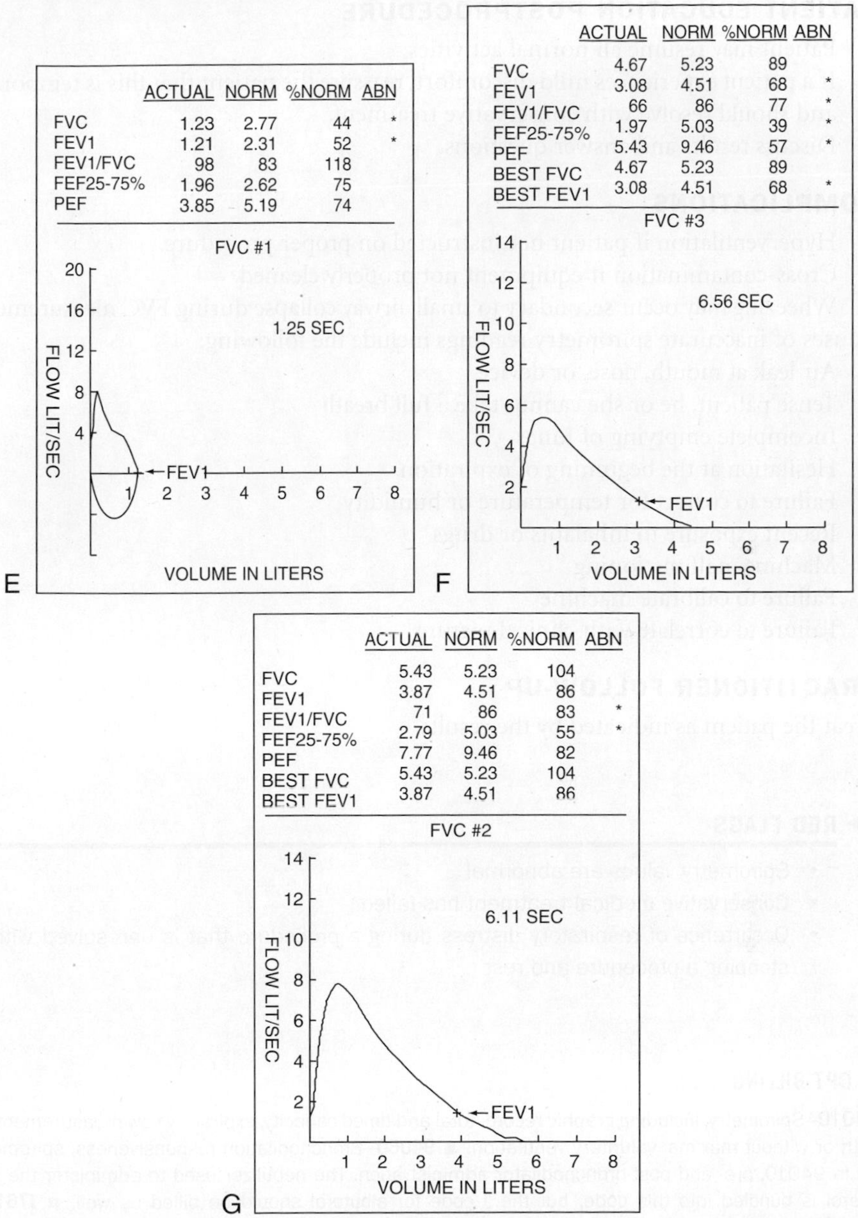
ACTUAL NORM %NORM ABN
FVC 1.23 2.77 44 *
FEV1 1.21 2.31 52 *
FEV1/FVC 98 83 118
FEF25-75% 1.96 2.62 75
PEF 3.85 5.19 74
FVC #1
1.25 SEC
FLOW LIT/SEC
FEV1
VOLUME IN LITERS
E
ACTUAL NORM %NORM ABN
FVC 4.67 5.23 89
FEV1 3.08 4.51 68 *
FEV1/FVC 66 86 77 *
FEF25-75% 1.97 5.03 39 *
PEF 5.43 9.46 57 *
BEST FVC 4.67 5.23 89
BEST FEV1 3.08 4.51 68 *
FVC #3
6.56 SEC
FLOW LIT/SEC
FEV1
VOLUME IN LITERS
F
ACTUAL NORM %NORM ABN
FVC 5.43 5.23 104
FEV1 3.87 4.51 86
FEV1/FVC 71 86 83 *
FEF25-75% 2.79 5.03 55 *
PEF 7.77 9.46 82
BEST FVC 5.43 5.23 104
BEST FEV1 3.87 4.51 86
FVC #2
6.11 SEC
FLOW LIT/SEC
FEV1
VOLUME IN LITERS
G

FIGURE 4-2, cont'd **E,** Severe restriction. The FEV_1/FVC is normal, so obstruction does not exist. The FVC, however, is only 44% of normal, indicating severe restriction. The FEV_1 is also decreased, but to a lesser degree than the FVC in restrictive disorders. Note the sharp peak and rapid, straight, and steep decline of the flow-volume curve. **F,** Before the use of a bronchodilator. **G,** After the use of a bronchodilator.

4

PATIENT EDUCATION POSTPROCEDURE

- Patient may resume all normal activities.
- If a patient experiences mild discomfort, reassure the patient that this is temporary and should resolve with conservative treatment.
- Discuss results and answer questions.

COMPLICATIONS

- Hyperventilation if patient not instructed on proper procedure.
- Cross-contamination if equipment not properly cleaned.
- Wheezing may occur secondary to small airway collapse during FVC measurement.

Causes of inaccurate spirometry readings include the following:

- Air leak at mouth, nose, or device
- Tense patient; he or she cannot take a full breath
- Incomplete emptying of lungs
- Hesitation at the beginning of expiration
- Failure to correct for temperature or humidity
- Recent exposure to inhalants or drugs
- Machine malfunctioning
- Failure to calibrate machine
- Failure to correlate with clinical picture

PRACTITIONER FOLLOW-UP

Treat the patient as indicated by the results.

RED FLAGS

- Spirometry values are abnormal
- Conservative medical treatment has failed
- Occurrence of respiratory distress during a procedure that is unresolved with stopping a procedure and rest

4

CPT BILLING

94010—Spirometry, including graphic record, total and timed capacity, expiratory flow measurement(s), with or without maximal voluntary ventilation. ■ **94060**—Bronchodilation responsiveness, spirometry as in 94010, pre- and post-bronchodilator administration. The nebulizer used to administer the albuterol is bundled into this code, but the J code for albuterol should be billed as well. ■ **J7613**—Albuterol 2.5 mg

If the visit is for spirometry only, there should be no additional E/M charge. The procedure code is the charge.

REFERENCES AND RELATED RESOURCES

McCarthy K, Dweik R: *Pulmonary function testing*. http://emedicine.medscape.com/article/303239-overview. Updated February 18, 2015. Accessed May 29, 2015.

Miller M, Hankinson J, Brusasco V, et al: Series "ATS/ERS task force: standardization of lung function testing," *Eur Respir J* 26:319–338, 2005.

Occupational and Health Administration: *Spirometry testing in occupational health programs: best practices for healthcare professionals*. https://www.osha.gov/Publications/OSHA3637.pdf. 2013. Accessed May 29, 2015.

Peak Flowmeter

DESCRIPTION

The peak flowmeter is a simple, portable handheld device that is used to objectively assess dynamic pulmonary function and patient response to therapy. It is commonly used in patients who are asthmatic, but may be helpful in other respiratory diseases as well. Peak flowmeters are relatively inexpensive and easy to use.

ANATOMY AND PHYSIOLOGY

The meter measures the peak expiratory flow rate (peak flow rate) as the maximum force and speed that can be exhaled from the lungs, after a maximum inhaled breath. Peak flow is measured in liters per minute, with patient results being compared with previous findings and normal predicted average peak expiratory flow for adults, adolescents, or children. The patient's use of a peak flowmeter can reduce the severity, frequency, and duration of asthma attacks.

INDICATIONS

- *Patients who have asthma:* Check peak flow at regular intervals to determine severity of asthma and response of therapy.
- *Patients who have COPD:* Check peak flow at the onset of acute exacerbations and following treatment.
- Peak flow measurement is also useful in other chronic and acute respiratory problems for detection of decreases in lung function.

CONTRAINDICATIONS

None, unless use of meter triggers respiratory distress or an asthma attack.

PRECAUTIONS

To obtain accurate results, proper instructions must be given to ensure the test is performed correctly. Limitations of the peak flowmeter include patient ability (skills) and motivation to use the device. Limitations also include the inability of younger children or patients who have special needs to understand instructions for using the device.

ASSESSMENT

Assess the patient's ability to cooperate and understand the procedure.

PATIENT PREPARATION

- Explain/demonstrate the procedure to the patient.
- Patient should be standing upright.

TREATMENT ALTERNATIVES

Spirometry is more sensitive and accurate for diagnosis, but tends to be more expensive and must be performed in the office.

EQUIPMENT

- Peak flowmeter with mouthpiece

4

Procedure

1. Explain the procedure to the patient.
2. Place mouthpiece over the peak flowmeter.
3. Move indicator to the lowest position.
4. Have patient stand, if possible, to achieve maximum chest expansion.
5. Hold the meter close to the mouth so indicator is not obstructed.
6. Have patient breathe in as deeply as possible.
7. Have patient close lips around the outside of the mouthpiece, making a tight seal, and blow out as hard and fast as possible for 1 to 2 seconds.
8. Note and record the indicator reading.
9. Repeat steps 5 through 8 to obtain three readings. Have the patient rest between readings if necessary.
10. Record the highest reading in the patient's chart and diary.
11. Routinely clean the meter according to manufacturer instructions.
12. Dispose of the mouthpiece after use.

PATIENT EDUCATION POSTPROCEDURE

- The patient should use the meter according to provider instructions, usually two or three times daily, at the same times each day. The patient should learn and know expected values and abnormal values requiring medical attention (Figure 4-3).
- The patient should be instructed to call the provider or return to the clinic for abnormal values.
- The patient should be instructed to notify the provider or return to the clinic if experiencing respiratory distress regardless of peak flowmeter values.

COMPLICATIONS

- Respiratory distress triggered by procedure.
- Peak flow meter should be kept clean to prevent microbial contamination.

PRACTITIONER FOLLOW-UP

Adjust treatment based on the results. Use peak flowmeter results to assist in adjusting the patient's treatment plan.

RED FLAGS

- Respiratory distress
- Peak flow results that are unimproved or worsened by prescribed treatment

CPT BILLING

There are no CPT codes for peak flow readings. They are considered part of the office visit.

REFERENCES AND RELATED RESOURCES

Bailey W, Gerald L: Patient information: how to use a peak flow meter (beyond the basics), *UptoDate* 2014, Wolters Kluwer. http://www.uptodate.com/contents/how-to-use-a-peak-flow-meter-beyond-the-basics. Updated April 4, 2014. Accessed May 29, 2015.

Neuspiel D: *Peak flow rate measurement*, 2014. http://emedicine.medscape.com/article/1413347-overview. Updated January 30, 2014. Accessed May 29, 2015.

Pesola G, Otolorin L: Peak flow meter characteristics and asthma, *Internet Journal of Asthma, Allergy and Immunology* 7(2):2008. http://ispub.com/IJAAI/7/2/6572. Accessed May 29, 2015.

Predicted Values – Adult

Normal Adult Predicted Average Peak Expiratory Flow (LPM)

Data From: Leiner GC, et al.: Expiratory peak flow rate. Standard values for normal subjects. Use as a clinical test of ventilatory function. *Am Rev Resp Dis* 88:644, 1963.

Age (yrs)	Men Height					Women Height				
	60"	65"	70"	75"	80"	55"	60"	65"	70"	75"
20	554	602	649	693	740	390	423	460	496	529
25	543	590	636	679	725	385	418	454	490	523
30	532	577	622	664	710	380	413	448	483	516
35	521	565	609	651	695	375	408	442	476	509
40	509	552	596	636	680	370	402	436	470	502
45	498	540	583	622	665	365	397	430	464	495
50	486	527	569	607	649	360	391	424	457	488
55	475	515	556	593	634	355	386	418	451	482
60	463	502	542	578	618	350	380	412	445	475
65	452	490	529	564	603	345	375	406	439	468
70	440	477	515	550	587	340	369	400	432	461

Predicted Values – Child

Data From: Polger, G, Promedhat V: *Pulmonary function testing in children: Techniques and standards.* Philadelphia, Saunders, 1971.

Normal Child & Adolescent Predicted Average Peak Expiratory Flow (LPM)

Height (inches)	LPM	Height (inches)	LPM
43	147	56	320
44	160	57	334
45	173	58	347
46	187	59	360
47	200	60	373
48	214	61	387
49	227	62	400
50	240	63	413
51	254	64	427
52	267	65	440
53	280	66	454
54	293	67	467
55	307		

Note: These tables are averages and are based on tests with a large number of people. An individual's PEFR may vary widely. Further, many individuals' PEFR values are consistently higher or lower than the average values. It is recommended that PEFR objectives for therapy be based upon each individual's "personal best," which is established after a period of PEFR monitoring while the individual is under effective treatment.

The above note, normal adult and normal child & adolescent tables from: "Guidelines for the Diagnosis and Management of Asthma," U.S. Department of Health and Human Services, Public Health Service, National Institutes of Health, Publication No. 91-3042, August 1991.

FIGURE 4-3 Normal values for peak flow rates. (From *Guidelines for the diagnosis and management of asthma*, Bethesda, MD, 1991, US Department of Health and Human Services, Public Health Service, National Institutes of Health, NIH publication No. 91-3042.)

4

5

Cardiovascular Procedures

Kent D. Blad and Sabrina Jarvis

Electrocardiography and *continuous electrocardiographic monitoring* are diagnostic procedures used primarily to evaluate ischemic coronary artery disease (CAD) or to confirm the diagnosis in intermittent arrhythmias.

The *ankle-brachial index* (ABI) test is used to screen and diagnose lower extremity peripheral artery disease (PAD) in patients with one or more of the following: non-healing leg wounds, exertional leg symptoms, age 65 years or older, or age 50 years or older with a medical history of diabetes or smoking.

ANATOMY AND PHYSIOLOGY

Atherosclerosis in general and CAD are discussed here. Information specific to PAD is given in the procedure.

The myocardium receives its blood supply from the coronary arteries, which form a system of small arteries that branch from the aorta (Figure 5-1).

The atherosclerotic process refers to the buildup of plaque in blood vessels, which can occur throughout the body. Critical arteries often affected are the coronary arteries (CAD), cerebral vascular arteries (stroke), renal arteries (renal failure), and peripheral arteries (PAD). Vascular endothelial function affects vascular tone, platelet adhesion, thrombogenicity, and cell proliferation. This contributes to the development of atherosclerosis. Fatty streaks form on the artery wall and progress to fatty plaques. The plaque may develop an internal hemorrhage, which then leaks to the surface and may cause vessel occlusion (Figure 5-2).

CAD or ischemic heart disease is the leading cause of death in industrialized societies.

ASSESSMENT

History is crucial to the diagnosis of CAD. *Angina* is usually described as a heavy substernal pressure or pain, which may radiate to the left arm. It is brought on by exertion and often relieved by rest. The sensation may be described as tightness, squeezing, gas, indigestion, or a vague discomfort in the chest. The pain/discomfort may be located anywhere from the lower jaw to the epigastrium. It may radiate to the right arm in addition to the left. Older adults and patients who are diabetic are less likely to experience pain and more likely to present with shortness of breath and other symptoms. Female patients often present with gastrointestinal symptoms

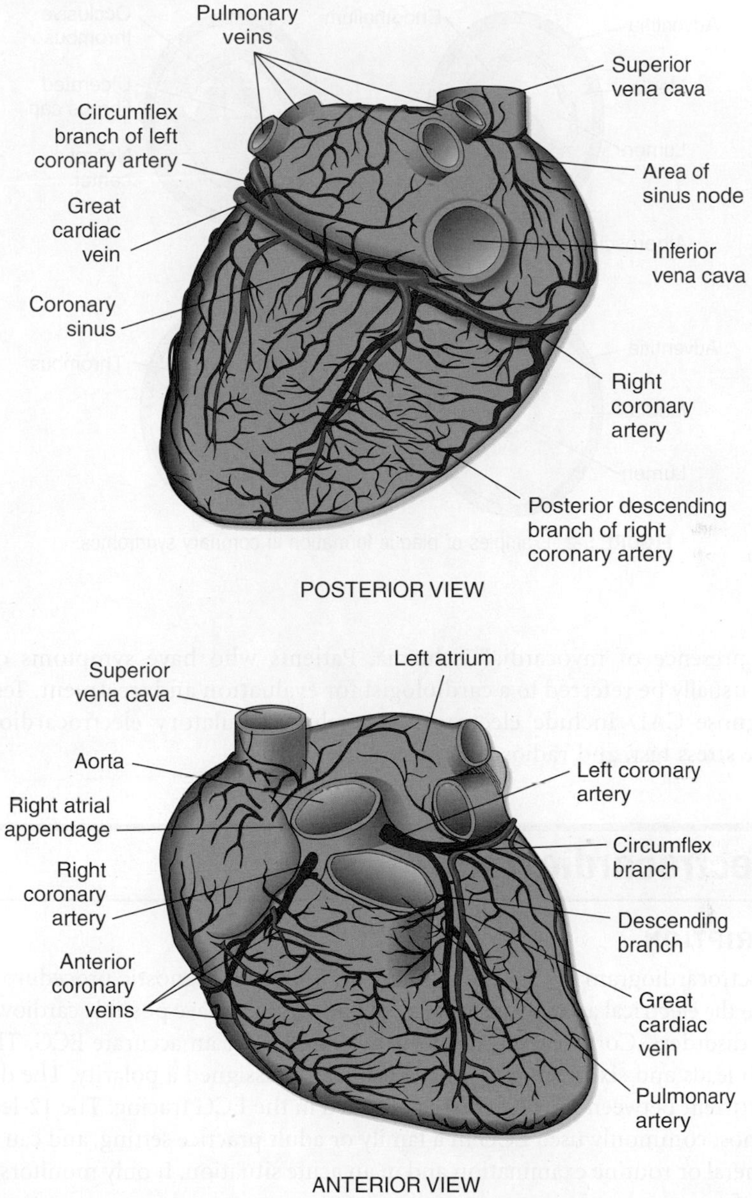

FIGURE 5-1 Anterior and posterior surfaces of the heart, illustrating the location and distribution of the peripheral coronary vessels. (From Koeppen BM, Stanton BA: *Berne & Levy physiology*, ed 6, updated, Philadelphia, 2010, Mosby.)

5

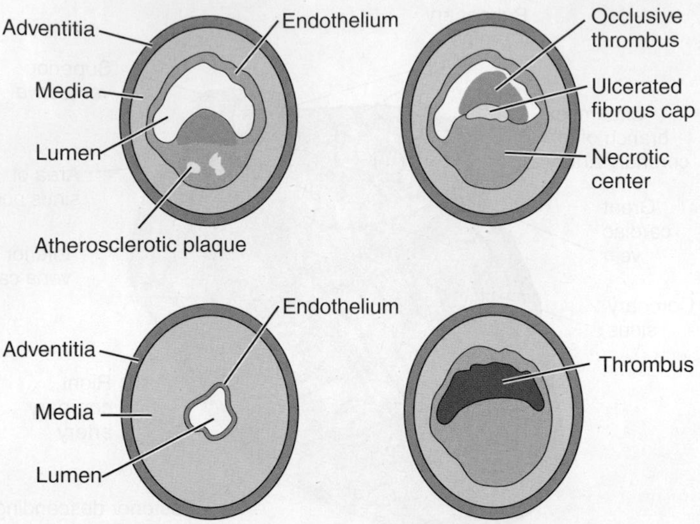

FIGURE 5-2 Examples of plaque formation in coronary syndromes.

in the presence of myocardial ischemia. Patients who have symptoms of CAD should usually be referred to a cardiologist for evaluation and treatment. Tests used to diagnose CAD include electrocardiography, ambulatory electrocardiography, exercise stress test, and radioscopic imaging.

Electrocardiography

DESCRIPTION

The electrocardiogram (ECG) is a routine, noninvasive diagnostic procedure used to evaluate the electrical activity of the heart in patients who have possible cardiovascular-related disorders. Correct lead placement is essential for an accurate ECG. There are six limb leads and six precordial leads. Each lead is assigned a polarity. The direction of the current between the polarities is reflected in the ECG tracing. The 12-lead ECG is the most commonly used ECG in a family or adult practice setting, and can be used in a general or routine examination and in an acute situation. It only monitors cardiac activity for a moment in time.

ANATOMY AND PHYSIOLOGY

The ECG is a recording of the electrical activity of the heart.

INDICATIONS

- Chest pain
- Follow-up of cardiovascular disease
- Preoperative evaluation
- Differential diagnosis of:
  - Ischemic heart disease

- Myocardial infarction (MI)
- Cardiomyopathy
- Arrhythmias
- Pericarditis
- Electrolyte abnormalities
- Endocarditis
- Drug toxicity

- Chest trauma
- Pacemaker function
- Use before defibrillation/cardioversion

CONTRAINDICATIONS

There are none; it is a noninvasive procedure.

PRECAUTIONS

- Accurate findings depend on correct lead placement (Figure 5-3).
- It is important that practitioners become familiar with the equipment in their facility. The manufacturer's instruction manual should be read.
- A normal ECG does not rule out CAD.
- A trained expert must be involved in the proper reading of the ECG.

ASSESSMENT

- Take a complete history.
- Conduct a complete cardiac examination.
- Look for risk factors for MI/CAD.

PATIENT PREPARATION

- The procedure requires patients to lie still on the back for several minutes.
- The ECG is noninvasive; it will not hurt or shock the patient.

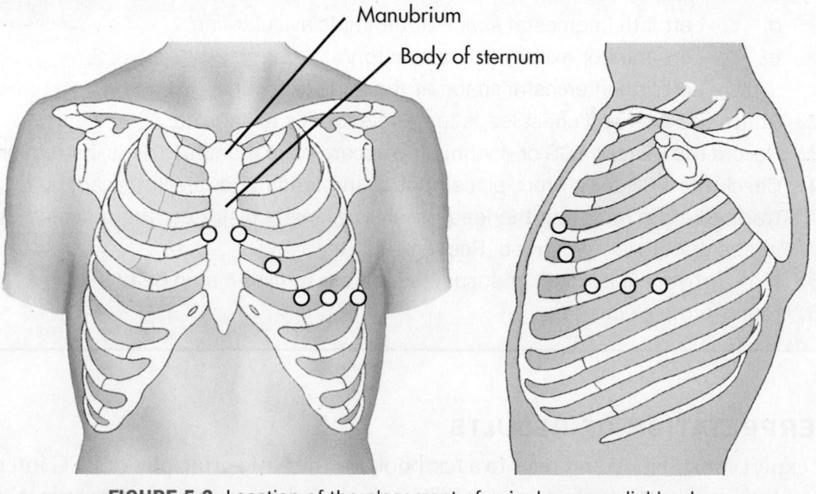

FIGURE 5-3 Location of the placement of unipolar precordial leads.

EQUIPMENT

- ECG machine with limb and chest leads and cables
- ECG paper
- Electrodes
- Grounded safe electrical outlet or charged battery

Procedure

1. Place the patient in a flat, supine position.
2. Plug in the machine.
3. Enter the patient's identification according to manufacturer's instructions.
4. Set the speed at 25 mm/sec and the sensitivity at 10 mm/mV.
5. Prepare the skin by cleaning it with an alcohol wipe if it is dirty or oily.
6. If the patient has so much hair on the chest that it prevents good electrical contact, clip hair, wipe area with alcohol, and dry.
7. Place the electrode onto the extremities and the chest. Figure 5-3 shows the correct placement.

LIMB LEADS

1. Avoid muscular and bony prominences.
2. On the legs, place the electrode on the distal third of the lower legs on the anterior medial surface.
3. On the upper extremities, place the lead on the volar surfaces of the distal third of the forearms.
4. If artifact is persistent, move lead closer to trunk.

CHEST PLACEMENT FOR ELECTROCARDIOGRAPHIC LEADS

1. Place leads V_1 through V_6 (see Figure 5-3).
   a. V_1—Fourth intercostal space at the right sternal border
   b. V_2—Fourth intercostal space at the left sternal border
   c. V_3—Halfway between V_2 and V_4
   d. V_4—Left fifth intercostal space at the midclavicular line
   e. V_5—Left anterior axillary line lateral to V_4
   f. V_6—Left fifth intercostal space at the midaxillary line
2. Attach the limb and chest leads to the electrodes as labeled.
3. Record the 12-lead ECG or rhythm strip according to manufacturer's instructions.
4. Check the ECG for correct placement of the leads and check the adequacy of tracing before removing the leads. If the tracing is distorted, the machine may not be adequately grounded. Recheck and try again.
5. If an arrhythmia is noted or suspected, obtain a rhythm strip (lead II).
6. Remove the electrodes.

INTERPRETATION OF RESULTS

Seek expert consultation and refer to a textbook for the basic principles of ECG interpretation. A typical pattern of a normal ECG is included to assist with determination of whether leads have been placed correctly (Figure 5-4). Computer-aided interpretation

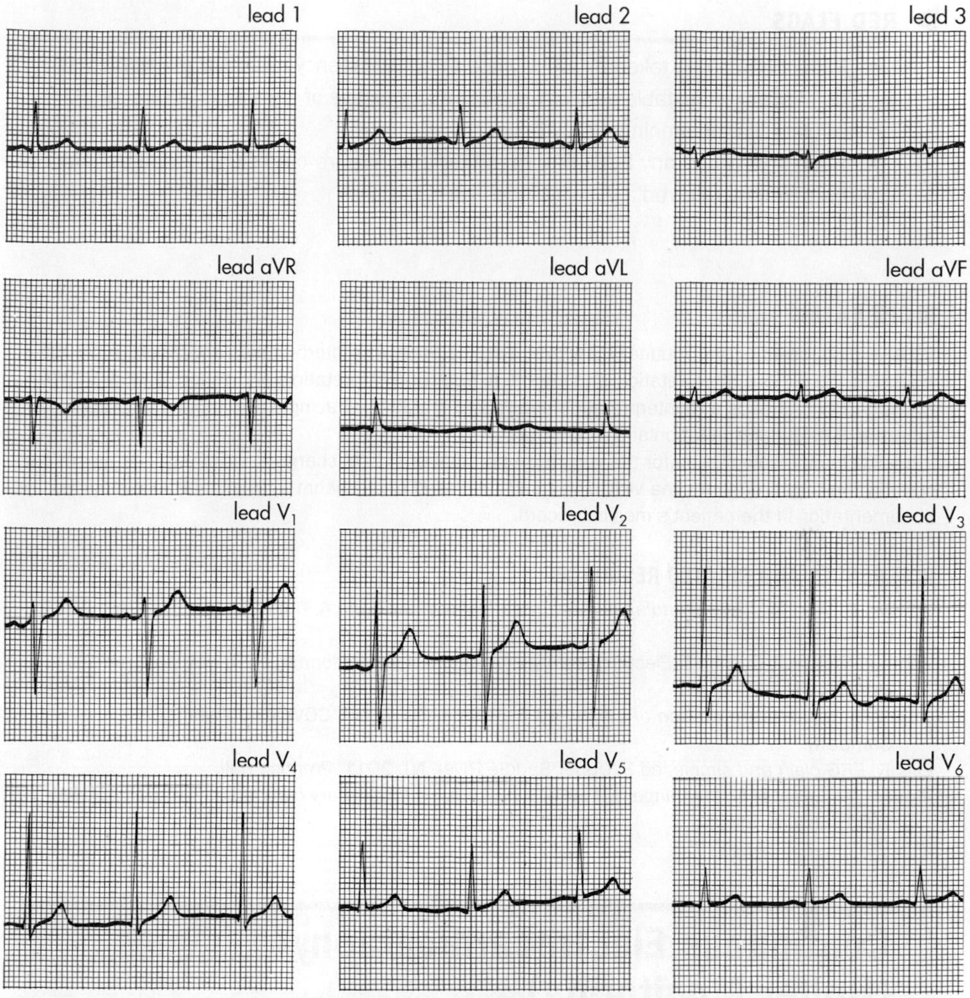

FIGURE 5-4 Normal 12-lead electrocardiogram.

of ECGs is widespread and reliable, but should be validated by an expert who is trained in ECG interpretation.

PATIENT EDUCATION POSTPROCEDURE

- Reassure the patient.
- Review the results and their implications with the patient.

COMPLICATIONS

- To eliminate erroneous tracings and misinterpretation of the ECG, correct electrode placement must be ensured.
- Check the ECG by looking for erroneous configurations.

PRACTITIONER FOLLOW-UP

Review ECG results with the patient and determine whether the patient needs consultation with a cardiologist.

RED FLAGS

- Patient should be taken by ambulance to an emergency room if a medical condition becomes unstable and/or the ECG is suggestive of myocardial infarction (MI) or other life-threatening dysrhythmias.
- Patient who has any ECG abnormalities that require cardiology consult should be promptly referred.

CPT BILLING

93000—Electrocardiogram, routine ECG with at least 12 leads; with interpretation and report ■ **93005**—Tracing only, without interpretation and report ■ **93010**—Interpretation and report only ■ **93040**—Rhythm ECG, 1-3 leads with interpretation and report ■ **93041**—Tracing only without interpretation or report ■ **93042**—Interpretation and report only

If the ECG is the sole reason for the visit, then no additional E/M charge is indicated. The procedure code is the only charge for the visit. The need for the ECG or rhythm strip should be supported by documentation in the patient's medical record.

REFERENCES AND RELATED RESOURCES

Beasley B, West M: *Understanding EKGs: a practical approach*, ed 4, Upper Saddle River, NJ, 2013, Prentice Hall.

Booth K, DeiTos P, O'Brien T: *Electrocardiology for health care personnel*, ed 3, New York, NY, 2011, McGraw-Hill.

Dubin D: *Rapid interpretation of EKG's*, ed 6, Tampa, FL, 2000, COVER Publishing Company.

Ellis K: *EKG plain and simple*, ed 3, Upper Saddle River, NJ, 2011, Prentice Hall.

Pfenninger J, Fowler G: *Pfenninger & Fowler's procedures for primary care*, ed 3, Philadelphia, PA, 2011, Elsevier Mosby.

Continuous Electrocardiography (Holter Monitoring)

DESCRIPTION

Holter monitoring involves 24-hour monitoring of a patient's ECG. The purpose is to document episodes of abnormal cardiac electrical behavior in the patient who is ambulatory. It is a standard monitoring procedure for frequently occurring arrhythmias. Holter monitoring can also be used to identify silent ischemia, drug effects on the heart, and pacemaker function.

ANATOMY AND PHYSIOLOGY

Myocardial ischemia and cardiac arrhythmias may be prompted at different times of the day or night by food, activity, or stress. Sometimes a continuous tracing, correlated with an activity diary, will help in the diagnosis of troublesome symptoms. In addition, patients who are taking medications that can have cardiac side effects and those who use pacemakers can be monitored continuously for brief periods of time.

INDICATIONS

- Evaluation of patients who have periodic symptoms such as chest pain, dizziness, palpitations, or syncope.
- Further evaluation of patients who have an abnormal ECG or a history suggestive of ischemic disease or arrhythmias.
- Evaluation of an antiarrhythmic drug treatment or pacemaker function.
- Evaluation of patients who have cardiac disease and a possible correlation between cardiac events and daily activities.

CONTRAINDICATIONS

Patients whose history or physical examination is suggestive of acute ischemia should receive emergency treatment.

PRECAUTIONS

- A standard 12-lead ECG should be obtained before ambulatory electrocardiography is performed.
- In order to correctly diagnose the patient, correct placement of the electrodes is necessary, especially for the detection of myocardial ischemia.
- Caution: This test can be expensive, so cost should be a consideration when ordering this procedure.
- Some patients develop strong emotional reactions or fears to this type of testing.

ASSESSMENT

- Evaluate patient's radial and apical pulse.
- Listen to heart sounds with stethoscope and evaluate rate, rhythm, and pattern of any irregularity.

PATIENT PREPARATION

- Explain the importance of keeping an event diary.
- Give the patient an event diary with columns for time, symptom or feeling, and activity.
- The patient should record the time and describe the symptom if he or she experiences the target symptom or any other episode of chest pain, dizziness, palpitation, syncope, or unusual symptom.
- The patient should keep a record of the time and his or her activities even if no symptoms are experienced.
- If the patient is unable to keep a diary, he or she should enlist the help of a caregiver.
- Instruct the patient to not take a shower or bath during the 24 hours the monitor is in use.

TREATMENT ALTERNATIVES

Holter monitors are appropriate for patients for whom primary care monitoring seems safe and who are able to follow directions and cooperate. Most monitors use a continuous 24-hour recording. Also available are intermittent records, which record only a limited number of episodes, when the patient is experiencing the symptom in question.

EQUIPMENT

- Holter monitor with new batteries
- Case with strap
- Cable and lead wires (lead attachment kit)
- Printer, paper, ink, and extra cassettes
- Razor or clippers
- Alcohol wipes
- Electrode
- Extra batteries
- Activity diary or logbook

Procedure

1. Refer to the manufacturer's instruction manual supplied with the machine.
2. Install fresh batteries and a new tape in the machine.
3. Prepare the skin using alcohol wipes.
4. Clip or shave hair where electrodes will be placed, if necessary.
5. Position patient in an upright, sitting position.
6. Apply electrodes by removing the backing material, pressing them firmly in place, and attaching the leads to the chest (Figure 5-5).
7. Attach the cables to the monitor.
8. Ensure that the monitor is working correctly by printing out a sample rhythm strip.
9. Place the monitor strap around the patient's neck.
10. Place the monitor in a case and put the case on the patient.
11. Place leads/cables through the front of the patient's shirt or blouse.
12. Give the patient a diary to take home to record symptoms.
13. Have the patient return in 24 hours to have the Holter monitor removed and obtain a copy of the patient's activity diary.

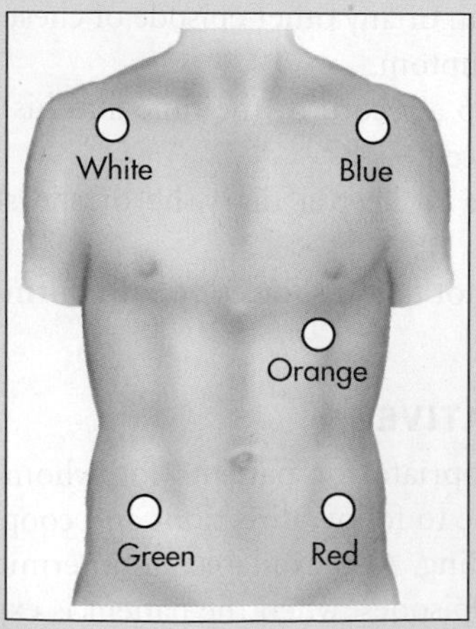

FIGURE 5-5 Lead placement for a Holter monitor.

INTERPRETATION OF RESULTS

- Interpretation of the results of Holter monitoring is beyond the scope of this book; it requires a specialist's review and interpretation.
- It is important to look for correlations between symptoms and arrhythmias.
- Premature ventricular contractions (PVCs) are common in the general population and increase in frequency with increasing age. The presence of PVCs alone does not necessarily indicate heart disease.

PATIENT EDUCATION POSTPROCEDURE

- Give general information to the patient about when the results will be available. Definitive interpretation will be provided by a cardiologist in a written report.
- Wear loose-fitting clothes.
- Avoid getting electrodes or Holter monitor wet.
- Avoid magnets, metal detectors (in airports), and high-voltage areas.
- Instruct the patient to return to the clinic if the monitor lead is dislodged.

COMPLICATIONS

There are none.

PRACTITIONER FOLLOW-UP

Review Holter monitor results with the patient.

▶ RED FLAG

Patients should be referred to a cardiologist if significant abnormalities are found on the Holter monitor recording.

■ CPT BILLING

93224—External electrocardiographic recording up to 48 hours by continuous rhythm recording and storage; includes recording, scanning analysis with report, review and interpretation by a physician or other qualified health care professional.

REFERENCES AND RELATED RESOURCES

Booth K, DeiTos P, O'Brien T: *Electrocardiology for health care personnel*, ed 3, New York, NY, 2011, McGraw-Hill.

Colyar M, Ehrhardt C: *Ambulatory care procedures for the nurse practitioner*, ed 2, Philadelphia, PA, 2004, F.A. Davis Company.

Mathur N, Seutter R, Levine G: Holter monitors, event monitors, ambulatory monitors, and implantable loop recorders. In *Cardiology secrets*, ed 4, St. Louis, MO, 2013, W.B. Saunders Company, 60–67.

Pfenninger J, Fowler G: *Pfenninger & Fowler's procedures for primary care*, ed 3, Philadelphia, PA, 2011, Elsevier Mosby.

Ankle-Brachial Index

DESCRIPTION

The ankle-brachial index (ABI) is a noninvasive vascular screening test used in the initial screening to help objectively assess for the presence of lower extremity PAD.

The ABI measurement is obtained by recording the brachial artery systolic pressure of each arm and the systolic pressures for the posterior tibial and dorsalis pedis arteries for each ankle. The result is reported as a ratio with the ankle systolic pressure in the numerator and the higher brachial pressure in the denominator. The ABI is calculated for both legs, and the lower of the two values is recorded in the patient's results.

ANATOMY AND PHYSIOLOGY

The normal arteries in the leg are shown in Figure 5-6.

Atherosclerosis is the primary cause of PAD. Arterial plaques obstruct the normal arterial blood flow to the extremities. This is generally part of systemic arteriosclerosis. Patients who have PAD usually have plaque disease in the arteries of the brain, heart, kidneys, and other vasculature regions in the body.

INDICATIONS

- Aids in the diagnosis of chronic venous insufficiency and deep venous thrombosis
- Aids in the diagnosis of peripheral arterial insufficiency and arterial occlusion
- Monitor clients who have had an invasive arterial procedure and/or clients who have undergone arterial reconstruction and bypass grafts

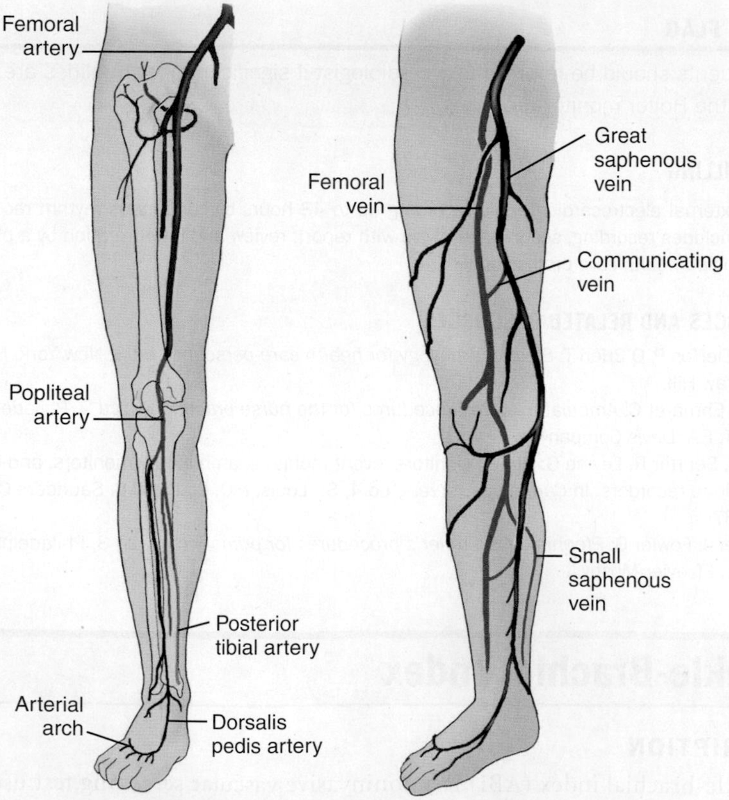

FIGURE 5-6 Normal arteries and veins in the leg.

- In a patient who is asymptomatic, perform a vascular examination and assess for PAD risk factors.

CONTRAINDICATIONS

- Patients who are unable to lie supine for the length of the procedure
- Patients in whom use of an occlusive sphygmomanometer may worsen an extremity injury
- Acute deep vein thrombophlebitis

PRECAUTIONS

- May fail to detect mild arteriosclerotic plaques and smaller thrombi
- May fail to detect major calf vein thrombosis, so the practitioner should be alert for other signs and symptoms
- May fail to detect abnormalities in patients who have obese legs or extensive leg swelling
- Is invalid in patients who have calcified vessels, as in some patients who are diabetic
- A cold room will cause vasoconstriction and invalidate the results

ASSESSMENT

- Symptoms of PAD
  - Intermittent claudication, progressing to resting limb pain, gangrene, and amputation
  - Pain provoked by predictable exercise and relieved by cessation of activity within 2 to 3 minutes
  - Nocturnal leg cramps that are not vascular in origin
  - However, resting limb pain, especially when legs are elevated (when gravity is not aiding the blood to the limbs), may be a symptom of severe PAD
- Physical examination
  - Palpate pulses.
  - Auscultate for bruits (neck and abdomen).
  - Elevate the legs; ask the patient to alternately dorsiflex and plantarflex both feet for 30 to 60 seconds. Inspect for pallor.
  - Then have the patient place his or her feet hanging down and observe for return of color (delayed in PAD) to the skin. Rubor (redness) on dependency and pallor or cyanosis on elevation are characteristic of PAD. Coldness, delayed color return, and venous filling may also be found in PAD.
  - Examination of the feet may reveal ischemic ulcers, fissures, calluses, tinea, and/or xanthomas.
  - The skin may be thin, shiny, and atrophic with a loss of hair.
  - Examine for other signs of generalized cardiovascular disease, including palpation of abdominal aorta.
- It should be noted that approximately 12% of the population has a congenital absence of a dorsal pedal pulse. However, if a patient does not have a palpable posterior tibial pulse, then he or she is likely to be diagnosed with PAD.

PATIENT PREPARATION

The patient may experience light pressure from the blood pressure cuff and transducer, but he or she will not feel the sound waves.

The patient lies supine on the examination table with a small pillow under the head.

TREATMENT ALTERNATIVES

In patients who have noncompressible vessels (e.g., long-standing diabetes) or are unable to undergo ABI testing, then other vascular diagnostic testing may be performed. This includes duplex sonography, leg segmental pressure measurements, magnetic resonance angiogram (MRA), or arteriogram.

EQUIPMENT

- Doppler with probe
- Water-soluble conduction jelly
- Appropriate size sphygmomanometer with arm and thigh cuffs

Procedure

1. Place the patient supine with the head slightly elevated for a minimum of 10 minutes before the procedure. The patient should be relaxed and comfortable. The patient's legs should be slightly abducted and externally rotated, with the knees slightly flexed.
2. Apply cuff to upper arm with the bottom edge 2.5 cm above the antecubital space. Arm should be relaxed and at the heart level (Figure 5-7).

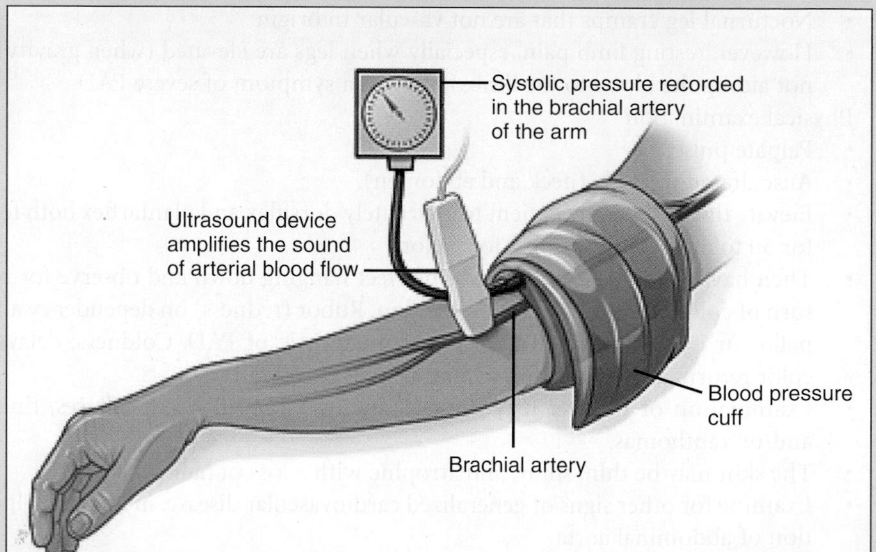

FIGURE 5-7 Brachial systolic blood pressure. (From National Heart, Lung, and Blood Institute: *How is peripheral arterial disease diagnosed?* US Department of Health and Human Services National Institutes of Health, August 2, 2011. http://www.nhlbi.nih.gov/health/health-topics/topics/pad/diagnosis. Accessed March 3, 2015.)

5

3. Palpate the brachial artery to determine its location.
4. Set the Doppler volume control on the lowest setting.
5. Apply the conduction gel over the pulse site.
6. Hold the Doppler probe against the skin at a 45-degree angle, pointing it toward the heart, until a pulse signal is obtained.
7. Inflate the cuff to 20 to 30 mm Hg above the point that the pulse is no longer audible.
8. Deflate the cuff at a rate of 2 to 3 mm Hg/sec, noting the manometer reading at which the first pulse signal is heard, and record the brachial systolic pressure.
9. Remove the cuff and clean the gel from the skin.
10. Repeat the procedure on the other arm.
11. Apply the appropriate size blood pressure cuff to ankle with bottom of cuff approximately 2.5 cm above the malleolus (Figure 5-8).
12. Measure both the dorsalis pedis and posterior tibial artery pressures in each leg. The higher and stronger pressures will be used to calculate the ABI.
13. Apply conduction gel over the pulse site.
14. Place the Doppler probe at a 45-degree angle, pointing it toward the knee, until a pulse signal is obtained.
15. Inflate the cuff to 20 to 30 mm Hg above the point the pulse is no longer audible.
16. Deflate the cuff at a rate of 2 to 3 mm Hg/sec, noting the manometer reading at which the first pulse signal is heard, and record the systolic pressure.
17. Remove the cuff and clean the gel from the skin.
18. Repeat the procedure on the other arm.

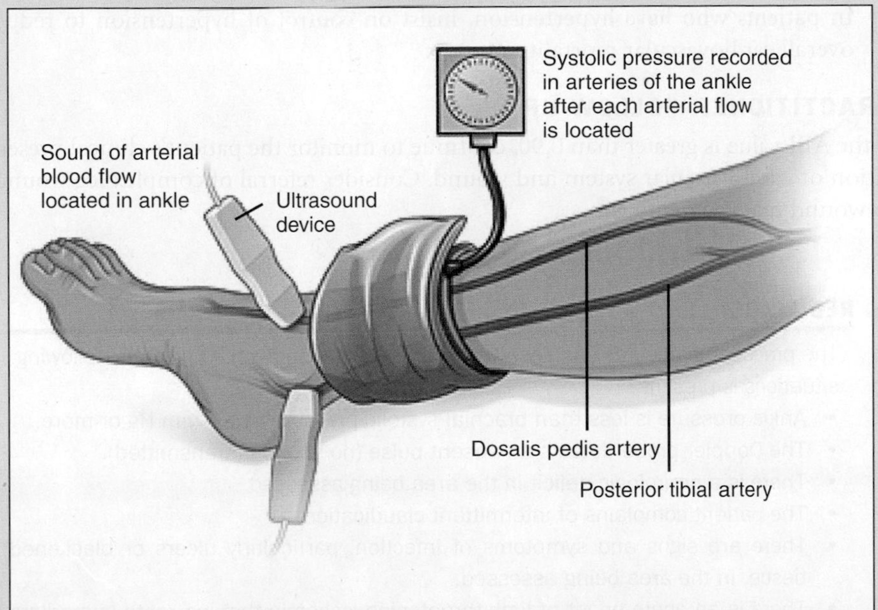

FIGURE 5-8 Ankle systolic blood pressure. (From National Heart, Lung, and Blood Institute: *How is peripheral arterial disease diagnosed?* US Department of Health and Human Services National Institutes of Health, August 2, 2011. http://www.nhlbi.nih.gov/health/health-topics/topics/pad/diagnosis. Accessed March 3, 2015.)

INTERPRETATION OF RESULTS

- Venous flow—Normal flow is continuous and equal bilaterally.
- Arterial flow—Normal ankle pressure is equal to or slightly greater than the brachial pressure. Calculate the ABI for both ankles by dividing the ankle systolic pressure by the brachial systolic pressure. An ABI value within 1.00 to 1.40 is considered normal, 0.91 to 0.99 is borderline, and 0.90 or less is abnormal. An ABI value greater than 1.40 is interpreted as noncompressible with severely calcified vessels.
- Note any differences between the extremities (>5-10 mm Hg). In particular if there is a greater than 15 to 20 mm Hg difference between the upper arm systolic pressures, which may suggest subclavian stenosis.

PATIENT EDUCATION POSTPROCEDURE

- For patients who have documented venous insufficiency:
  - Recommend the use of support stockings.
  - Instruct the patient to keep his or her legs elevated whenever possible.
  - Warn the patient to avoid constrictive clothing.
- For patients with documented arterial insufficiency:
  - Encourage gentle exercise, such as walking, to aid in the development of collateral circulation.
- Strongly encourage patients to stop smoking and provide smoking cessation interventions. If the patient has diabetes mellitus, encourage glycemic control, because this may slow the development of peripheral neuropathy.
- Encourage dietary control of cholesterol and weight reduction.
- In patients who have hypertension, insist on control of hypertension to reduce overall cardiovascular mortality rates.

PRACTITIONER FOLLOW-UP

If the ABI value is greater than 0.90, continue to monitor the patient's clinical presentation of cardiovascular system and wound. Consider referral of complex leg wounds to wound management team.

RED FLAGS

The practitioner should consider referral to a vascular surgeon if any of the following situations is present:

- Ankle pressure is less than brachial systolic pressure by 30 mm Hg or more.
- The Doppler probe detects an absent pulse (no sound is transmitted).
- There is a neurologic deficit in the area being assessed.
- The patient complains of intermittent claudication.
- There are signs and symptoms of infection, particularly ulcers or blackened tissue, in the area being assessed.
- There is an acute onset of limb-threatening ischemia that warrants immediate attention by a vascular surgeon. These patients usually present with severe, acute pain; an absence of pulse; coldness; pallor; and impaired motor and sensory function of the affected limb.

■ CPT BILLING

93922—Limited bilateral noninvasive physiologic studies of upper or lower extremity arteries (e.g., for lower extremity: ankle/brachial indices at distal posterior tibial and anterior tibial/dorsalis pedis arteries plus bidirectional, Doppler waveform recording and analysis at 1-2 levels, or ankle/brachial indices at distal posterior tibial and anterior tibial/dorsalis pedis arteries plus volume plethysmography at 1-2 levels, or ankle/brachial indices at distal posterior tibial and anterior tibial/dorsalis pedis arteries with, transcutaneous oxygen tension measurement at 1-2 levels).

When only one arm or leg is available for study, report 93922 with modifier 52 for a unilateral study when recording 1-2 levels. Report 93922 when recording 3 or more levels or performing provocative functional maneuvers.

Report 93922 only once in the upper extremity(s) and/or once in the lower extremity(s). When both the upper and lower extremities are evaluated in the same setting, 93922 may be reported twice by adding modifier 59 to the second procedure.

93965—Noninvasive physiologic studies of extremity veins, complete bilateral study ■ **93970**—Duplex scan of extremity veins including responses to compression and other maneuvers; complete bilateral study ■ **93971**—Unilateral or limited study

REFERENCES AND RELATED RESOURCES

Al-Qaisi M, Nott D, King D, Kaddoura S: Ankle brachial pressure index (ABPI): an update for practitioners, *Vasc Health Risk Manag* 5:833–841, 2009.

Khan T, Farooqui F, Niazi K: Critical review of the ankle brachial index, *Curr Cardiol Rev* 4:101–108, 2008.

Park C: *Ankle-brachial index measurement*, 2013. http://emedicine.medscape.com/article/1839449. Accessed May 29, 2015.

Rooke T, Hirsch A, Misra S, et al: 2011 ACCF/AHA focused update of the guideline for the management of patients with peripheral artery disease (updating the 2005 guideline), *Circulation* 124:2020–2045, 2011.

Wound Ostomy and Continence Nurses Society: *Ankle-brachial index: best practice for clinicians* 2005. http://www.qsource.org/toolkits/pressureUlcer/docs/articles/whitePapers/abi.pdf. Accessed May 29, 2015.

5

6

Gastrointestinal Procedures

Joanne Rolls

This chapter contains a variety of procedures for the *gastrointestinal* (GI) *tract.* The two upper GI procedures share the common requirement of the insertion of a *nasogastric tube* (NGT). The three lower intestinal procedures require similar evaluations of the rectal area to make a diagnosis. Thus an explanation of both relevant upper and lower GI anatomy is helpful in understanding these procedures.

ANATOMY AND PHYSIOLOGY

Upper Gastrointestinal Tract

At the beginning of the GI tract, the mouth opening into the *pharynx* is about 12.5 cm (or 5 inches) long and is divided into three portions: the nasopharynx, oropharynx, and laryngopharynx. The uppermost portion of the tube just behind the nasal cavities is the *nasopharynx;* the portion behind the mouth is the *oropharynx;* and the last or lowest portion is the *laryngopharynx.*

The pharynx as a whole serves to pass food to the stomach and air to the lungs. Air enters the pharynx from two nasal cavities and the mouth and exits via the larynx; food enters the pharynx from the mouth and is moved downward into the esophagus. The epiglottis partially covers the opening into the larynx, closing off the larynx during swallowing to prevent food from entering into the trachea (Figure 6-1).

Lower Gastrointestinal Tract

At the lower end of the GI tract, the *anus* is the final structure, opening out of the body. The anus is connected to the *rectum,* the lower 10 to 15 cm of the large intestine (Figure 6-2).

The *valves of Houston,* which are in the rectum, are not true valves, but prominent mucosal folds. The dentate or pectinate line divides the squamous epithelium from the mucosal or columnar epithelium. There are four to eight anal glands that drain into the crypts of Morgagni at the level of the dentate line, and the glands are the site of most rectal abscesses and fistulas. The dentate line also marks the end of sensory fibers. Above (proximal to) the dentate line, the rectum has nerve fibers for stretch, but not the fibers that carry pain. Thus many surgical procedures can be performed without anesthesia above the dentate line; however, there is extreme sensitivity beneath the dentate line because the perianal area is one of

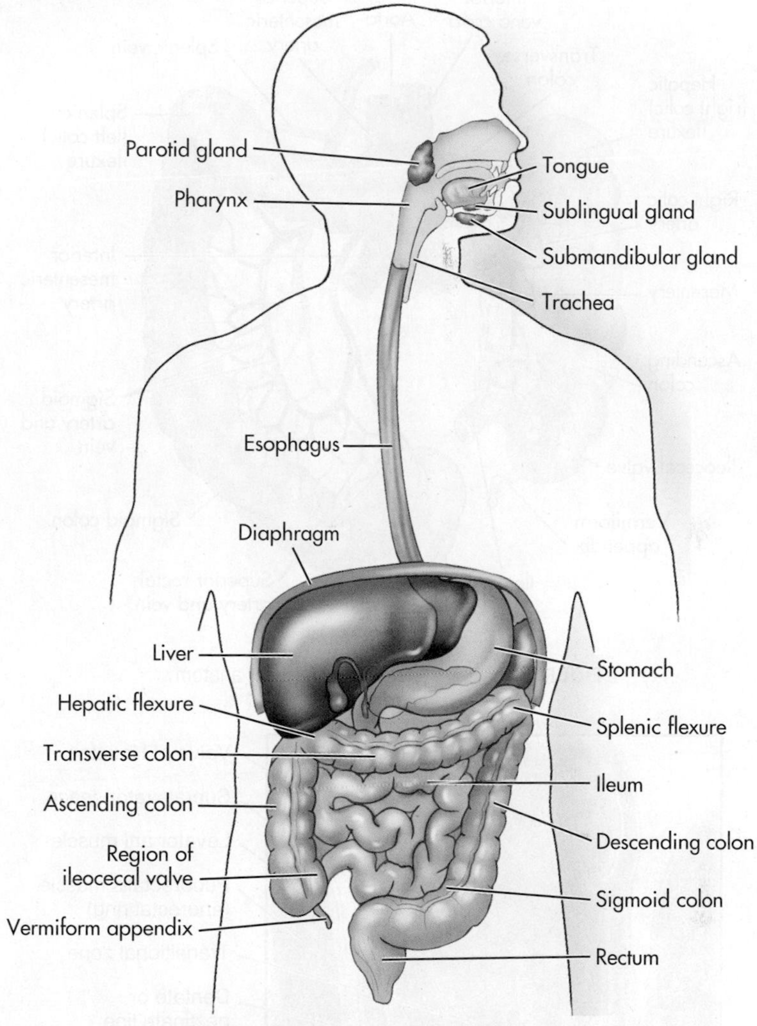

FIGURE 6-1 Gastrointestinal tract anatomy.

the more sensitive areas of the body. Muscles of both the involuntary internal sphincter and voluntary external sphincter are involved in the evacuation of bowel contents.

The *anal canal* (Figure 6-3) is created by invagination of the ectoderm and the rectum by invagination of the endoderm. The resultant anatomic differences are important in the evaluation and treatment of anorectal disorders. The anal canal is lined with anoderm, a continuation of the external skin; the rectal lining is composed of red, glistening glandular mucosa. At the superior boundary of the anal canal is the *anorectal junction* (pectinate line, mucocutaneous junction, dentate line), the location of 8 to 12 anal crypts and 5 to 8 papillae. The crypts provide the environment for the development of anorectal abscesses and fistulas.

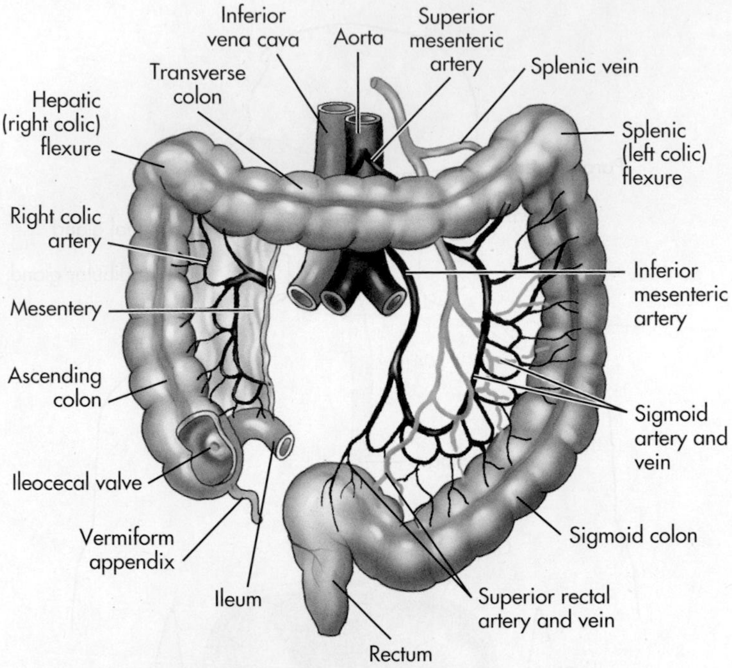

FIGURE 6-2 Lower gastrointestinal tract anatomy.

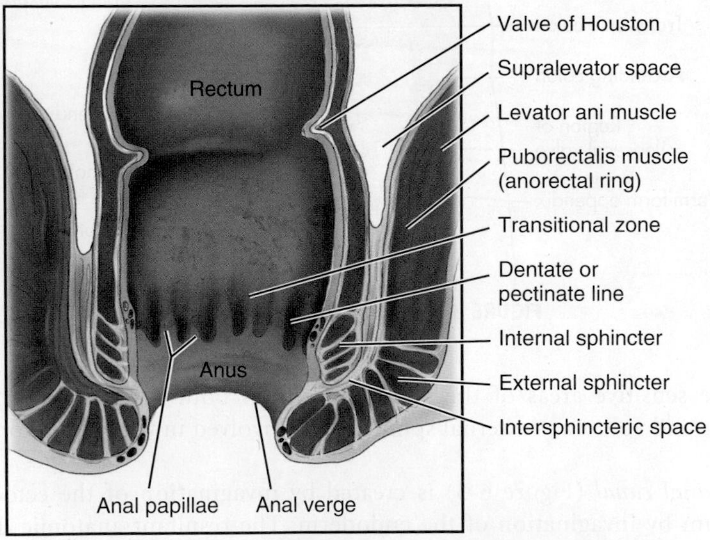

FIGURE 6-3 Anatomy of the anal canal.

The *sphincteric ring* encircling the anal canal is composed of the fusion of the internal sphincter, the central portion of the levators, and the components of the external sphincter. Anteriorly, it is more vulnerable to trauma, which can result in incontinence. The muscular sling around the rectum is called the *puborectalis*, and it provides support and assistance in defecation.

The venous and lymphatic distribution in the rectal area explains how malignant disease and infection are easily spread. Venous drainage above the anorectal junction occurs through the portal system; the anal canal is drained through the caval system. The area of the anorectal junction can drain into both the portal and caval systems. Lymphatics from the anal canal (Figure 6-4) pass to the internal iliac nodes, the posterior vaginal wall (in women), and the inguinal nodes, whereas lymphatic return from the rectum occurs along the superior hemorrhoidal vascular pedicle to the inferior mesenteric and aortic nodes.

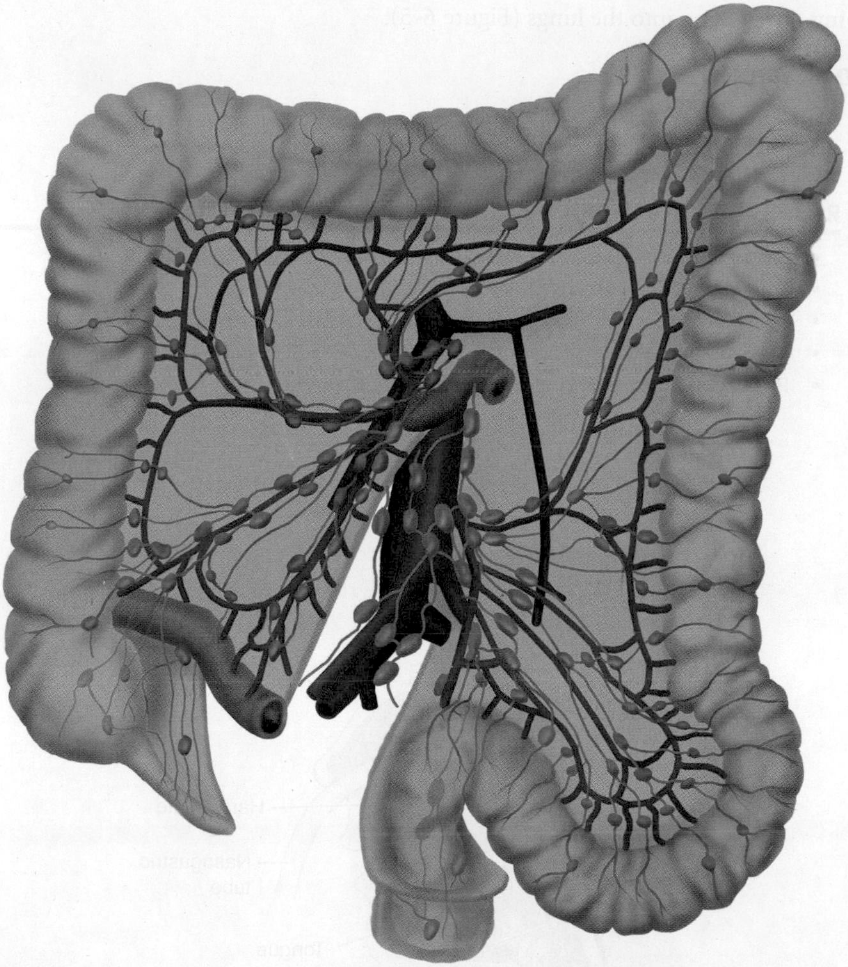

FIGURE 6-4 Efferent lymph vessels and regional lymph nodes of the vermiform appendix, cecum, colon, sigmoid, and superior part of the rectum. (From Földi M et al: *Földi's textbook of lymphology*, ed 3, 2012, © Elsevier GmbH, Urban & Fischer, Munich.)

Nasogastric Tube Insertion and Removal

DESCRIPTION

The placement of an NGT is a clean procedure that is used for both diagnosis and therapy. The basic procedures for the placement of an NGT and its removal are described here. Gastric lavage using an NGT is discussed in the following procedure.

ANATOMY AND PHYSIOLOGY

As long as the epiglottis is closed, the NGT can easily be passed from either the nose or the mouth and down into the stomach. Care must be exerted to ensure that the tubing does not go into the lungs (Figure 6-5).

INDICATIONS

- Aspiration of stomach contents
- Administration of feedings or medications, if gastric lavage is indicated.

RED FLAGS: SITUATIONS WARRANTING EMERGENCY EVALUATION

- Poisoning with corrosive agents, such as acid and alkali poisoning
- Poisoning with hydrocarbons and petroleum distillates
- Acute seizure
- Maxillofacial or skull trauma
- Possible misplacement of NGT, especially aspiration risk

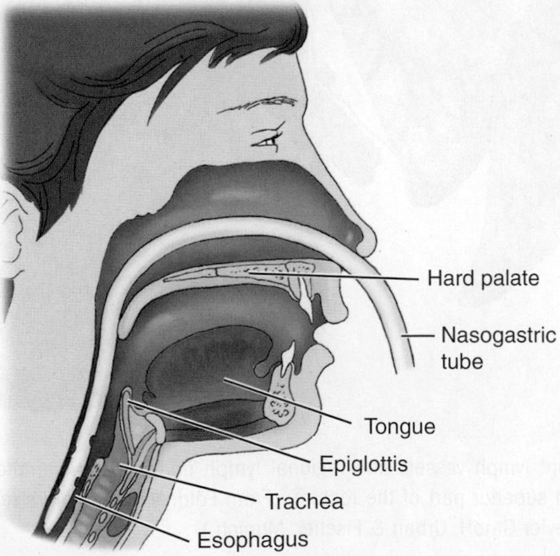

FIGURE 6-5 Anatomy of the pharynx, showing the course of the nasogastric tube.

PRECAUTIONS

- Esophageal perforations and submucosal passage of the NGT are more likely to occur if the NGT is forced during advancement.
- Aspiration potential can be decreased by maintaining the head of the bed at an angle of greater than 30 degrees.
- Mucosal ulcerations of the nose, pharynx, and stomach are less likely to occur if the tube is periodically rotated and irrigated and secured in place without placing pressure on the nose. Pressure occurs when the tube is sharply bent upward as soon as it exits the nostril and is taped down over the nose.
- Proper placement of the NGT should be ascertained before any solutions are administered.
- Head flexion and slow advancement timed with the patient's repeated swallowing help prevent the NGT from entering the larynx and lungs.
- The use of a water-soluble lubricant decreases the risk for lung infection if aspiration should occur.
- Keep the patient nothing by mouth (NPO) and place the patient in a semi- to high Fowler's position for aspiration and lavage.

ASSESSMENT

A relevant history and physical examination should be completed for the patient before the procedure. Careful assessment is also made after the procedure to ensure that the NGT is properly placed in the GI tract and not in the lungs.

PATIENT PREPARATION

Sensations likely to be experienced include gagging (with possible vomiting), tearing, and nasal discomfort. Practitioners should review the methods used to ease NGT insertion with the patient. These include mouth breathing, swallowing, and head flexion or hyperextension. Practitioners should reassure the patient that tissues and an emesis basin are readily available for use as needed.

TREATMENT ALTERNATIVES

- Referral to surgery

EQUIPMENT

- NGT (No. 6, 8, or 12 Levin or No. 14 to 16 French for an adult, a No. 10 French for a child)
- Water-soluble lubricant or 2% viscous lidocaine gel
- Penlight or flashlight
- Waterproof pad or towel
- Stethoscope
- 1-inch hypoallergenic cloth tape
- Safety pin (optional)
- Rubber band (optional)
- Tissues
- Two plastic emesis basins (one for ice and/or warm water in which to soak the NGT, and one in which to empty the gastric contents)
- A 60-ml catheter-tipped syringe with piston
- Clean gloves
- Goggles (optional)
- Glass of water and straw
- Connecting tubing and suction equipment (optional)
- pH paper (optional)
- Clamp for NGT (optional)
- One or two 1-L bottles of sterile normal saline irrigating solution

6

Procedure

1. If the NGT is made of rubber, place it in the plastic basin on ice for at least 5 minutes before insertion. This will increase the tube's rigidity, allowing for easier advancement. If the NGT is made of plastic, however, place it in the basin in warm water. This increases the tube's pliability, making insertion easier.
2. Place a waterproof pad or towel across the patient's chest, and, if possible, elevate the head of the bed to at least 45 degrees.
3. Remove any ill-fitting dentures.
4. Have the patient hyperextend his or her head. Use the penlight or flashlight to observe the nostrils for patency. In addition, occlude each nostril separately and have the patient breathe through the unoccluded nostril. Select the nostril with the best airflow for NGT insertion.
5. Estimate the distance the NGT will need to be inserted for it to reach the stomach by placing the distal end of the NGT at the tip of the nose, extending the tube across to the tip of the earlobe, and then continuing on to the tip of the sternum's xiphoid process. Mark the site on the tube using tape.
6. Lubricate the first 4 inches of the NGT with the water-soluble jelly and coil the tube around your fingers for a few seconds to help stiffen the tube for easier insertion. In addition, the use of a topical anesthetic in the nostril or oropharynx can aid in insertion and certainly improve patient comfort.
7. With the patient's head upright to hyperextended, insert the distal end of the tube into the nostril with the tube curvature following the natural curvature at the nasopharyngeal junction. Gently advance the NGT along the nostril floor and downward toward the patient's ipsilateral ear until the oropharynx is reached. This is when resistance and gagging are encountered (Figure 6-6).

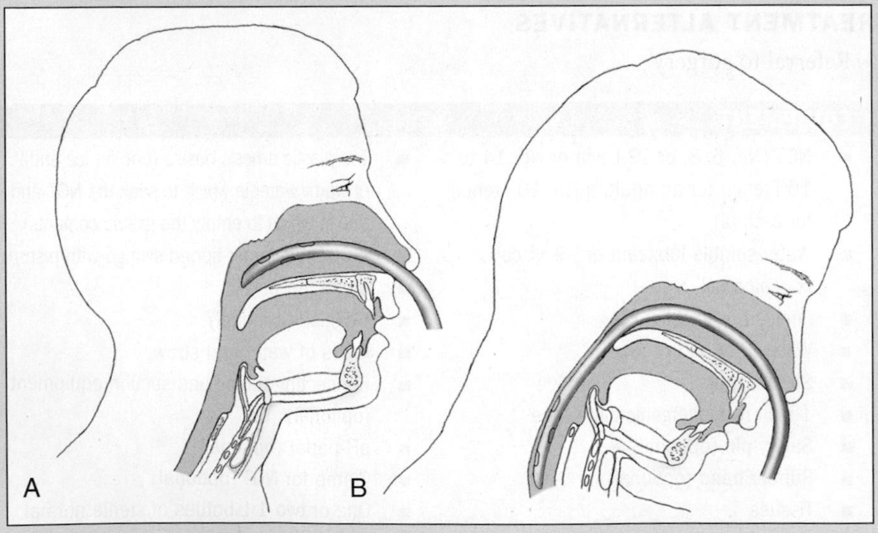

FIGURE 6-6 A, Nasogastric tube insertion. **B,** Have the patient flex the head and gently advance the tube; then, ask the patient to swallow.

8. At this point, have the patient flex his or her head slightly forward and rotate the tube medially 180 degrees toward the contralateral nostril. Have the patient begin swallowing repeatedly (if the patient is not NPO, give him or her the glass of water and straw from which to drink) as the tube is slowly being advanced. Time the advancement attempts with each swallow so that no more than 3 to 5 inches of tubing is advanced with each swallow. Too rapid advancements can lead to NGT coiling in the oropharynx and exiting the mouth. Keep in mind that resistance may be encountered on NGT advancement behind the cricoid cartilage, behind the bifurcation of the bronchus, and at the esophagogastric sphincter.
9. Whenever the patient starts to gag, stop advancing briefly and observe for NGT coiling in the oropharynx or signs of respiratory distress. If any signs of respiratory distress, such as dyspnea or inability to talk, occur, withdraw the tube and reattempt insertion when the patient is not experiencing respiratory distress. When excessive gagging is encountered, have the patient breathe or take small sips of water without advancing the tube to calm the gag reflex.
10. Continue advancing the NGT as previously described once the gag reflex has diminished until the tape mark on the tube reaches the tip of the nose. At this point, temporarily secure the tube in place with tape and check for correct placement of the NGT via x-ray or clinical confirmation.
11. First, aspirate a small amount of fluid to determine whether there are gastric contents present. The fluid should have a pH of less than 7, look clear to yellow, and have mucus present. Gastric contents may be difficult if not impossible to aspirate when a small-bore NGT is inserted.
12. Next, draw up 10 ml of air using the plastic syringe, attach the syringe to the proximal end of the NGT, and place the diaphragm of the stethoscope over the epigastric/stomach area. Instill 10 ml of air and, using the stethoscope, auscultate for a swooshing sound or rush of air, indicating that the tube is likely in the stomach (Figure 6-7).

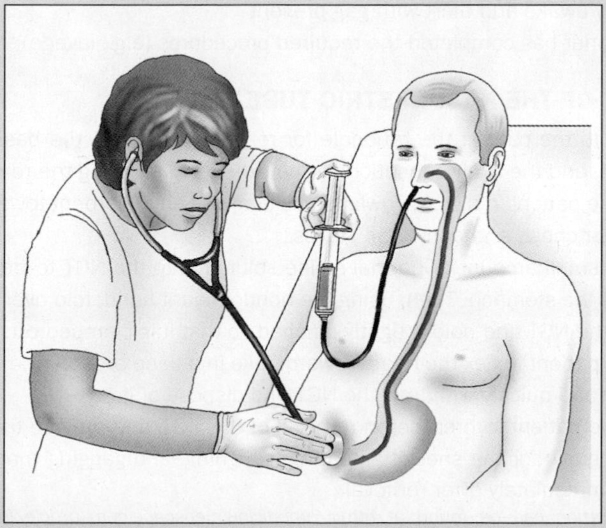

FIGURE 6-7 Injection of air into the nasogastric tube and auscultation help to confirm proper placement of the tube.

13. Then, either leave the syringe attached to the proximal end of the NGT and clamp the NGT, or attach it to suction.
14. Tear off a 4-inch piece of cloth tape and split 2 inches of it vertically. Replace the temporary tape with this tape by placing the unsplit end over the bridge of the nose and wrapping the chevron ends underneath and around the NGT in opposite directions while keeping the NGT straight down from the nose.
15. Finish securing the NGT by wrapping a piece of cloth tape or the rubber band around the tube near the proximal end and pinning it to the patient's gown or clothing OR, if the facility uses a commercial product to secure NGTs, apply it now.
16. Proceed with any other necessary procedures such as gastric emptying, lavage, medication, or feeding administration.
17. Maintain the NGT by periodically rotating and retaping the tube to minimize the potential for mucosal necrosis; keep the mouth, throat, and nostrils moist by using room humidity, throat lozenges or sprays, gum, or hard candy; and clean the nostrils and mouth, applying lubricant to the nostrils frequently. Note the amount, color, consistency, and presence of heme or clots in the gastric drainage/aspirate, residual volumes, and any resistance encountered on flushing or instilling solutions. Note the presence of any abdominal distention, bowel sounds, bowel movements, flatus, nausea, vomiting, and abdominal pain.

CRITERIA FOR REMOVAL OF A NASOGASTRIC TUBE (AS APPLICABLE)

- Decrease in gastric drainage
- Normoactive bowel sounds or flatus
- Absence of abdominal distention
- Ability to tolerate the NGT clamped or straight, and drainage that is without nausea, vomiting, or abdominal distention
- Ability to tolerate sips of clear liquids without nausea, vomiting, or abdominal distention
- Swallowing without difficulty
- Mentally awake and alert with gag present
- Practitioner has completed the required procedures (e.g., lavage)

REMOVAL OF THE NASOGASTRIC TUBE

1. Explain to the patient the rationale for removing the NGT, the basic method of removal, and the likely sensations to be experienced during the removal.
2. Place the patient in a semi-Fowler's position with an absorbent towel or pad over his or her chest, and don clean gloves.
3. Instill a small amount of normal saline solution into the NGT to free it from the lining of the stomach. Then, using the nondominant hand, fold over the proximal end of the NGT and hold it tightly pinched so that it is clamped off.
4. Ask the patient to flex the head forward, take in a deep breath, and hold it. Then, steadily and quickly withdraw the NGT and dispose of it.
5. Allow the patient to breathe on removal of the NGT, and provide tissues and an emesis basin for the sneezing, tearing, coughing, and gagging that are likely to ensue immediately after removal.

Video of insertion can be found at http://emedicine.medscape.com/article/80925-overview under "Multimedia Library."

Additional video can be found at https://www.youtube.com/watch?v=fwEx9C7r9gg.

COMPLICATIONS

- Submucosal, intracranial, or pulmonary passage of the NGT
- Esophageal perforation
- Mucosal ulcerations of the nose, pharynx, or stomach
- Aspiration of stomach contents into the lungs, leading to pneumonia

PRACTITIONER FOLLOW-UP

Monitor the patient for the next 48 hours for nausea, vomiting, abdominal distention, and food intolerance.

■ CPT BILLING

There are no CPT codes for insertion of an NG tube unless it requires a physician's skill and fluoroscopic guidance.

REFERENCES AND RELATED RESOURCES

Ellett M: What is known about methods of correctly placing gastric tubes in adults and children, *Gastroenterol Nurs* 27(6):253–259, 2004.

Metheny N, Meert K, Clouse R: Complications related to feeding tube placement, *Curr Opin Gastroenterol* 23(2):178–182, 2007.

Shlamovitz G: *Nasogastric intubation*, 2014. http://emedicine.medscape.com/article/80925-overview. Accessed January 12, 2015.

St. George's AVMS: *Nasogastric tube insertion, clinical skills series*, 2013. http://www.youtube.com/watch?v=fwEx9C7r9gg. Accessed January 12, 2015.

Gastric Lavage

DESCRIPTION

Gastric lavage is the process of washing the stomach of its contents (i.e., blood and toxins) for purposes of arresting bleeding or decreasing the systemic absorption of poisonous substances. Lavage is used to prepare the stomach for a diagnostic procedure or to obtain gastric washing specimens for analysis.

ANATOMY AND PHYSIOLOGY

At times, the contents of the stomach have to be removed, either for diagnostic analysis or because they contain substances that would be harmful to the body. The lower esophageal sphincter at the bottom of the esophagus is easily penetrated so that the stomach itself can be easily assessed (Figure 6-8).

INDICATIONS

- Upper GI bleeding
- Poisoning with a noncorrosive agent, especially within 1 hour of ingestion
- Drug overdose, especially within 1 hour of ingestion
- Acquisition of fresh gastric washing specimens for cytology and analysis
- Preparation for diagnostic testing (e.g., endoscopy)

CONTRAINDICATIONS

- Poisoning with corrosive agents (e.g., acid and alkali poisoning)
- Poisoning with hydrocarbons and petroleum distillates
- Poisoning when agent identification is unclear

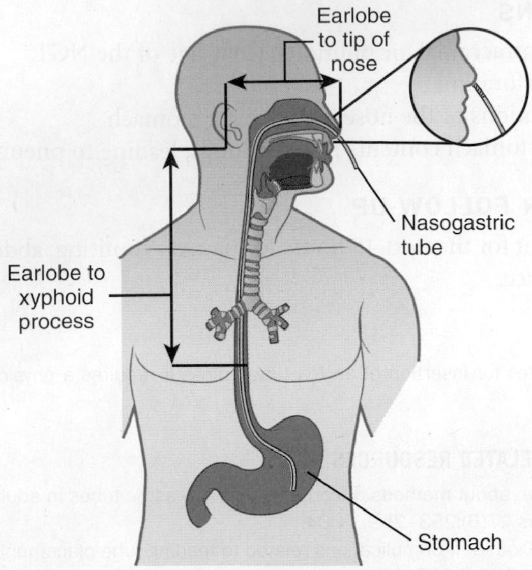

FIGURE 6-8 Stomach contents are removed in lavage.

- Acute seizure
- Any airway compromise
- Patient who has bowel obstruction, ileus, and/or perforation

RED FLAGS

- Hemodynamic instability
- Suspected central nervous system depression or airway compromise
- Suspected upper GI bleeding

PRECAUTIONS

- Proper placement of the NGT should be ascertained before the administration of any solutions.
- There is substantial debate about the use of gastric lavage in patients who are poisoned when risks are compared with its possible benefits.

ASSESSMENT

- Take a medical history and conduct a physical examination to determine potential sites of bleeding and to ascertain the type of poison ingested. Relevant past and present medical histories should be obtained, such as a history of congestive heart failure. In poisoning, the timing, type and amount of the substance ingested, and the age, weight, and gender of the patient can help determine the appropriate treatment.

PATIENT PREPARATION

- The patient should be kept NPO and placed in a semi- to high Fowler's position for aspiration and lavage.
- Sensations likely to be experienced include gagging (with possible vomiting) and nasal discomfort.

TREATMENT ALTERNATIVES

- Monitor the patient
- Supportive care
- Use of antidote to counter the effects of the poison

EQUIPMENT

- NGT (No. 6, 8, or 12 Levin or a No. 14 to 16 French for an adult; No. 10 French for child)
- Equipment to insert tube (see "Nasogastric Tube Insertion and Removal, Procedure")
- A plastic emesis basin in which to empty the gastric contents
- A 60-ml catheter-tipped syringe with piston
- Clean gloves
- Connecting tubing and suction equipment (optional)
- pH paper (optional)
- Clamp for the NGT (optional)
- One or two 1-L bottles of sterile normal saline irrigating solution
- Any antidotes, absorbents, or cathartics indicated
- Activated charcoal (1 g/kg maximum dose of 50 g) for poisonings ingested in the past 1 to 2 hours and will bind to activated charcoal; Poison Control may be contacted at 1-800-222-1222 for help in determining whether a substance binds to activated charcoal

Procedure

1. Place the NGT via the nose or mouth of the patient and lower to the epigastric/stomach region (see "Nasogastric Tube Insertion and Removal, Procedure").
2. Check for correct placement of the NGT. First, aspirate a small amount of fluid to determine whether it is gastric contents and obtain a specimen. The fluid should have a pH of less than 7, look clear to yellow, and have mucus present. Gastric contents may be difficult, if not impossible, to aspirate when small-bore NGTs are placed. Aspiration is performed by pulling back on the syringe piston after connecting it to the proximal portion of the NGT; therefore, using the plastic syringe, draw up 10 ml of air, attach the syringe to the proximal end of the NGT, and place the diaphragm of the stethoscope over the epigastric/stomach area. Instill the 10 ml of air and, using the stethoscope, auscultate for a swooshing sound or rush of air, indicating the tube is likely to be in the stomach. Then, either leave the syringe attached to the proximal end of the NGT and clamp the NGT or attach it to suction.
3. Secure the NGT. Tear off a 4-inch piece of cloth tape and split 2 inches of it vertically. Replace the temporary tape with this tape by placing the unsplit end over the bridge of the nose and wrapping the chevron ends underneath and around the NGT in opposite directions while keeping the NGT straight downward from the nose. Finish securing the NGT by wrapping a piece of cloth tape or the rubber band around the tube near the proximal end and pinning it to the patient's gown or clothing OR if the facility uses a commercial product to secure NGTs, apply it now.

6

4. Proceed with the lavage: Instill the iced saline in 50- to 60-ml increments, up to a maximum of 200 ml, before aspirating back or suctioning out the stomach contents. Overfilling of the stomach can lead to regurgitation and/or aspiration of the instilled solution and stomach contents. Be sure to let the cool solution sit in the stomach for at least 1 or 2 minutes before aspirating or suctioning so that the vasoconstriction desired to arrest the bleeding can occur. Continue the process until the returns are essentially clear.
5. When the lavage is complete, the stomach may be left empty or an antidote, a cathartic, or an absorbent may be instilled as indicated by the underlying causative poisonous agent. Cathartics facilitate the transition of the poison through the intestines, whereas absorbents are instilled to limit the amount of absorption of the poison.

COMPLICATIONS

- Submucosal, intracranial, or pulmonary passage of the NGT
- Esophageal perforation
- Mucosal ulcerations of the nose, pharynx, or stomach
- Aspiration of stomach contents into the lungs, leading to pneumonia

PRACTITIONER FOLLOW-UP

- During and after the lavage, monitor the patient's vital signs, hydration, and mental, renal, respiratory, and cardiovascular status; administer intravenous fluids and blood products as necessary.
- In cases of poisoning, pay particular attention to signs and symptoms of mucosal destruction, such as increased burning and pain, drooling, and dysphagia.
- Monitor the patient for the next 48 hours for nausea, vomiting, abdominal distention, and food intolerance.

■ CPT BILLING

43753—Gastric intubation and aspiration(s) therapeutic, necessitating physician's skill (e.g., for gastrointestinal hemorrhage), including lavage if performed ■ **43754**—Gastric intubation and aspiration, diagnostic; single specimen

REFERENCES AND RELATED RESOURCES

Cooper G, et al: A randomized clinical trial of activated charcoal for the routine management of oral drug overdose, *QJM* 98:655–660, 2005.

Tucker JR: Indications for, techniques of, complications of, and efficacy of gastric lavage in the treatment of the poisoned child, *Curr Opin Pediatr* 12:163, 2000.

Position Paper: Whole bowel irrigation, *J Tox Clin Tox* 42(6):843–854, 2004.

Position Paper: Gastric lavage, *J Tox Clin Tox* 42(7):933–943, 2004.

Anoscopy

DESCRIPTION

Anoscopy can be used to evaluate the patient who reports perianal and anal discomfort.

ANATOMY AND PHYSIOLOGY

The anal canal is accessed through the rectal sphincter. The specific anatomic structures that are visible during an anoscopy are shown in Figure 6-3.

INDICATIONS

- Anal or perianal pain
- Rectal prolapse (see "Rectal Prolapse Reduction, Procedure")
- Hemorrhoids
  - Minimal bright red blood per rectum
  - Abnormal anal exfoliative cytology in screening in men patients who have sex with men

CONTRAINDICATIONS

- Symptoms of an acute abdomen

PRECAUTIONS

- Acute cardiovascular condition

ASSESSMENT

- An anorectal assessment consists of inspection, palpation, and an anoscopic examination. Position the patient in the left lateral decubitus position and drape the patient (Figure 6-9). This position is much more comfortable for the patient than the traditional head-down, "jack-knife" position, yet it still allows adequate visualization and access for the examiner.
- Spread the glutei to provide adequate visualization of the anus. The patient can assist, if necessary, by raising the right gluteal area with the right hand to better expose the perianal area.
- Examine the perianal area. An external inspection may reveal fissures, fistulas, perianal dermatitis, masses, thrombosed hemorrhoids, condyloma, and other growths and may help the examiner anticipate internal rectal findings.

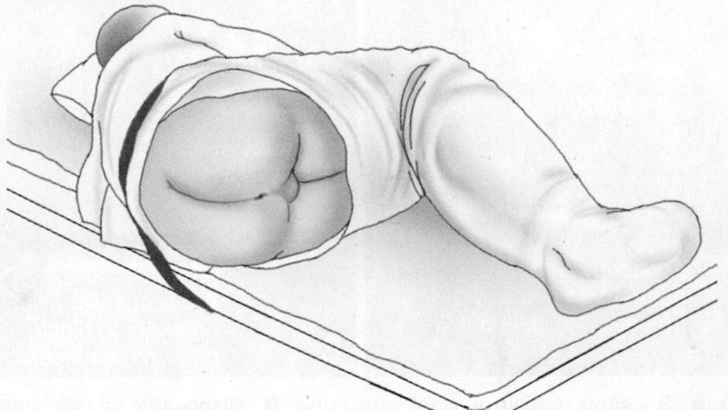

FIGURE 6-9 Placement of the patient for anoscopy, in the left lateral decubitus position (Sim's position). Digital examination, flexible sigmoidoscopy, and most anorectal procedures can be performed in this position.

- Have the patient bear down. Observe for prolapse of hemorrhoids or of the rectum.
- Perform a digital rectal examination unless the patient is experiencing extreme pain.
- Sweep the finger through all 360 degrees of the anal canal and define any palpable mass. Because of the redundant mucosa, small tumors may not be visualized even with the anoscope, but often can be detected by palpation.
- In *men,* the prostate should be palpated in addition to the digital assessment of the anal canal.

TREATMENT ALTERNATIVES

- Examination using flexible sigmoidoscopy and/or colonoscopy may be indicated in individual patients.
- Referral to GI.

PATIENT PREPARATION

- Although preparation with an enema is not usually necessary before an anoscopy, it can improve visualization and may be aesthetically more acceptable to the examiner and to the patient.
- Practitioners should explain that this procedure will be uncomfortable, but should not be very painful and should give the patient an estimate of the total time for the procedure.

EQUIPMENT

- Anoscope (Figure 6-10)
- Light source
- Gloves
- Lubricant
- Cotton swabs

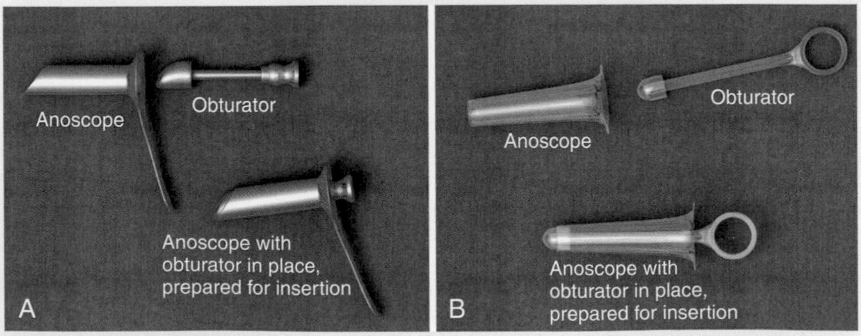

FIGURE 6-10 A, Reusable stainless steel anoscope. **B,** Disposable plastic anoscope. (From Roberts JR, Custalow CB, Thomsen TW, eds: *Roberts and Hedges' clinical procedures in emergency medicine,* ed 6, Philadelphia, 2014, Elsevier.)

Procedure

1. Choose an anoscope with good visualization. Some small plastic anoscopes are available, but visualization with them is often difficult.
2. Lubricate the anoscope with the obturator in place.
3. Insert the anoscope slowly in the direction of the umbilicus.
4. Remove the obturator.
5. Observe one fourth of the mucosa as the anoscope is slowly removed.
6. Remove fecal material with a swab, as necessary.
7. Remove the anoscope slowly, observing the mucosa.
8. Reinsert the obturator, and then rotate the instrument 90 degrees. Then, repeat step 7.
9. The procedure is performed four times to visualize the entire circumference of the anal canal.
10. Identify lesions. It is rare to see a polyp or carcinoma; more likely are erythema and edema at the distal 8 to 10 cm, particularly anteriorly.

PATIENT EDUCATION POSTPROCEDURE

Discuss findings and follow-up plans with the patient.

COMPLICATIONS

Sometimes a small amount of bleeding occurs.

PRACTITIONER FOLLOW-UP

Patients should be evaluated for abrasion or tearing of the perianal skin or mucosa or for hemorrhoidal tissue.

■ CPT BILLING

46600—Anoscopy; diagnostic, including collection of specimen(s) by brushing or washing, when performed ■ **46604**—With dilation (e.g., balloon, guide wire, bougie) ■ **46606**—With biopsy, single or multiple ■ **46608**—With removal of foreign body ■ **46610**—With removal of single tumor, polyp, or other lesion by hot biopsy forceps or bipolar cautery ■ **46611**—With removal of single tumor, polyp, or other lesion by snare technique ■ **46612**—With removal of multiple tumors, polyps, or other lesions by hot biopsy forceps or bipolar cautery or snare technique ■ **46614**—With control of bleeding (e.g., injection, bipolar cautery, unipolar cautery, laser, heater probe, stapler, plasma coagulator) ■ **46615**—With ablation of tumor(s), polyp(s), or other lesion(s) not amenable to removal by hot biopsy forceps, bipolar cautery, or snare technique

REFERENCES AND RELATED RESOURCES

Machalek D, et al: Anal human papillomavirus infection and associated neoplastic lesions in men who have sex with men: a systematic review and meta-analysis, *Lancet Oncol* 13(5): 487–500, 2012.

National Institutes of Health (NIH), U.S. National Library of Medicine, MedlinePlus: *Anoscopy* (Cowles, R, updated). http://www.nlm.nih.gov/medlineplus/ency/article/003890.htm. Last updated October 24, 2014. Accessed January 12, 2015.

Roberts JR, Hedges JR, editors: *Clinical procedures in emergency medicine*, ed 5, Philadelphia, 2009, Saunders Elsevier, chapter 45.

6

Rectal Prolapse Reduction

DESCRIPTION

Prolapse is a protrusion of the rectum through the anus. The types of rectal prolapse are listed in Box 6-1. Transient, minor prolapse of just the rectal mucosa often occurs in otherwise normal infants. Mucosal prolapse in adults persists and may progressively worsen.

Procidentia is complete prolapse of the entire thickness of the rectum. Abnormal anterior displacement of the rectum resulting from elongation of the mesorectum is probably the primary cause. Most patients are women who are older than 60 years.

ANATOMY AND PHYSIOLOGY

Complete rectal prolapse is a relatively rare, but serious disorder that is most often seen in infants or older adults (see Box 6-1). It is more common in women than in men. Factors that predispose rectal prolapse include the following:

- Chronic constipation
- Severe chronic diarrhea
- Obstetric injury
- Neurologic disease, such as multiple sclerosis
- Weakness of the external rectal sphincter
- Rectal intercourse, including sexual abuse

INDICATIONS

Reduction is required when prolapse is chronic or severe.

CONTRAINDICATIONS

When episodes of recurrences increase and the tissue becomes prone to excoriation and ulcerations and at risk for strangulation, surgery should be considered; however, the surgical options so far are not extremely successful in preventing or alleviating fecal incontinence.

PRECAUTIONS

Once a complete rectal prolapse is diagnosed, conservative methods should be tried before surgical intervention. If the prolapse is small and limited to the mucosa, a high-fiber diet and reeducation on bowel habits to prevent straining may control the problem.

BOX 6-1 Types of Rectal Prolapse

PARTIAL

The rectal mucosa protrudes for 1 to 3 cm beyond the anal sphincter. In mucosal prolapse, the mucosal folds are radial, the anus is inverted, and there is no sulcus groove between the anus and the protruding tissue.

COMPLETE

There is an intussusception of all three layers of the rectum through the anal opening. The mucosal folds are concentric, the anus is in a normal anatomic position, and there is a sulcus between the anus and protruding bowel tissue.

INTERNAL

Patients have symptoms of rectal prolapse, but tissue cannot be demonstrated to protrude through the anal canal.

ASSESSMENT

- Take a thorough history. There usually is no pain; the presence of pain indicates incarceration with impending strangulation or some other condition not related to the prolapse.
- Rectal bleeding can occur, and incontinence is frequent. The most prominent symptom is protrusion, which occurs only while straining (in mild cases) or while walking or standing (in more advanced cases).
- Diagnosis is made on inspection and demonstration of the prolapse. The patient should be examined while standing or squatting, and while straining to determine the full extent of the prolapse. Ask patients to strain. This pressure should reveal a full-thickness rectal prolapse as it mushrooms through the anal sphincters. If straining does not produce a prolapse, have the patient squat or have him or her sit on the toilet to produce the prolapse. Differentiate between hemorrhoid, mucosal (partial) prolapse, or rectal (complete) prolapse by visual examination.
- Diminished anal sphincter tone is usually present. Sigmoidoscopy and barium enema radiography of the colon may be performed to confirm diagnosis or search for other colon or intrinsic disease. Primary neurologic disorders must be ruled out. Rectal procidentia must be distinguished from hemorrhoids.
- A colonoscopy should be performed when recommended by current guidelines.

TREATMENT ALTERNATIVES

- Conservative treatment is usually indicated in infants and children. Correct any underlying nutritional disorders to try to reduce any causes of straining. Spontaneous resolution of prolapse in children is sometimes accomplished by firmly strapping the buttocks together between bowel movements.
- For simple repetitive mucosal prolapse in adults, excess mucosa can be excised or ligated with a rubber band (see "Treatment for Hemorrhoids, Description").
- For procidentia, surgical repair with elevation and posterior fixation of the rectum to the sacrum to correct anterior displacement or a low posterior fixation of the rectum may be required.
- In patients who are older adults and are frail or in generally poor health, a wire or synthetic plastic loop may be inserted at the sphincteric ring (Thiersch's procedure). This procedure provides external support to the sagging mucosa and holds it in place so that it cannot protrude.
- Multiple surgical techniques can effectively treat rectal prolapse if conservative therapy fails.

PATIENT PREPARATION

Place the patient in a left lateral position. Have tissues available if the patient reports urinary stress incontinence.

EQUIPMENT

- Sterile gauze
- Normal saline
- Disposable absorbent pads/tissues
- Anoscope
- Water-soluble lubricant

Procedure

1. Assist patients into a left lateral decubitus position (left side lying, knee-to-chest position); this position allows the abdominal viscera to fall cephalad, which may pull the extruded bowel back through the anus and reduce the prolapse.
2. Place a saline-soaked gauze over the prolapse to prevent it from drying.
3. Apply very gentle pressure with the saline-moistened gauze to guide the protruding tissue through the relaxed sphincter.

PATIENT EDUCATION POSTPROCEDURE

- Patient should lie down and apply pressure to the area if the prolapse recurs.
- Provide counseling regarding diet, fluid, and exercise to help prevent recurrent prolapse, which will lead to continuous prolapse, fecal incontinence, and surgery.
- Instruct the patient to increase fiber in the diet. Fiber absorbs water and increases stool bulk, stimulating peristalsis and bowel emptying. Uncooked fruits and vegetables are good sources of bulk. Cereal fiber is a more effective stool softener than fruits and vegetables. Prunes have a laxative effect in some people.
- Instruct the patient that 2000 to 2500 ml or 2 quarts per day of fluid intake will help keep the stool soft. Space the fluid at intervals throughout the day so that it does not diminish the appetite.
- Instruct the patient to select a consistent time of day to attempt defecation. The gastrocolic reflex that occurs 20 to 40 minutes after eating would make this an optimal time. Also, the gastrocolic reflex is stronger after a hot meal, so a regular habit may be established after a hot breakfast or dinner rather than after a regular cold lunch. Because the optimal physiologic position for defecation is the squat, patients who must use a built-up toilet seat should be advised to elevate the feet on a footrest and to bend forward when attempting a bowel movement.
- If these measures do not relieve constipation, order a bulk-forming laxative, such as Metamucil, or a stool softener, such as Colace, to facilitate stool transit through the colon.

COMPLICATIONS

- Inability to reduce prolapse
- Tearing of tissue
- Strangulation of tissue

PRACTITIONER FOLLOW-UP

- Patients who have a complete rectal prolapse should be referred after reduction for proctoscopy and barium enema or endoscopy to confirm the diagnosis and to exclude other lesions. Children should be carefully evaluated to rule out sexual abuse.
- Make a follow-up referral for rectal prolapse that is considered to be either partial or complete. Patients should be instructed that they may anticipate biopsy, sigmoidoscopy, or a barium enema for a complete evaluation.
- If conservative therapy is recommended in patients who have a complete prolapse, anal sphincter function should be assessed regularly to ensure that there is no deterioration.
- Assess for complications by noting progression: increases in recurrences, decreases in anal sphincter tone, development of fecal incontinence, or presence of pain.

- Refer for surgical intervention if the patient's condition deteriorates.
- After surgical intervention, the patient should be observed for the following complications: hemorrhage, bowel obstruction, pelvic abscess, fecal impaction, and recurrent prolapse.

CPT BILLING

45900—Reduction of procidentia (separate procedure) under anesthesia

If no anesthesia was administered, use the appropriate E/M code.

REFERENCES AND RELATED RESOURCES

Felt-Bersma RJ, Cuesta MA: Rectal prolapse, rectal intussusception, rectocele, and solitary rectal ulcer syndrome, *Gastroenterol Clin North Am* 30:199, 2001.

Peters WA 3rd, Smith MR, Drescher CW: Rectal prolapse in women with other defects of pelvic floor support, *Am J Obstet Gynecol* 184:1488, 2001.

Pfenninger JL, Zainea GG: Common anorectal conditions: part I. symptoms and complaints, *Am Fam Physician* 63:2391-2398, 2001.

Yildirim W, Koksal HM, Baykan A: Incarcerated and strangulated rectal prolapse, *Int J Colorectal Dis* 16:60, 2001.

Treatment for Hemorrhoids

DESCRIPTION

Hemorrhoids are varicosities of the veins of the hemorrhoidal plexus that are often complicated by inflammation, thrombosis, and bleeding. When the varicosities are thrombosed, significant pain may develop. Primary care treatment involves conservative therapy, then pushing the hemorrhoids back up into rectum or ligating them with a rubber band. Rubber band ligation involves placing a small rubber band at the base of the internal hemorrhoid with a special applicator. The rubber band cuts off the blood supply to the hemorrhoid, and the hemorrhoid falls off in about 4 to 5 days. There is generally minimal or no discomfort associated with this procedure.

ANATOMY AND PHYSIOLOGY

External hemorrhoids are derived from the external hemorrhoidal plexus beneath the dentate line and are covered by squamous epithelium. *Internal hemorrhoids* are derived from the internal hemorrhoidal plexus located above the dentate line and are lined by rectal mucosa (Figure 6-11). Hemorrhoids typically occur in the right anterior, right posterior, and left lateral zones and universally affect adults and children. They are often caused by chronic constipation or diarrhea, pregnancy, heredity, faulty bowel function, and straining during bowel movements. The tissues supporting the veins stretch and dilate, and their walls become thin and bleed. The weakened veins protrude if the process continues.

Hemorrhoids are classified as the following:

- First degree: No prolapse
- Second degree: Prolapses, which reduce spontaneously
- Third degree: Reduces with manual reduction
- Fourth degree: Permanently prolapsed; will not reduce

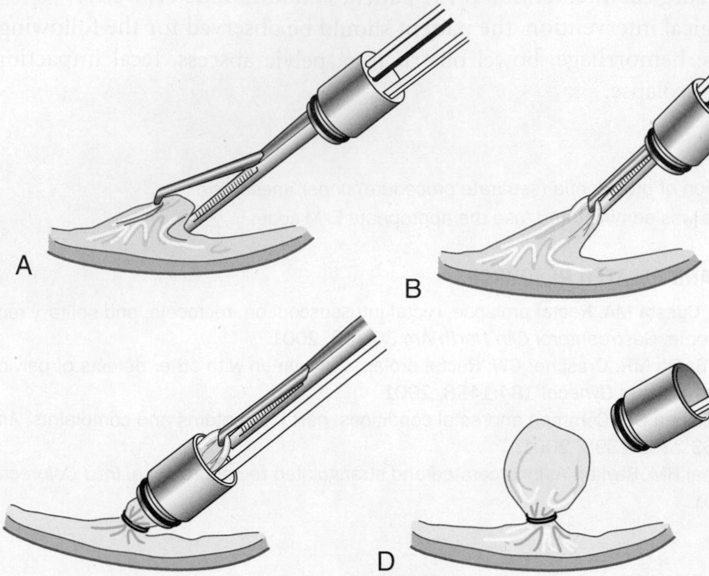

FIGURE 6-11 Rubber band ligation technique for hemorrhoids. **A** and **B,** The hemorrhoid is grasped and firmly tethered. **C** and **D,** The tissue is drawn into the drum, and two rubber bands are released. If the patient tolerates the grasping of the hemorrhoid with forceps, ligation can be performed with minimal or no discomfort.

The recognition of a sliding anal canal lining and the knowledge that hemorrhoidal cushions are a normal part of the anal anatomy should encourage symptom control rather than radical removal of tissue.

INDICATIONS

- Most symptomatic internal hemorrhoids, degrees 1 through 3, can be treated successfully with medical management or office-based procedures.
- Techniques that tack the anal canal hemorrhoidal cushions back in position can be performed in outpatient clinics with reasonable success rates. When required, surgery should be aimed at symptomatic hemorrhoids that have resisted medical management.
- If the patient requires sedation, then the patient needs to have the procedure performed in an emergency department or hospital where airway support can be provided.

CONTRAINDICATIONS

- Infection
- Active bleeding
- Bleeding disorders

PRECAUTIONS

Hemorrhoidectomy is performed infrequently for bleeding hemorrhoids. If the hemorrhoids are primarily external, hemorrhoidectomy is required.

Hemorrhoids in pregnancy often resolve after delivery and should be treated conservatively.

ASSESSMENT

- Assessment of the patient who has hemorrhoids should include collecting an excellent focused history, performing an abdominal and complete rectal examination, and anoscopy.
- Hemorrhoids are often asymptomatic, but may present with bleeding, itching, protrusion, and/or pain. Research suggests that the most common causes of rectal bleeding are hemorrhoids, fissures, and polyps; however, rectal bleeding should be attributed to hemorrhoids only after more serious conditions are excluded. Hemorrhoidal bleeding, which typically follows defecation and is noted on toilet tissue, rarely leads to anemia or severe hemorrhage.
- External and internal hemorrhoids can protrude; they may regress spontaneously or may require manual reduction. Less commonly, internal hemorrhoids cause mucus discharge and a sensation of incomplete evacuation, and external hemorrhoids may cause difficulty in cleansing the anal region.
- Pain is the hallmark of thrombosed or ulcerated hemorrhoids. A thrombosed hemorrhoid presents as a perianal protrusion with pain varying from nonexistent to severe. Ulcerated, edematous, or strangulated hemorrhoids are usually associated with severe pain.
- Thrombosed hemorrhoids and ulcerated edematous strangulated hemorrhoids can be readily diagnosed on inspection and palpation of the rectum. Examination after straining when stool is present or a phosphate enema is used often reveals the extent of the patient's hemorrhoidal pathology. Use of an anoscopy is essential in evaluating painless hemorrhoids.

PATIENT PREPARATION

- Obtain written informed consent from the patient.
- Explain the procedure to the patient.
- Give the patient time to consider the pros and cons of the procedure before beginning.
- Put the patient in the lithotomy position and visualize the area with adequate lighting.

TREATMENT ALTERNATIVES

- Conservative therapies for the treatment of hemorrhoids include diet, lifestyle changes, and hydrotherapy, which require a high degree of patient compliance to be effective. There are several over-the-counter topical agents available for hemorrhoids; numerous creams and suppositories (e.g., Proctofoam HC or Anusol) can help relieve irritation and pain symptoms. Conservative therapy should always be considered and education on diet and lifestyle changes provided to prevent further episodes.
- Ulcerated edematous strangulated hemorrhoids can be managed conservatively because pain and swelling are likely to resolve rapidly; the thromboses are reabsorbed over 4 to 8 weeks. Incapacitating pain that fails to resolve with analgesics, sitz baths, topical compresses, and other conservative measures may be treated by (1) injection of a local anesthetic agent that contains hyaluronidase, followed by

rubber band ligation of the internal hemorrhoids and multiple thrombectomies or (2) hemorrhoidectomy.

- When conservative hemorrhoid therapy is ineffective, a variety of other nonsurgical specialized modalities are available, such as injection sclerotherapy, cryotherapy, manual dilation of the anus, infrared photocoagulation, bipolar diathermy, direct current electrocoagulation, or rubber band ligation. Nonsurgical modalities require the practitioner to be specially trained, own specialized equipment, and assume associated risks. If a nonsurgical approach fails, the patient is often referred to a surgeon.
- Oral dietary supplementation assists in the traditional treatment of hemorrhoids. Because the loss of vascular integrity is associated with the pathogenesis of hemorrhoids, some botanical extracts may improve microcirculation, capillary flow, and vascular tone and to strengthen the connective tissue of the perivascular amorphous substrate. Oral supplementation with *Aesculus hippocastanum, Ruscus aculeatus, Centella asiatica, Hamamelis virginiana,* and bioflavonoids may assist in the treatment of hemorrhoids.
- Stool softeners or bulking agents (e.g., psyllium) may reduce constipation and straining, thus allowing hemorrhoids to resolve. Standard treatment for a thrombosed hemorrhoid includes reassurance, warm sitz baths, anesthetic ointments, or witch hazel *(H. virginiana)* compresses. Bleeding hemorrhoids can be treated by injection sclerotherapy with 5% phenol in vegetable oil. After these treatments, bleeding should cease at least temporarily.
- Infrared photocoagulation is useful for ablating small internal hemorrhoids, hemorrhoids that cannot be ligated with a rubber band because of pain sensitivity, or hemorrhoids that are not cured with rubber band ligation. Modalities of unproven efficacy include laser destruction and various types of electrodestruction.
- Infrequently, simple incision and evacuation of the clot may relieve pain rapidly. Circular stapling may also assist in pain control.

EQUIPMENT

- Gloves
- Drapes
- Anoscope to dilate area and aid in visualization of the hemorrhoid
- McGivney ligator with rubber bands
- Alligator forceps

Procedure

1. Larger internal hemorrhoids or those that fail to respond to injection sclerotherapy are treated by rubber band ligation. With mixed internal and external hemorrhoids, only the internal component should be rubber band ligated. Rubber band ligation is useful for second-degree and small third-degree hemorrhoids.
2. Load the ligating drum with two bands. The ¼-inch-diameter elastic bands are dilated to about ⅜ inch. A small amount of soapy water on the cone will facilitate the loading of the rubber bands.
3. Insert the anoscope and obtain good visualization of the hemorrhoid to be ligated. One person is usually required to hold the anoscope in place.

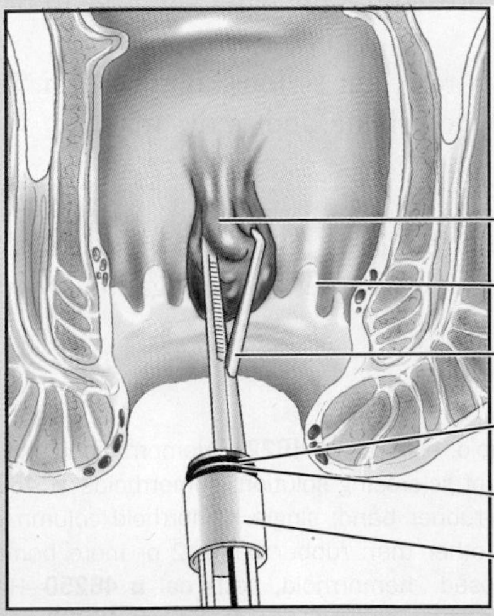

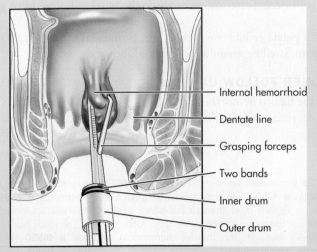

FIGURE 6-12 Close-up view of rubber band ligation of internal hemorrhoid. An alligator forceps grasps the hemorrhoid. The forceps passes through the drum of the ligator. Squeezing on the ligator handle pushes the outer drum over the inner drum, displacing the bands onto the base of the hemorrhoid. Choose the ligating point well above the dentate line to minimize pain.

4. Another person should use an alligator forceps to draw the hemorrhoidal tissue into the ligating drum. To reduce the pain experienced by the patient, grasp the hemorrhoid tissue proximally (Figures 6-11 and 6-12).
5. Grasp the handle of the ligator with the other hand and push forward slightly, and then squeeze the handle. The outer drum slides over the inner drum, displacing the rubber bands around the hemorrhoid.
6. Reposition and repeat in one other hemorrhoidal area, or withdraw the anoscope.
7. Limit treatment to two hemorrhoidal areas at one time. Subsequent treatments can be performed at 4- to 6-week intervals.

Video: https://www.youtube.com/watch?v=z2hqoeSOoXA

PATIENT EDUCATION POSTPROCEDURE

- Emphasize the helpfulness of a high-fiber diet, ingestion of fluid, exercise, and use of sitz baths for 20 to 30 minutes three or four times a day for the next 2 to 3 days after the procedure.
- Instruct the patient that mild analgesics, such as acetaminophen, may be used to control the mild aching discomfort after the procedure. There may be increased pain if the ligation area is close to the anus. A dull ache may continue for 2 days after the procedure, but it may last as long as 7 to 10 days.
- Instruct the patient to report any bleeding, dysuria, fever, inability to urinate, or increasing pain.
- Follow up in 3 to 4 weeks for reexamination and further banding if needed.

COMPLICATIONS

- Bleeding of hemorrhoids often occurs 1 to 2 weeks after the procedure, when the hemorrhoidal tissue sloughs off. This bleeding can be significant.

- If severe pain occurs after the procedure, the band will have to be removed with scissors.
- Sepsis with pelvic cellulites is a rare, but serious complication. Watch for fever, perineal pain, swelling, inability to urinate, and/or dysuria.

PRACTITIONER FOLLOW-UP

The status of the ligated hemorrhoid should be monitored every 2 weeks to determine the extent of necrosis and sloughing and whether further ligation procedures are indicated.

■ CPT BILLING

46083—Incision of thrombosed hemorrhoid, external ■ **46221**—Hemorrhoidectomy, internal, by rubber band ligation(s) ■ **46500**—Injection of sclerosing solution, hemorrhoids ■ **46945**—Hemorrhoidectomy, internal, by ligation other than rubber band; single hemorrhoid column/group ■ **46946**—Hemorrhoidectomy, internal, by ligation other than rubber band; 2 or more hemorrhoid columns/groups ■ **46320**—Excision of thrombosed hemorrhoid, external ■ **46250**—Hemorrhoidectomy, external, 2 or more columns/groups (For single column, use 46999) ■ **46999**—Unlisted procedure, anus ■ **46255**—Hemorrhoidectomy, internal and external, single column/group ■ **46260**—Hemorrhoidectomy, internal and external, 2 or more columns/groups

REFERENCES AND RELATED RESOURCES

Acheson AG, Scholefield JH: Management of haemorrhoids, *BMJ* 336(7640):380–383, 2008.

AmerraMedical: *Rubber band ligation for hemorrhoids, 3D medical animation*, 2012. https://www.youtube.com/watch?v=z2hqoeS0oXA. Accessed January 13, 2015.

Hulme-Moir M, Bartolo DC: Hemorrhoids, *Gastroenterol Clin North Am* 30:183, 2001.

MacKay D: Hemorrhoids and varicose veins: a review of treatment options, *Altern Med Rev* 2:126, 2001.

Mounsey A, Halladay J, Sadiq T: Hemorrhoids, *Am Fam Physician* 84(2):204–210, 2011.

Pfenninger JL, Zainea GG: Common anorectal conditions: part I. symptoms and complaints, *Am Fam Physician* 63:2391-2398, 2001.

7

Orthopedic Procedures

Christy L. Crowther-Radulewicz and Jared Spackman

Orthopedic procedures are commonly required in primary care. Regardless of whether the patient ultimately requires referral to an orthopedist, the patient often first seeks medical care in the primary care office. Thus the clinician should have a basic understanding of musculoskeletal anatomy and physiology.

ANATOMY AND PHYSIOLOGY

As a whole, the musculoskeletal system provides form to the body, produces heat, enables movement, and helps protect underlying organs and structures. Knowledge of surface anatomy allows the practitioner to identify certain abnormalities in underlying structures.

Muscles are specialized soft tissues attached to the skeleton by fibrinous cords known as *tendons;* muscle contraction and relaxation allow for movement and performance of work by the body and help maintains posture. *Ligaments* attach bone to bone and stabilize joints by limiting their movement to appropriate planes. The skeleton provides form to the body via a rigid scaffold to which muscles attach. In addition to locomotion, the skeletal system also provides protection to certain internal organs and is involved in mineral homeostasis and the production of blood components.

For example, hand injuries are often seen in primary care. The *metacarpal* bones make up the hand just as the phalanges make up the digits. The *proximal phalanges* articulate with the metacarpals, forming the *metacarpophalangeal* (MCP) joints. The bases of the middle phalanges form the *proximal interphalangeal* (PIP) joints by articulating with the distal ends of the proximal phalanges. Finally, the distal phalanges articulate with the distal ends of the middle phalanges, forming the *distal interphalangeal* (DIP) joints of the hand (Figure 7-1).

Tendons of the hand are numerous. The flexor tendons lie on the *volar,* or palmar aspect of the hand; the extensor tendons lie along the dorsal aspect. The combined, coordinated functions of flexor and extensor tendons enable smooth movement of each digit and their joints.

Both the wrist and hand have an abundance of ligamentous support. Broad *dorsal* and *palmar radiocarpal* ligaments that run from the distal radius to the carpal bones join the joints of the wrist and strengthen them. The palmar, or volar, ligaments are generally clinically more important than the dorsal ligaments. The *distal radioulnar* joint has both dorsal and palmar ligaments (Figure 7-2).

Other joints have similar anatomy with regard to osseous and soft tissue structures. As with the hand, the bones of the ankles and feet are made up of smaller bones that work together to provide the foot with stability and flexibility. The foot is made up of

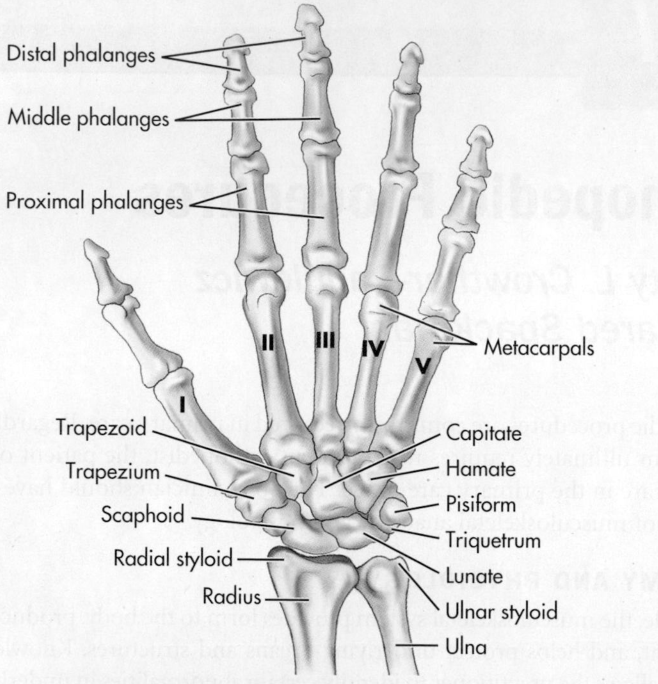

FIGURE 7-1 Bony anatomy of the wrist and hand.

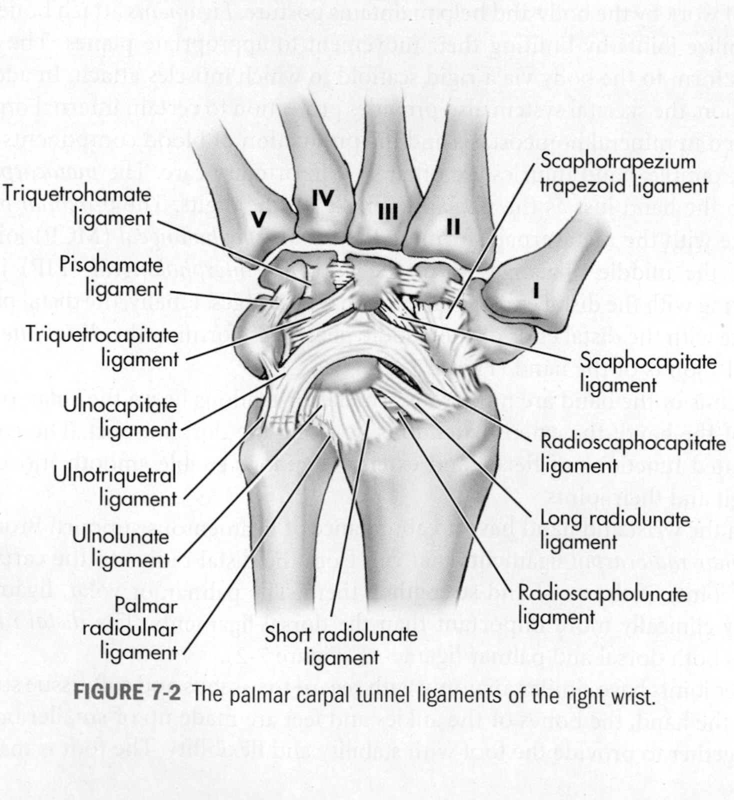

FIGURE 7-2 The palmar carpal tunnel ligaments of the right wrist.

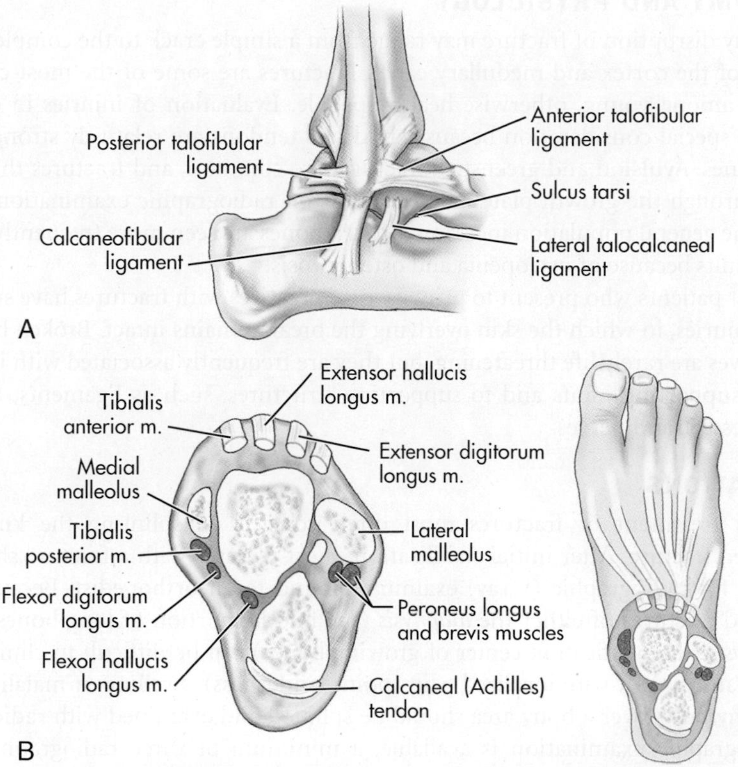

FIGURE 7-3 The ankle. **A,** The lateral collateral ligaments of the ankle. **B,** The relationship of tendons and osseous structures at the ankle joint.

the tarsal bones (calcaneus [or os calcic], talus, cuboid, and three cuneiform bones), the metatarsals, and the phalanges. Commonly, these areas are referred to as the hindfoot (the talus and calcaneus), the midfoot (the navicular, cuboid, and cuneiform bones), and the forefoot (the metatarsals and phalanges). The talus, in combination with the distal tibia and distal fibula, forms the ankle joint. It is a saddle-type joint, stabilized by the collateral ligaments of the ankle (Figure 7-3).

Basic anatomic knowledge is important in helping to determine what underlying musculoskeletal structure(s) is responsible for an individual's complaint or concern. In concert or individually, the most common complaints of acute ankle and foot pain are due to inflammation, autoimmune and systemic disease, degradation of soft tissue, fractures, sprains, and strains.

Fracture Immobilization

Christy L. Crowther-Radulewicz

DESCRIPTION

A *fracture* is a break in the integrity of a bone. Immobilization is required to achieve adequate healing and pain reduction.

ANATOMY AND PHYSIOLOGY

The bony disruption of fracture may range from a simple crack to the complete transection of the cortex and medullary canal. Fractures are some of the most common injuries among young, otherwise healthy people. Evaluation of injuries in children requires special consideration because children's tendons are relatively stronger than their bones. Avulsion and greenstick fractures are common, and fractures that occur solely through the growth plate may not show on radiographic examination. As the age of the general population increases, broken bones are seen more frequently among older adults because of osteopenia and osteoporosis.

Most patients who present to primary care practices with fractures have sustained *closed* injuries, in which the skin overlying the break remains intact. Broken bones by themselves are rarely life threatening, but they are frequently associated with injury to nearby supporting joints and to supporting structures, such as ligaments, tendons, blood vessels, and nerves.

INDICATIONS

Primary treatment of fractures most often consists of splinting the known or suspected fracture. After initial stabilization, most patients with a fracture should be referred for radiographic (x-ray) examination and to an orthopedist. Because nondisplaced fractures of either the *diaphysis* (the middle portion of long bones) or the *metaphysis* (the ossification center of growing bones) can be difficult to clinically diagnose, any patient with localized pain (point tenderness), swelling or malalignment, and ecchymosis over a bony area should be splinted and examined with radiography. If radiographic examination is available, a minimum of three radiographic views (anteroposterior, lateral, and oblique) of the injured extremity should be obtained.

RED FLAGS/CONTRAINDICATIONS

There are few absolute contraindications to splinting, but care should be taken if there is an open wound or any type of skin breakdown where the splint is to be applied. Open fractures, in which the injured bone is in contact with the outside environment, should be covered with a sterile dressing, carefully immobilized, and emergently referred to a hospital. In the case of obvious fracture with severe limb deformity, gentle manual traction to straighten the limb may be applied by trained personnel, but splinting without any attempt to straighten the bone and emergently referring to an orthopedist is appropriate.

PRECAUTIONS

Although contraindications to splinting are few, precautions are numerous:

- The practitioner must be aware that the early complications of fracture include damage to nerves and blood vessels, ligament disruption with associated joint instability, and skin breakdown.
- If there is any indication of neurovascular compromise, such as markedly diminished sensation, absence of pulse, or pallor in the affected extremity, the individual should be immediately referred to an orthopedic surgeon.
- Compartment syndrome may occur with any long bone fracture, although it is most common with lower leg trauma. An elastic bandage applied too tightly will increase any elevated compartment pressures.
- Unstable fractures may require surgical reduction. Improper splinting may aggravate or induce complications. Radiographs should be obtained after the splint has been placed.

- Patients with a known or suspected fracture that is displaced or a fracture that is near an articular surface should always be referred to an orthopedist for definitive care.
- In children, fractures that involve the growth plate also warrant special attention. Red Flag: Known or suspected growth plate fractures should be referred to an orthopedic surgeon.
- Patients should be splinted before they are referred out of the primary care office.

ASSESSMENT

After clinically assessing the patient and determining the likelihood of fracture, the clinician should decide whether radiographs are necessary. For ankles, well-validated guidelines (Ottawa ankle rules) are often utilized. Ottawa ankle rules state that radiographs are indicated if:

- There is pain over the malleolar or midfoot zone.
- There is bone tenderness over the lateral or medial malleolus, the base of the fifth metatarsal, or the tarsal navicular.
- There is an inability to bear weight for four steps both immediately after the injury and in the clinical setting.

For other areas of injury, clinical judgment is indicated, but radiographs are generally low-cost, rapid, and effective diagnostic tools.

PATIENT PREPARATION

- Explain that splinting and immobilization of the injured area is a temporary intervention to reduce pain and the risk of further damage.
- The splinting material (either plaster or fiberglass) is placed in water to begin the chemical reaction that will harden the material. As the splint hardens, it becomes warm, but the warmth is temporary.
- The splint is to remain in place at all times, unless the patient is instructed by the practitioner to remove it.

EQUIPMENT

- Casting tape (fiberglass or plaster of Paris) or preformed, cut-to-length splinting material (such as Orthoglass)
- Stockinette (optional)
- Synthetic cast padding
- Bandage scissors
- Gloves (nonsterile)
- Elastic bandage (e.g., Ace wrap)
- Bucket of water

Procedure

1. Begin by explaining the procedure to the patient.
2. Measure out the length of the stockinette so that it extends several centimeters past the planned length of the splint, and then cover the injured limb with the stockinette.
3. Using the roll of cast padding, measure out a length long enough to include the joint distal to the injury. The joint proximal to the injury should also be included

if appropriate (e.g., casts for nondisplaced distal radius fractures do not usually have to include the elbow).

4. Layer the padding to create four to six layers. Cut or tear another single layer of padding the same length.
5. Don gloves. Dip the splinting material in the water for 10 to 15 seconds. Gently wipe or blot excess water from the splinting material with a towel. Do not wring out the material.
6. Repeat the layering process with fiberglass splinting material; this should be four to six layers thick for the upper extremities and eight to ten layers thick for the lower extremities.
7. Place the single layer of padding over the fiberglass to form a "sandwich" of thick padding-splinting material-single layer of padding.
8. Place the heavily padded side of the splint against the limb while maintaining the limb in anatomic alignment (if used, fold the edges of the stockinette back to cover the raw edge of the splinting material). Wrap the splint with the Ace bandage in a distal-to-proximal direction. Do not stretch the elastic bandage while wrapping the splint because this may result in neurovascular compromise. The splint will harden and dry in 10 to 15 minutes. Secure the elastic bandage with tape, metal clips, or the attached Velcro.

NOTE: If using cut-to-length preformed splinting material (such as Orthoglass), there is no need to provide additional padding. The material should be moistened, and then applied and secured with an elastic bandage.

PATIENT EDUCATION POSTPROCEDURE

- The splint is temporary, but should not be removed by the patient.
- The patient may shower with a fiberglass splint, but should take care not to get the inside of the splint wet. The patient may not shower with a plaster splint in place.
- Instruct the patient to notify the provider if the pain significantly worsens or if swelling, numbness, coldness, or tingling of the splinted area occurs.

COMPLICATIONS

Complications include neurovascular damage (including compartment syndrome) and skin breakdown due to either the original injury or poor splinting technique, which may compromise circulation. Inadequate immobilization due to excessive padding may allow for movement of the affected area. Itching beneath a splint is common.

PRACTITIONER FOLLOW-UP

Patients who have a documented fracture should be referred to an orthopedist for definitive care. If radiographs are unavailable or inconclusive, patients should be referred to an orthopedist within 24 to 48 hours. If the radiographic examination was performed in the primary care office, the films should accompany the patient to the orthopedic surgeon's office.

■ CPT BILLING

An individual who applies the initial cast, strap, or splint and also assumes all of the subsequent fracture, dislocation, or injury care cannot use the application of casts and strapping codes as an initial service, since the first cast/splint or strap application is included in the treatment of fracture and/or dislocation codes. A temporary cast/splint/strap is not considered to be part of preoperative care and the use of modifier 56 is not applicable. Additional evaluation and management services are reportable only if significant, separately identifiable services are provided at the time of the cast application or strapping.

The listed procedures apply when the cast application or strapping is a replacement procedure used during or after the period of follow-up care, or when the cast application or strapping is an initial service performed without a restorative treatment or procedure(s) to stabilize or protect a fracture, injury, or dislocation and/or to afford comfort to a patient. Restorative treatment or procedures(s) rendered by another individual following the application of the initial cast/splint/strap may be reported with a treatment of fracture and/or dislocation code.

If cast application or strapping is provided as an initial service (e.g., casting of a sprained ankle or knee) in which no other procedure or treatment (e.g., surgical repair, reduction of a fracture, or joint dislocation) is performed or is expected to be performed by an individual rendering the initial care only, use the casting, strapping, and/or supply code (99070) in addition to an evaluation and management code as appropriate.

Listed procedures include removal of cast or strapping. Codes for cast removals should be employed only for casts applied by another individual.

29105—Application of long arm splint (shoulder to hand) ■ **29125**—Application of short arm splint (forearm to hand); static ■ **29126**—Application of short arm splint (forearm to hand); dynamic ■ **29505**—Application of long leg splint (thigh to ankle or toes) ■ **29515**—Application of short leg splint (calf to foot)

REFERENCES AND RELATED RESOURCES

Boss SE, Mehta A, Maddow C: Critical orthopedic skills and procedures, *Emerg Med Clin N Am* 31: 261–290, 2013.

Boyd AS, Benjamin HJ, Asplund C: Principles of casting and splinting, *Am Fam Physician* 79(1): 16–22, 2009.

Polzer H, Kanz KG, Prall WC, et al: Diagnosis and treatment of acute ankle injuries: development of an evidence-based algorithm, *Orthop Rev (Pavia)* 4:22–32, 2012.

Splinting: Wrist and Hand

Christy L. Crowther-Radulewicz

DESCRIPTION

Splinting is a commonly used therapeutic procedure performed in the primary care setting for the management of hand and wrist injuries. Splinting is a temporary or adjunct therapy that is used to stabilize an injured limb. Although splinting in general does not provide sufficient support to immobilize forearm or wrist fractures, it is an important initial procedure in fracture care.

ANATOMY AND PHYSIOLOGY

See "Fracture Immobilization."

INDICATIONS

- Any injury to the wrist or hand that involves torn or stretched tendons or ligaments

- Stable fractures
- Congenital or acquired deformities (radial club hand, arthritis)
- Conditions that require temporary immobilization to reduce inflammation (e.g., carpal tunnel syndrome, tendinitis)

CONTRAINDICATIONS

Uncontrolled bleeding

PRECAUTIONS

Splinting is a temporary therapy. Improper or inordinately long periods of splinting may result in functional limitation or deformity of the affected area. Some preformed splints are difficult to apply snugly enough to ensure a proper fit.

The practitioner can often accurately diagnose hand injuries by obtaining a thorough patient history and performing a complete physical examination of the hand. When the severity of injury is uncertain, immobilization in a splint with next-day referral is appropriate. Immediate consultation should be obtained in the presence of nerve or vascular damage, fracture-dislocation injuries, open fractures, substantial skin loss, or flexor tendon injuries at or distal to the wrist.

ASSESSMENT

Once the patient history, including mechanism of injury and any associated conditions, and physical examination suggest bone, tendon, or ligament injury, splinting is indicated. Inspect the skin for any breaks in integrity; do not apply a splint over major open wounds.

Fingers

- Before splinting, examine the finger carefully for evidence of rotational deformity; this can be accomplished by having the patient sit opposite the practitioner. The patient then places his or her palms up and flexes the MCP joints to 90 degrees. The practitioner examines the digits from the distal end and notes the orientation of the nail beds and distal finger pads. Normally, the nail beds should be in approximately the same plane as those on the opposite hand.
- Instruct the patient to "make a fist" while keeping the PIP and DIP joints straight; if there is overriding or underriding of a digit that is different from the contralateral hand, there is evidence of rotational deformity. Immediately refer these patients to a hand specialist or an orthopedist.

PATIENT PREPARATION

- Inform the patient of the reason for the splinting, how his or her wrist or hand is to be positioned as the splint is applied, when the splint may be removed (if at all) by the patient, the expected duration of the splinting, and how to keep the splint clean and dry.
- While the splint is being applied, explain to the patient that as the splinting material hardens (if it is plaster or fiberglass), it becomes quite warm. The heat given off is temporary and will not cause a burn; the heat subsides within a few minutes.

EQUIPMENT

- Rigid or semirigid material 3 to 4 inches wide (fiberglass, preformed splinting material, or plaster casting tape), padded aluminum splints (for fingers), or preformed splints
- Padding material
- Water
- Gloves (nonsterile)
- Scissors
- Elastic bandage (such as Ace wrap); usually 2-inch width is appropriate for hand or wrist
- Tape (¼-inch adhesive or silk) or metal clips

Procedure

WRIST

1. Measure the patient's arm from the MCP joints to 1 inch distal to the elbow (Figure 7-4). Unroll the cast padding to that same length, creating six to eight layers. Create one additional layer of padding the same length, and set it aside.
2. Don gloves. Dip the casting tape into the water for 10 to 15 seconds; gently squeeze excess water from the tape.
3. Unroll four to six layers of casting tape on top of the layered padding. Place the final single layer of padding on top of the casting tape.
4. With the wrist in the appropriate position (generally straight or in slight dorsiflexion), place the layered padding side of the splint against the volar surface of the skin and secure it with an Ace wrap. Do not stretch the Ace wrap while securing the splint.
5. Once the splint is in place, use the palm of your hand to mold the splint to the patient's wrist and arm. The splint will harden in about 10 minutes.

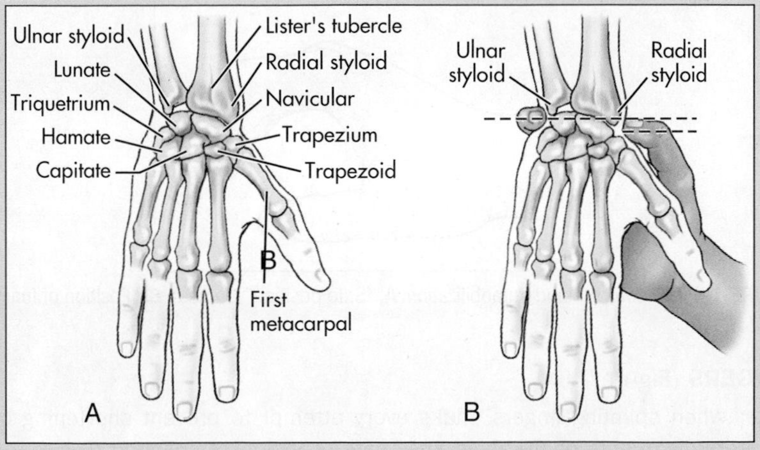

FIGURE 7-4 Bones of the wrist. **A,** Bones of the wrist (dorsal aspect). **B,** Reference points in palpation of the wrist. The radial styloid process is more distal than the ulnar styloid.

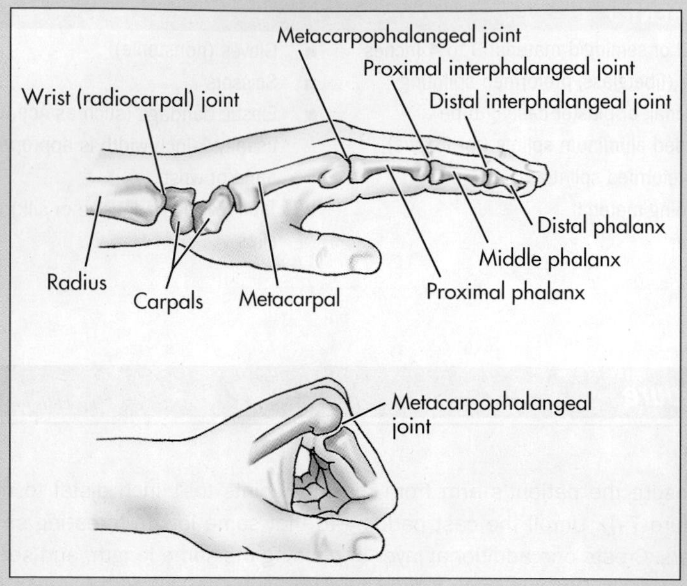

FIGURE 7-5 Carpal bones of the hand.

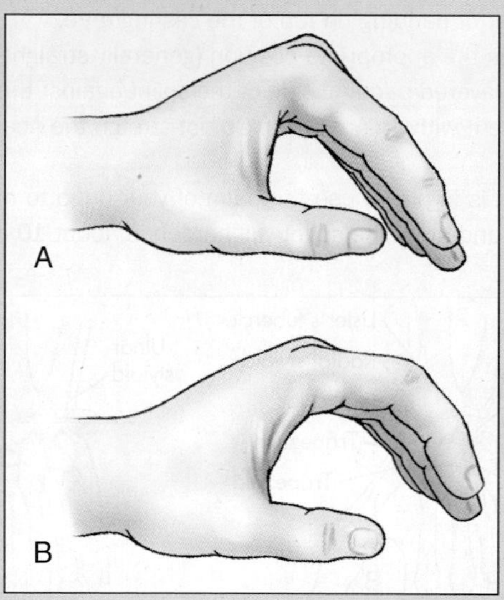

FIGURE 7-6 Positions of hand immobilization. **A,** "Safe position" (James). **B,** "Position of function."

FINGERS (Figure 7-5)

Note: When splinting fingers, make every attempt to prevent shortening of the collateral ligaments of the digit. The "safe" position of splinting (Figure 7-6, A) maintains the MCP joint in 70 to 90 degrees of flexion and the PIP joint in 10 to 20 degrees of flexion. The "position of function" used in the splinting of finger fractures and sprains may result in a loss of hand function secondary to collateral ligament shortening (see Figure 7-6, B).

1. Using the contralateral uninjured digit as a template, measure from the tip of the finger to the heel of the hand.
2. Using scissors, cut a padded aluminum splint to this length. Splints may be applied to either the dorsal or volar surface of the digit; if in doubt, the volar surface is generally safe.
3. Again using the contralateral digit as a guide, place the affected digit in the "safe" position. The splint is applied to the palmar surface of the finger.
4. Once the splint is appropriately bent, attach it to the injured finger with ¼-inch tape. If additional security is necessary, "buddy tape" the splinted digit to the adjacent digit.

PATIENT EDUCATION POSTPROCEDURE

- Instruct the patient as to signs of neurovascular compromise and/or pressure areas.
- The patient may loosen the Ace wrap if throbbing, pain, or swelling increases.
- Instruct the patient to contact the primary care practitioner if the acts of loosening the Ace wrap and elevating the wrist do not relieve symptoms.

COMPLICATIONS

- Complications of improper splinting include skin breakdown beneath the splint, contracture, functional deficit, and decreased circulation.
- Flexor or extensor tendon tears of the fingers that are improperly or inadequately splinted may result in a permanent loss of function.

PRACTITIONER FOLLOW-UP

- Follow-up should be determined on the basis of the type and severity of the injury. The patient with a known or suspected fracture should be referred to an orthopedist within 1 to 2 days of the injury.
- Patients who have a tendon injury must be immediately referred to an orthopedist or a hand specialist.

■ CPT BILLING

29130—Application of finger splint; static ■ **29131**—Application of finger splint; dynamic

The codes for treatment of fractures and joint injuries (dislocations) are categorized by the type of manipulation (reduction) and stabilization (fixation or immobilization). These codes can apply to either open (compound) or closed fractures or joint injuries.

26600—Closed treatment of metacarpal fracture, single; without manipulation, each bone ■ **26750**—Closed treatment of distal phalangeal fracture, finger or thumb; without manipulation, each bone ■ **25622**—Closed treatment of carpal scaphoid (navicular) fracture; without manipulation ■ **25630**—Closed treatment of carpal bone fracture (excluding carpal [scaphoid]); without manipulation, each bone ■ **25650**—Closed treatment of ulnar styloid fracture ■ **25500**—Closed treatment of radial shaft fracture; without manipulation ■ **25530**—Closed treatment of ulnar shaft fracture; without manipulation ■ **25600**—Closed treatment of distal radial fracture (e.g., Colles or Smith type) or epiphyseal separation, includes closed treatment of fracture of ulnar styloid, when performed without manipulation

REFERENCES AND RELATED RESOURCES

Borchers JR, Best TM: Common finger fractures and dislocations, *Am Fam Physician* 85(8):805–810, 2012.

Chow J, Hsu S, Kwok D, Reagh J: Application techniques for plaster of Paris back slab, resting splint, and thumb spica using ridged reinforcement, *J Emerg Nurs* 39(5):e79–e81, 2013.

Gaston RG, Chadderdon C: Phalangeal fractures: displaced/nondisplaced, *Hand Clin* 28(3):395–401, 2012.

Splinting: Ankle Sprains

Christy L. Crowther-Radulewicz

7

DESCRIPTION

Sprains are the most common injury to the ankle for which a patient is seen in the emergency department or by a primary care practitioner. *Simple sprains,* although common, are frequently inappropriately treated because many practitioners have a limited understanding of ankle anatomy and physiology. Proper assessment and treatment of ankle injuries are essential to promoting return of motion and function.

ANATOMY AND PHYSIOLOGY

Any stretching or tearing of the lateral or medial ligaments surrounding the joint as the result of excessive force being applied by inversion, eversion, or hyperextension may result in an ankle sprain. Inversion injuries to the ankle are most common and result in damage to the lateral ligaments. Ankle injuries occur in every age population, but are more prevalent in childhood through late middle age.

The ankle joint is primarily stabilized by two sets of ligaments: the *lateral collateral ligaments* (made up of the anterior talofibular, calcaneofibular, and posterior talofibular ligaments) and the *medial* or *deltoid ligaments.* The most commonly injured ligament of the ankle is the *anterior talofibular* ligament; this occurs when an inversion stress is applied, often when the foot is plantar flexed. The *calcaneofibular* ligament joins the so-called upper and lower ankle joints; this is the second most commonly injured ligament. The *posterior talofibular* ligament is the strongest of the three and is least likely to be injured in a common lateral malleolar sprain (Figure 7-7). Damage to the posterior talofibular ligament tends to be associated with higher impact-type activities that often involve a rotational component to the injury.

Eversion injuries, which result in damage to the medial ligaments, are much less common than *inversion* injuries. The deltoid ligament is the broadest and thickest

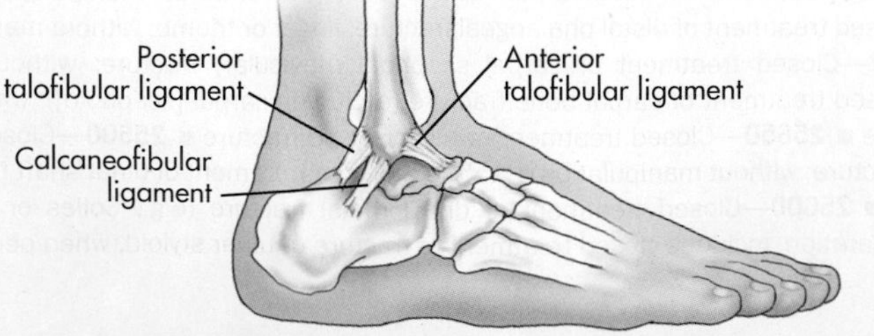

FIGURE 7-7 Three important ligaments of the lateral aspect of the ankle.

ligament in the ankle, so it is more difficult to sustain excessive stress to this ligament. Medial malleolar sprains may result in an avulsion of the distal medial tip of the tibia (the medial malleolus). As force is continued in an eversion injury, the inferior tibiofibular ligament and interosseous membrane may tear (Figure 7-8).

INDICATIONS

- Ankle sprains are classified into three grades, based on pathology, function, and instability (Table 7-1):
  - **Grade I** injuries are those that result from minor stretching without tearing of the involved ligament or ligaments and do not involve joint instability.
  - **Grade II** sprains consist of partial tearing of the involved ligaments with some joint instability. This is a moderate injury, which results in some compromise of function.
  - **Grade III** injuries are marked by significant swelling, ecchymosis, and instability of the joint. These are the result of a complete tear of the ligament.

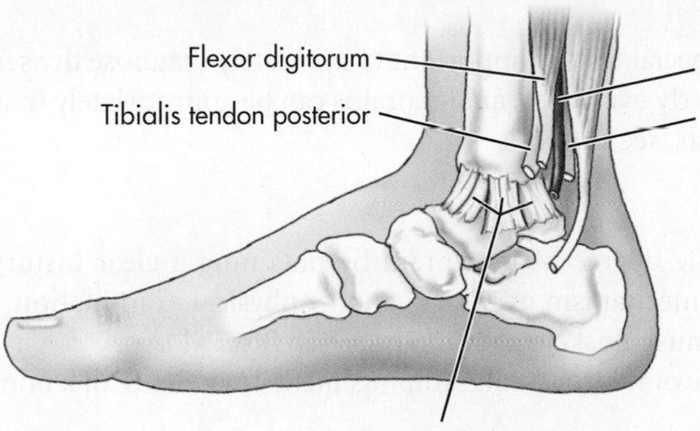

FIGURE 7-8 Deltoid ligament.

TABLE 7-1 Clinical Diagnosis of Ligament Injury

	FIRST-DEGREE SPRAIN	SECOND-DEGREE SPRAIN	THIRD-DEGREE SPRAIN
Synonym	Mild sprain	Moderate sprain	Severe sprain
Etiology	Direct or indirect trauma to joint	Same	Severe direct or indirect trauma to joint
Symptoms	Pain, mild disability	Pain, moderate disability	Pain, severe disability
Signs	Mild point tenderness; no abnormal motion; little or no swelling	Point tenderness; loss of function; slight to marked abnormal motion; visible swelling	Moderate point tenderness; moderate abnormal motion; loss of function; obvious localized deformity/swelling; radiographs demonstrate abnormal motion
Pathology	Minor tearing of ligament	Partial tearing of ligament	Complete tearing of ligament
Complications	Tendency to recur	Persistent instability; recurrence; aggravation	Persistent traumatic arthritis instability; traumatic arthritis

Modified from Standard nomenclature of athletic injuries, American Medical Association, 1976, Chicago. In American Academy of Orthopaedic Surgeons: *Athletic Training and Sports Medicine,* ed 2. Rosemont, IL, 1991, American Academy of Orthopaedic Surgeons, p. 413.
Czaijka CM, Tran E, Cai AN, DiPreta JA: Ankle sprains and instability, *Med Clin North Am* 98:313-329, 2014.
Papaliodis DN, Vanushkina MA, Richardson NG, DiPreta JA: The foot and ankle examination, *Med Clin North Am* 98:181-204, 2014

- Patients presenting with signs of grade III sprains should immediately be referred to an orthopedic surgeon. Some grade I sprains may be treated by the primary care practitioner, but it is more prudent to refer these patients to an orthopedic surgeon.

CONTRAINDICATIONS

Open wounds or open fractures.

PRECAUTIONS

- Careful evaluation of the ankle must be made before any splinting.
- A patient with any ankle instability should be referred to an orthopedist.
- Other possible causes of ankle pain and swelling are:
  - Fractures of the foot (proximal fifth metatarsal)
  - Syndesmosis rupture
  - Achilles tendon rupture
  - Infection (osteomyelitis, septic joint)
  - Osteochondritis desiccans of the talus
  - Tumor
- Knowledge of a few special tests is important to accurately diagnose the severity of the injury. Once properly evaluated, ankle sprains can be appropriately treated. For specific evaluation tests, see Box 7-1.

ASSESSMENT

- Evaluate and grade the degree of the sprain by obtaining a clear history of the injury (including the mechanism of injury) and by physical examination.
- Perform a thorough musculoskeletal evaluation (see Box 7-1).
- Assess for any evidence of neurovascular impingement or evidence of a bony injury.

PATIENT PREPARATION

- Patients should be informed about the purpose of splinting and its expected duration.

BOX 7-1 Specific Tests

Anterior drawer test (Figure 7-9): This test is used to increase stress on the anterior talofibular ligament. If straight anterior movement of the talus occurs, it indicates both medial and lateral ligament insufficiency. If only one side moves forward, there is ipsilateral insufficiency.

Talar tilt test (Figure 7-10): This test is used to determine whether the calcaneofibular ligament is torn. The patient lies on his or her side while the examiner holds the foot in anatomic alignment with the leg parallel to the floor. The talus is then tilted from side to side. The calcaneofibular ligament is stressed when the foot is tilted into adduction.

Thompson test (Figure 7-11): This test measures the integrity of the Achilles tendon. The patient kneels on a chair with his or her feet hanging over the front of the seat. The practitioner compresses the calf muscles; if there is no plantar flexion of the foot, the test is positive for Achilles tendon rupture.

Radiographic examination: Ideally, three views of the ankle should be taken to rule out fracture or dislocation.

Anteroposterior view: Anteroposterior viewing allows for examination of the joint space and any obvious fracture of the distal tibia or fibula should be visible. This view also allows evaluation of the talus.

Lateral view: A lateral viewing allows for a better view of the talus and calcaneus; it is easier to see a spiral fracture of the distal fibula.

Mortise view: A mortise view is similar to the anteroposterior view, but the foot and ankle are internally rotated 15 to 30 degrees. This is the best view for evaluating the ankle mortise.

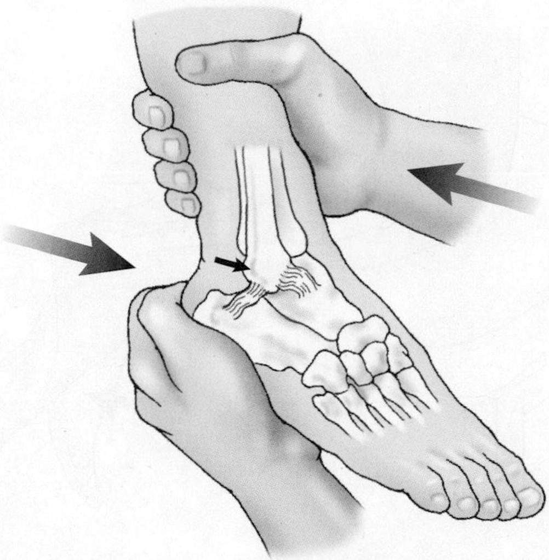

FIGURE 7-9 The calcaneus (and talus). The calcaneus and talus move anteriorly beneath the tibia when there is ligamentous disruption of the ankle joint. This is a positive "anterior drawer" sign.

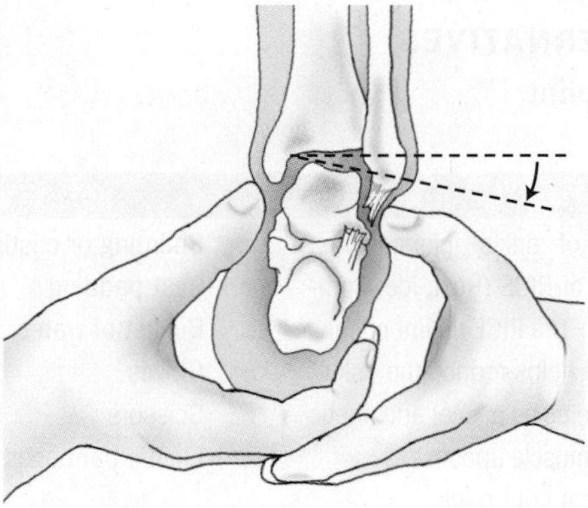

FIGURE 7-10 Talar tilt test. If both the anterior talofibular and calcaneofibular ligaments are disrupted, the ankle is unstable on talar tilt testing.

- Splinting and immobilization of the injured area is a temporary intervention to reduce pain and the risk of further damage to adjacent soft tissues.
- Explain that the casting tape will be placed in some water to begin the chemical reaction that will harden the fiberglass or plaster. As the splint hardens, it becomes warm, but the warmth is temporary.
- The splint is to remain in place at all times, unless the patient is instructed by a practitioner to remove it.
- Reassure the patient that this procedure should not hurt. A sprain may be as painful as a fracture, and immobilization will actually lessen the pain overall.
- Splinting will require the patient's cooperation in holding the proper position; it may take some time to complete the proper splinting procedure.

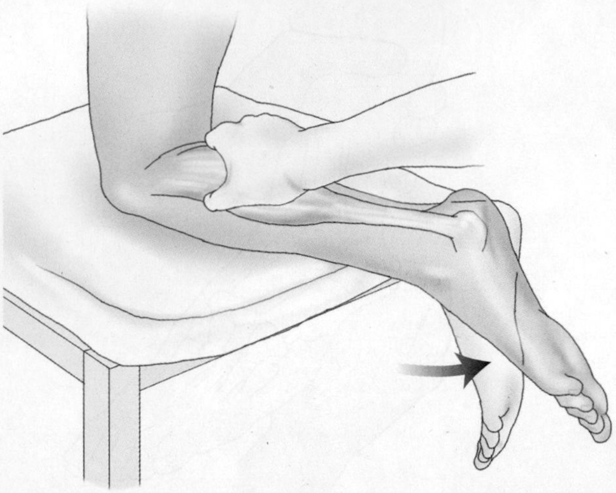

7

FIGURE 7-11 Thompson test. Squeezing the muscles in the calf should elicit plantar flexion of the foot when the Achilles tendon is intact. This Thompson test is most useful when there is prominent heel and calf pain and pain prevents adequate examination of the Achilles apparatus. A negative (normal) Thompson test in this case provides reassurance that the Achilles tendon is not ruptured.

TREATMENT ALTERNATIVES

- Air-stirrup-type splint

EQUIPMENT

The initial treatment of ankle injuries (first 24-48 hours) consists of RICE (Rest, Ice, Compression, and Elevation). The RICE regimen limits soft tissue swelling and helps reduce the risk of further injury. Ice also helps as a local anesthetic and may relieve some muscle spasm.

- Ice bag or chemical cold pack
- Ankle immobilizer (Aircast or other)
- Splinting or casting material
- Cast padding
- Bucket of water
- Gloves
- Scissors
- Elastic bandages

Procedure

Elastic bandages alone are insufficient support for anything but a grade I sprain. Significant ankle sprains require support that is strong enough to prevent movement of the joint.

READY-MADE STIRRUP-TYPE SPLINT

1. Place the flat central piece of fabric beneath the patient's heel (the rounded edge of the calcaneal strap follows the contour of the heel).

2. Apply the semirigid medial and lateral supports to the ankle.
3. If the splint does not conform to the individual's anatomy, inflate the air bladders in each upright side piece to provide compression and support. The supports should feel snug to the patient, yet still be comfortable.
4. Fasten the Velcro straps.

SUGAR TONG (COAPTATION SPLIT OR U-SPLINT)

1. Have the patient lie prone on a table with the injured leg flexed to 90 degrees at the knee. (This also assists in maintaining a 90-degree angle at the ankle.)
2. Measure a length of cast padding along the posterior lower leg from the tip of the toes to just beneath the knee. The splinting material is placed posteriorly along the calf and sole of the foot to the toes. (The splint should be wide enough to extend from the medial to lateral calf, crossing under the heel.)
3. Unroll several layers of padding this same length (or wrap the foot and lower leg with padding).
4. Using the first measured length of padding as a guide, wet and unroll six to eight layers of casting tape to the same length.
5. Place the casting layers on the posterior leg and the entire bottom of the foot.
6. Secure with an elastic wrap, wrapping in a distal-to-proximal direction.

PATIENT EDUCATION POSTPROCEDURE

- Teach patients how and when to use ice, compression, elevation, moist heat, crutches, and physical therapy.
- *Cryotherapy:* Apply an ice pack to the joint for 10- to 20-minute periods three or four times a day. Ice should (in general) be discontinued after the first 24 to 48 hours postinjury. A compressive dressing, such as an Ace wrap, may also reduce swelling if the ankle is not splinted.
- *Crutches:* Crutches may be used for the first several days to avoid placing additional stress on an already damaged joint.
- Teach patients a three-point gait wherein both crutches and the nonsupportive leg go forward, then the good leg comes through. The crutches are immediately brought forward and the pattern is repeated.
- Proper sizing of the crutches to the patient is crucial to successful crutch walking. To ensure proper placement, place the crutch tips 6 to 8 inches from the outside of each foot (using a short forward placement of the crutches to maximize stability), and measure the upper pads for fit. They should be two or three fingerbreadths beneath the axilla, with the patient's elbows slightly bent.
- *Ice:* Use ice as long as there is swelling.
- *Physical therapy:* Physical therapy is begun as soon as pain-free exercise is possible, usually within 1 to 2 weeks of injury. Exercises begin with range of motion, and then isometric, isotonic, and isokinetic activities for dorsiflexion, plantar flexion, inversion, and eversion. Athletes and older adults should be directed to a formal physical therapy program, whereas many otherwise healthy, motivated people may use a home exercise program.

- Make sure the patient can reiterate the signs and symptoms of neurovascular impairment: tingling, numbness, and blanching of the skin.
- Pain control may be achieved through the use of common nonsteroidal antiinflammatory drugs, with high doses at regular intervals often required. Patients on nonsteroidal antiinflammatory drug therapy should be aware of the purpose, dosage, side effects, and toxicities of their particular medication.
- Inform patients that ankle sprains may take some time to heal. Even after 6 to 8 weeks of healing, there may be residual problems, such as increased joint size and increased sensitivity to barometric pressure changes.

COMPLICATIONS

There is potential for increased swelling and skin breakdown or neurovascular compromise if the splint is wrapped too tightly with the elastic bandage. If applied too loosely, the splint will fail to adequately immobilize the ankle. Additionally, if the splint is not adequately padded, especially over bony prominences, skin breakdown can occur.

PRACTITIONER FOLLOW-UP

- Complications of an ankle sprain include ankle instability and weakness; surgical repair of an ankle sprain is still controversial.
- Ankle pain or swelling that does not resolve over a week or two may be indicative of additional injury, such peroneal tendonitis or peroneal neuropathy, or fracture (talus and anterior calcaneal process fractures are frequently missed on initial evaluation).
- Recurrent sprains are associated with inadequate immobilization for a sufficient time while ligamentous healing occurs. Recurrent swelling is fairly common and may persist for many months.
- Patients are generally followed for 2 to 4 weeks, as needed. If symptoms of pain or joint instability persist on follow-up, the patient should be referred to an orthopedist.
- Without adequate care, acute ankle trauma can result in chronic joint instability. Use of a standardized protocol enhances the management of ankle sprains. In patients who have grade I or II sprains, emphasis should be placed on accurate diagnosis, early use of RICE (see "Splinting: Ankle Sprains, Equipment"), maintenance of range of motion, and use of an ankle support. Sprains that have complete tendon tears (grade III) may require surgical intervention. Although early motion and mobility are recommended, ligamentous strength does not return until months after an ankle sprain.

■ CPT BILLING

29540—Strapping ankle and/or foot ■ **29515**—Application of short leg splint (calf to foot)

REFERENCES AND RELATED RESOURCES

Czaijka CM, Tran E, Cai AN, DiPreta JA: Ankle sprains and instability, *Med Clin North Am* 98:313, 2014.

Jibri Z, Mukherjee K, Kamath S, Mansour R: Frequently missed findings in acute ankle injury, *Semin Musculoskelet Radiol* 17(4):416–428, 2013.

Lau LH, Kerr D, Law I, Ritchie P: Nurse practitioners treating and foot injuries use the Ottawa Ankle Rules: a comparative study in the emergency department, *Australas Emerg Nurs J* 16:110, 2013.

Papaliodis DN, Vanushkina MA, Richardson NG, DiPreta JA: The foot and ankle examination, *Med Clin North Am* 98:181, 2014.

Polzer H, Kanz KG, Prall WC, Haasters F, Ockert B, Mutschler W, Grote S: Diagnosis and treatment of acute ankle injuries: development of an evidence-based algorithm, *Orthop Rev (Pavia)* 4:22–32, 2012.

Tiemstra JD: Update on acute ankle sprains, *Am Fam Physician* 83:1170, 2012.

Reduction of Subluxated Radial Head

Christy L. Crowther-Radulewicz

DESCRIPTION

Radial head subluxation ("pulled elbow" or "nursemaid elbow") is a common emergency pediatric problem. It often results from a child being suddenly pulled up by the extended arm, causing excessive traction on the arm. Other mechanisms of injury include infants rolling over on their arm during sleep or direct trauma to the arm. The injury is an anterior subluxation of the radial head away from the capitellum through the annular ligament. This distortion in bone positioning may be reversed through steady pressure and manipulation of the bone into its proper alignment.

ANATOMY AND PHYSIOLOGY

A *subluxated radial head* is a tear in the distal attachment of the annular ligament through which the radial head protrudes. The proximal portion of the annular ligament slips into the radiohumeral joint. This injury primarily occurs in children 1 to 5 years of age, with about 50% presenting with severe pain and an inability to move the arm after a sudden pull on the child's extended arm. About one third of children presenting with this problem have had a prior episode.

INDICATIONS

- Obvious deformity and pain on movement
- Often a prior history of radial head subluxation

CONTRAINDICATIONS

Do not attempt to reduce a radial head subluxation where there is a possibility of a fracture or dislocation.

PRECAUTIONS

If swelling, ecchymosis, discoloration of the arm, crepitation, or other injury is noted, refer the patient to an orthopedic specialist.

ASSESSMENT

- Listen for a history consistent with a subluxated radial head (usually the history is one of a sudden upward pulling force on the child's extended arm).
- The child often presents carrying the injured arm against the body or supports the injured arm using the other hand.
- The forearm is usually pronated with the elbow slightly flexed.
- Tenderness may be palpated over the anterolateral aspect of the radial head.
- Passive flexion and extension of the elbow is tolerated within a 30- to 120-degree range.
- The child strongly resists passive supination of the forearm.
- Examination of the shoulder, wrist, and clavicle is unremarkable.
- Do not obtain unnecessary radiographs. The radiographs may appear normal even when the radial head is indeed subluxated. Associated fractures can occur, but are not common. If there is a question about the existence of a fracture, radiographs are warranted.

PATIENT PREPARATION

- Explain to the parents that their child's elbow is slightly out of place and that you are going to put it back in place. Warn them that this is going to hurt for a few minutes.
- Warn the child that there will be momentary discomfort.

Procedure

1. Place the patient in the parent's lap (Figure 7-12).
2. Support the elbow with your hand. Put your thumb over the head of the radius and press down while you smoothly and fully supinate the forearm and extend the elbow.
3. Complete the procedure by fully flexing the elbow while your thumb remains pressing against the radial head and the forearm remains supinated (Figure 7-13).
4. A click should be felt and may even be heard. This signals the reduction has taken place.

An alternative procedure is to hyperpronate the lower arm/wrist.

1. Place the child in the parent's lap.
2. While supporting the affected elbow with your hand, place your thumb over the radial head and smoothly pull the arm toward you while pronating the wrist and forearm. After the forearm is fully pronated, the elbow is passively flexed.
3. The practitioner should feel a click as the reduction occurs.

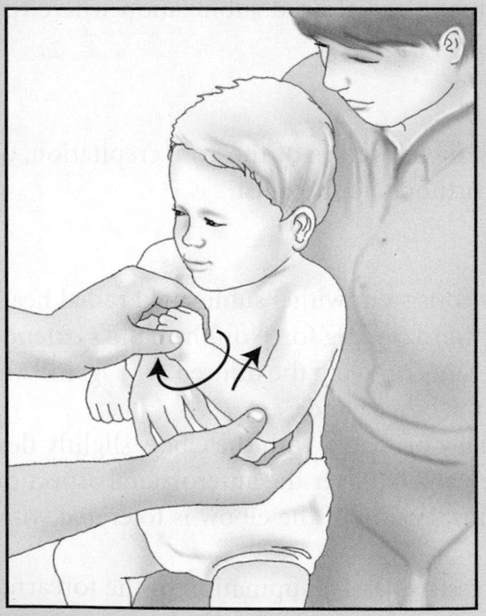

FIGURE 7-12 Positioning child for reduction of subluxated radial head. Maneuver involves gentle supination of the forearm and flexion of the elbow. The examiner's thumb can be placed over the child's elbow to help palpate the radial head during the reduction process.

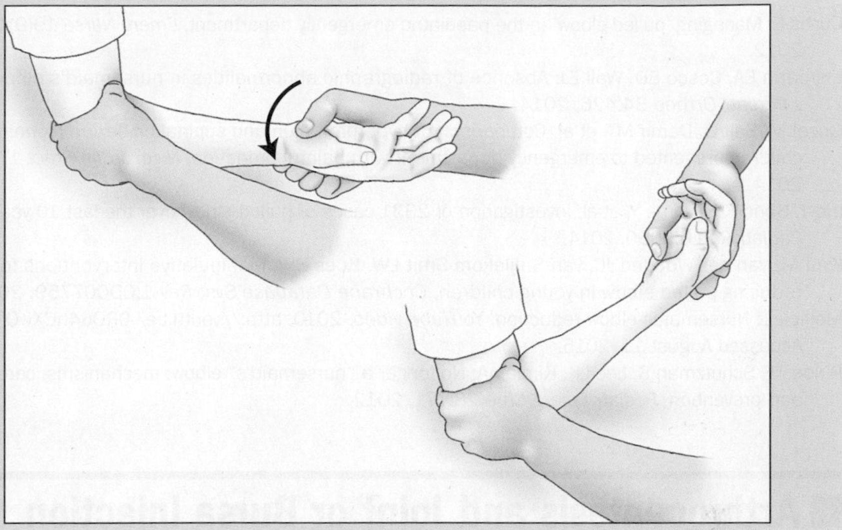

FIGURE 7-13 Hyperpronation technique for reduction of radial head subluxation.

PATIENT EDUCATION POSTPROCEDURE

- The child will usually scream or cry until the click is felt. Let the child calm down, and then reexamine to make sure the child has fully recovered.
- The child should begin to use his or her arm with full range of motion within 30 minutes. No sling or restraint is necessary.
- Instruct the patient to return for follow-up within 1 week.
- Educate the patient's parents against pulling on the child's hand.
- Instruct the patient's parents to watch for signs of restricted arm use or a repeated subluxation.
- Instruct the patient's parents to seek medical attention if fever, erythema, or edema occurs around the joint.

COMPLICATIONS

- Reoccurrence of subluxation.

PRACTITIONER FOLLOW-UP

- If the practitioner does not feel a click, the reduction is probably not complete.
- Failure to achieve or maintain reduction is more frequent in injuries less than 2 hours old.
- If full range of motion is not achieved, have the child wait 2 hours, and then repeat the procedure.
- Five percent of children will have recurrences; these patients should be referred to an orthopedic specialist.

■ CPT BILLING

24640—Closed treatment of radial head subluxation in child, nursemaid elbow, with manipulation
■ **24650**—Closed treatment of radial head or neck fracture; without manipulation

REFERENCES AND RELATED RESOURCES

Curtis E: Managing 'pulled elbow' in the paediatric emergency department, *Emerg Nurse* 19(9):24–27, 2012.

Eismann EA, Cosco ED, Wall EJ: Absence of radiographic abnormalities in nursemaid's elbows, *J Pediatr Orthop* 34:426, 2014.

Guzel M, Salt O, Demir MT, et al: Comparison of hyperpronation and supination-flexion techniques in children presented to emergency department with painful pronation, *Niger J Clin Pract* 17:201, 2014.

Irie T, Sono T, Hayama Y, et al: Investigation of 2331 cases of pulled elbow over the last 10 years, *Pediatr Rep* 6:5090, 2014.

Krul M, van der Wouden JC, van Suijlekom-Smit LW, Koes BW: Manipulative interventions for reducing pulled elbow in young children, *Cochrane Database Syst Rev* 1:CD007759, 2012.

Mellick L: Nursemaids elbow reduction, *YouTube video,* 2010. http://youtu.be/-0ROu4hCXwQ. Accessed August 11, 2015.

Ruloe TF, Schutzman S, Lee LK, Kimia AA: No longer a "nursemaid's" elbow: mechanisms, caregivers, and prevention, *Pediatr Emerg Care* 28:771, 2012.

7

Arthrocentesis and Joint or Bursa Injection

Christy L. Crowther-Radulewicz

DESCRIPTION

Arthrocentesis is the aspiration of fluid from a joint space for the purpose of diagnostic evaluation or to decrease inflammation. Bursal aspiration is also used for diagnostic evaluation or to reduce fluid accumulation from inflammation or blood. Corticosteroids are often injected to decrease inflammation and pain in either the joint or bursa. The use of in-office ultrasound machines to guide injections is becoming a more common practice among examiners.

ANATOMY AND PHYSIOLOGY

Joint spaces are surrounded by a synovial sac that is normally filled with a small amount of lubricating (synovial) fluid. Traumatic, autoimmune, or infectious processes can cause inflammation and excess fluid accumulation within the synovial sac. Excessive fluid within a joint is called an effusion. Joint effusions typically limit normal range of motion, particularly flexion.

Bursae lie closer to the surface and cover the bony prominences; normally, bursae are relatively flat, but when inflamed because of injury, infection, or other inflammatory processes, they can contain a large amount of fluid. Most bursae are extraarticular; as such, even when inflamed, they rarely interfere with range of motion.

Although corticosteroid injections are useful in relieving pain and inflammation, they should never be administered if there is any possibility of acute or untreated infection.

INDICATIONS

- Joint aspiration and injection are used therapeutically to reduce symptoms.
- As an adjunct to other rehabilitative therapies, function is improved by limiting pain and inflammation.
- Injection is recommended specifically for pain or swelling that causes limitation in range of motion, pain that affects usual daily activities, and pain that causes cessation of work activities.

- Joint injection also is a way of delivering pharmacologic agents directly into the joint space.
- Arthrocentesis also has a diagnostic function. It is often performed to obtain synovial fluid, which is helpful in the diagnosis of joint inflammation. The procedure is helpful in differentiating between local and referred joint or soft tissue pain.
- Local anesthetics can help differentiate between local and referred pain, provide fluid volume for the injection, and help distribute corticosteroids in large joints.

CONTRAINDICATIONS

- Active tumor at site
- Active infection, particularly cellulitis, at site
- Joint prosthesis in place
- Recent serious joint injury, especially if the skin is open over the injection site
- Patient is known to have bacteremia
- Patient is anticoagulated or has a major clotting disorder
- Unstable or inaccessible joints
- Weight-bearing tendons, such as Achilles tendon, patellar tendon, or posterior tibial tendon, directly overlie intended puncture site

PRECAUTIONS

- There are many relative contraindications to either arthrocentesis or injection, and the risk-benefit ratio should be taken into consideration for each patient. Consider carefully this procedure in patients with any of the following problems: diabetes, systemic immunosuppression or infection, osteoporosis, or history of steroid flare.
- Consider that the procedure may cause problems and potential problems caused by the corticosteroid agent itself. Allergic reactions to anesthetics are often related to preservatives. The use of a single-dose, preservative-free agent may decrease the risk of such an allergic reaction.
- Although the risk of tendon rupture is quite low, the potential for significant damage from this problem is high; therefore, direct tendon injection should be avoided. Any injections by primary care providers around the Achilles and patellar tendons are not recommended.
- The potential for injury to the cartilage from the corticosteroid injection is also high. Because of this, the number of injections at a single site should be limited. It has been observed that if three injections do not provide relief, it is unlikely that additional injections will make a difference.
- Because hypothalamic-pituitary-adrenal axis suppression can occur up to 4 days after an injection, inject only one large joint at a time.
- Patients are often very anxious about having a large needle inserted into their joints. When the clinician turns away from the patient to draw up the medication, the patient may be blocked from directly seeing the needle; this is often helpful in decreasing anxiety.

ASSESSMENT

- Perform a targeted physical examination aimed at detecting musculoskeletal pathology and identifying specific maneuvers that reliably provoke symptoms. This examination establishes a baseline on which therapeutic improvements may be measured.
- *Shoulder, rotator cuff (subacromial space):* Patient has pain with abduction and positive impingement maneuver.

- *Elbow, lateral epicondylitis:* Patient has localized pain over the lateral elbow that is exacerbated by resisted wrist extension.
- *Hip, greater trochanteric bursitis:* Patient has pain when sleeping on affected side and tenderness over the greater trochanter.
- *Knee:* Patient presents with effusion of joint or fluctuance and swelling of periarticular bursae.

PATIENT PREPARATION

- Explain procedure and obtain written informed consent.
- Both aspirations and injections will cause mild discomfort. Although lidocaine is used, it is not always injected to deaden the skin, but sometimes instead is injected with the corticosteroid after fluid is withdrawn.

TREATMENT ALTERNATIVES

- *Conservative treatment for mild problems:* RICE (see "Splinting: Ankle Sprains, Equipment").
- *Aggressive treatment:* Arthroscopic procedures.
- Refer the patient to an orthopedist for any potential infection, problems that require hand or wrist injection or injection into deep anatomic sites (hip; sacroiliac joint), or when there is any nerve involvement, tendonitis, lack of equipment, or lack of knowledge about how to perform the procedure.

EQUIPMENT

- Alcohol and povidone-iodine preps
- Sterile gloves
- One 3-ml, one 10-ml, and one or more 5- to 60-ml syringes
- One 25-gauge, 1½-inch needle for injection of local anesthetic agent
- One 22- to 25-gauge, 1½-inch needle for injection of corticosteroid
- 18-gauge, 1½-inch needles for injection of hyaluronic acid derivatives or aspiration of joint
- *Local anesthetic agents:* lidocaine HCl 1% and 2% solution **without** epinephrine or preservatives (in single-dose vial); bupivacaine HCl, or ethyl chloride or vapocoolant anesthesia spray
- Two sterile hemostats
- Culture tube and other laboratory supplies
- 4 × 4 sterile gauze pads
- Elastic bandages, 3 or 4 inches in width
- Tape
- *Therapeutic medications:* corticosteroids, hyaluronic acid derivatives (Table 7-2)
- Corticosteroids are classified as to their solubility and duration of action. High-solubility preparations have a shorter duration of action; low-solubility compounds have a longer duration.
- The dose of corticosteroid varies widely, depending on the injection site and the technique of the clinician.
- General rules include (1) decrease the dose for young patients, older adults, and those in poor health and (2) use caution with short-acting corticosteroids in patients who have diabetes because the drugs may exacerbate the disease.
- Short-acting steroids are used for quick relief in self-limiting disorders, such as bursitis. Intermediate-acting steroids are used to decrease inflammation and produce longer

TABLE 7-2 Comparison of Dosage, Solubility, and Relative Potencies of Corticosteroid Agents Used for Intraarticular Injections

CORTICOSTEROID	DOSE	SOLUBILITY	RELATIVE ANTIINFLAMMATORY POTENCY
Betamethasone sodium phosphate and acetate	4-8 mg (joint), 0.6 mg (bursa)	Low	20-30
Dexamethasone	0.3 mg (tendon)- 3.0 mg (large joints)	High	25
Hydrocortisone acetate	20 mg	High	1
Methylprednisolone acetate	4 mg (bursa), 20-60 mg (joint)	Medium	5
Prednisolone tebutate	5-10 mg	Medium	4
Triamcinolone acetonide	5-10 mg (joint)	Medium	5
Triamcinolone diacetate	12.5-25 mg		
Triamcinolone hexacetonide	20-60 mg (joint), 12.5-25 mg (bursa)		

Skedros JG, Hunt KJ, Pitts TC: Variations in corticosteroid/anesthetic injections for painful shoulder conditions: comparisons among orthopaedic surgeons, rheumatologists, and physical medicine and primary-care physicians. *BMC Musculoskelet Disord* 8:63, 2007.
Monseau AJ, Nizran PS: Common injections in musculoskeletal medicine. *Prim Care Clin Office Pract* 40:987, 2013.

relief. Long-acting steroids are used in chronic conditions, such as tendonitis and ganglion cysts.

- For individuals who have osteoarthritis of the knee and who do not respond to other pharmacologic or nonpharmacologic treatments, the knee may be injected with one of several hyaluronic acid derivatives. These products provide viscoelastic supplements that replace diseased synovial fluid of the osteoarthritic joint. Hyaluronate sodium is a natural substance that acts as both a lubricant and shock absorber in the joint. A series of hyaluronic acid injections given over a variable number of weeks can reduce joint pain from 1 week up to 1 year. The drugs are contraindicated in patients who have allergies to chicken because they are synthesized from chicken products.

Procedure

GENERAL ARTHROCENTESIS

Note:

The skin does not have to be anesthetized unless a large-diameter (18-gauge) needle is used. The anesthetic agent and corticosteroid can be mixed in the same syringe and injected simultaneously. As an option, the skin may be sprayed with a topical anesthetic, such as a vapocoolant spray, which provides sufficient anesthesia for a virtually painless entry.

1. Position the client comfortably with the affected joint well illuminated by light.
2. Take time to identify structural landmarks.
3. Maintain sterile procedure for injection site and needle tip.

4. Mark the injection site with your thumbnail or indent the skin with the end of the plastic needle cap.
5. Cleanse the area with alcohol pledgets, and then with povidone-iodine-soaked gauze.
6. Don sterile gloves.
7. If using a local anesthetic, use a 25- or 27-gauge needle, inject into the cutaneous layer of skin to form a superficial wheal, and then inject into deeper subcutaneous tissue without entering the joint or bursa. Avoid injecting large volumes of air by carefully loading the syringe.
8. Using the 5-ml syringe with an 18-gauge needle, insert the needle through the skin and into the intraarticular space.
9. Do not move the needle from side to side because this may damage articular surfaces. Aspirate slowly to minimize trauma.
10. If more fluid needs to be aspirated, stabilize the needle hub with the hemostat, remove the filled syringe, and replace it with an empty sterile syringe and then reaspirate the fluid.
11. Inject obtained fluid into tubes (depending on indications, complete cell count with differential, Gram stain and culture, and crystal analysis might be appropriate).
12. When no more fluid can be aspirated, withdraw the needle, cleanse the skin again, apply a pressure dressing with the 4 × 4 gauze, and tape securely. Wrap the joint with an elastic bandage.

ARTHROCENTESIS AND INTRAARTICULAR CORTICOSTEROID INJECTION

1. Proceed as in steps 1 through 12 until all fluid is removed.
2. Using a 3-ml syringe and a 25-gauge needle, draw up 1% lidocaine and appropriate corticosteroid. Mix well by gently rotating the syringe back and forth.
3. Stabilize the needle with a sterile hemostat, and replace the first syringe with the second syringe that contains the lidocaine and steroid mixture.
4. Aspirate to make sure there is no blood, and then inject the medication steadily into the joint.
5. Do not inject medication against resistance. Medication should be injected into anatomic spaces; resistance may suggest that the needle tip may be in a ligament or tendon. Redirect the needle until minimal resistance is encountered.
6. Remove the syringe and needle.
7. Cleanse the skin again. Apply a pressure dressing with a 4 × 4 gauze, and apply an elastic bandage over the joint.
8. Ice may be applied to the area for 20 minutes to help limit soft tissue swelling and pain.

Note: Technique modifications: Some clinicians do not mix the anesthetic agent and corticosteroid in one syringe, but instead inject the anesthetic, and then change syringes to inject the corticosteroid.

CORTICOSTEROID INJECTION INTO BURSAE

- Procedure is the same as outlined except that the amount of both the aspirate and injected corticosteroid is much less. The following are site-specific guides for injection:

Shoulder-Rotator Cuff (Subacromial Space)

- For the treatment of rotator cuff tendonitis and shoulder impingement syndrome, palpate the posterior tip of the acromion, and insert the needle into the space between the acromion and the head of the humerus. Use the thumb of the nondominant hand on the tip of the acromion and place the index finger on the coracoid process to maintain a clear orientation. Insert the needle 1 to 2 cm beneath the thumb, aiming anteriorly on a slight angle toward the coracoid process. Once in the space, draw back on the syringe to ensure that the needle is not in a vascular structure (Figure 7-14).

Elbow-Lateral Epicondylitis or Olecranon Bursitis

- Epicondylar injection is to be considered after more conservative measures have been attempted. The lateral epicondyle is palpated; this area is quite pain sensitive, so take care not to hit the bone (Figure 7-15).
- *Olecranon bursitis:* Raise a cutaneous wheal with lidocaine and infiltrate the skin and soft tissues with an anesthetic. Inject the needle directly into the bursa and aspirate any fluid. Use the nondominant hand to "milk" the fluid. Because this

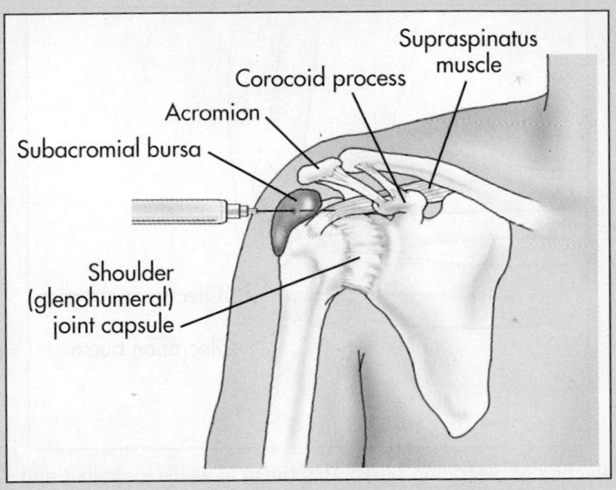

FIGURE 7-14 Sample injection process for rotator cuff (supraspinatus tendonitis).

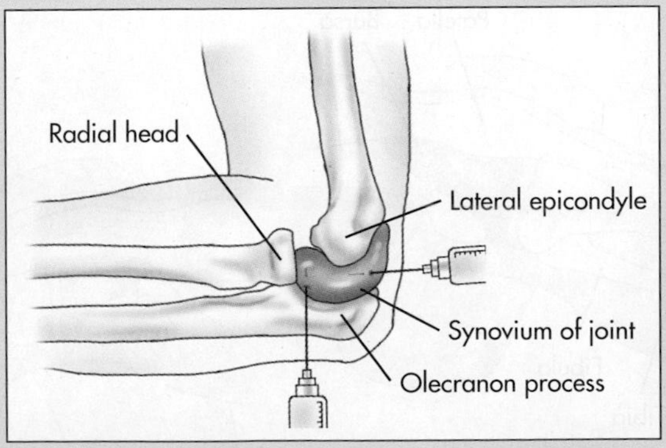

FIGURE 7-15 Injection for elbow-lateral epicondylitis. Flex the elbow 45 degrees. Identify the lateral epicondyle. Inject over the lateral epicondyle and superior to the olecranon process of the ulna.

bursa is fairly superficial and can easily become infected, use caution during this process (Figure 7-16).

- *Hip-greater trochanteric bursitis:* This is not usually treated by primary care clinicians.

Knee

- *Knee aspiration:* Patient may be seated or lie in the supine position with the knee slightly flexed with a pillow under the joint. A local anesthetic agent may be used for the skin and soft tissues down to the joint capsule. Palpate the superior lateral or medial aspect of the patella and insert the needle on an angle toward the posterior center of the patella and toward the femoral intercondylar notch (into the space between the patella and femur). This approach will enter the suprapatellar bursa, which directly communicates with the knee joint. Aspirate the fluid, taking care to massage or milk the suprapatellar spaces with the free hand to help compress any fluid and to aid in its withdrawal. Stabilize the needle with a hemostat, unscrew the syringe, and exchange it for the syringe containing the medication. Inject the medication, and then withdraw the needle (Figure 7-17).

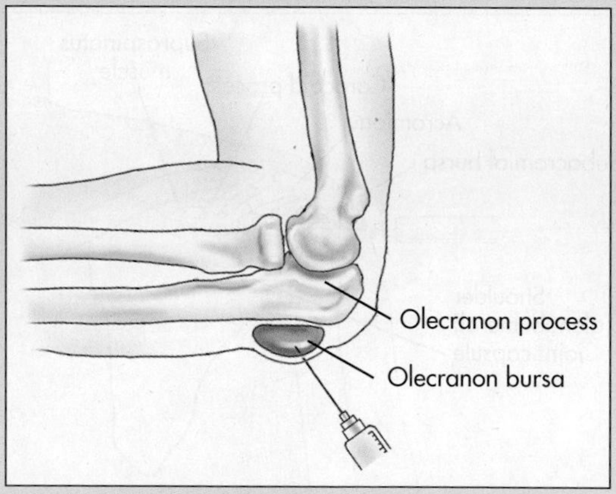

FIGURE 7-16 Injection of olecranon bursa. This bursa is easily identified and entered. Insert the needle directly into the bursa and aspirate until fluid is returned.

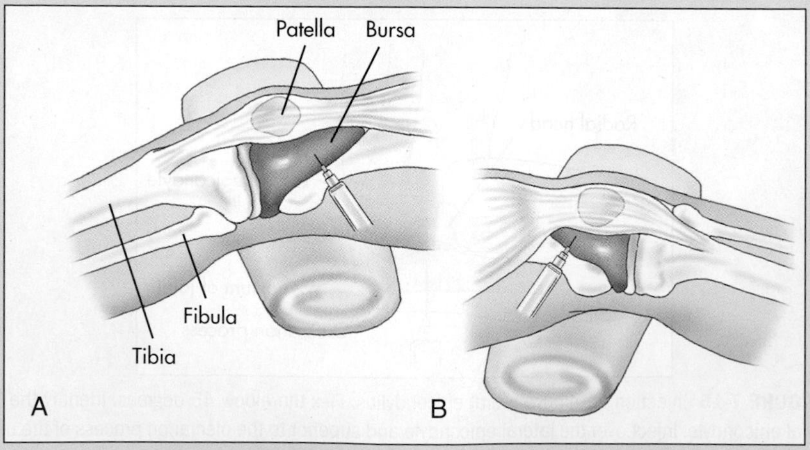

FIGURE 7-17 Aspiration of the knee joint. Position the slightly flexed knee with a towel in the popliteal space on an examination table. Either a lateral **(A)** or medial **(B)** approach may be used.

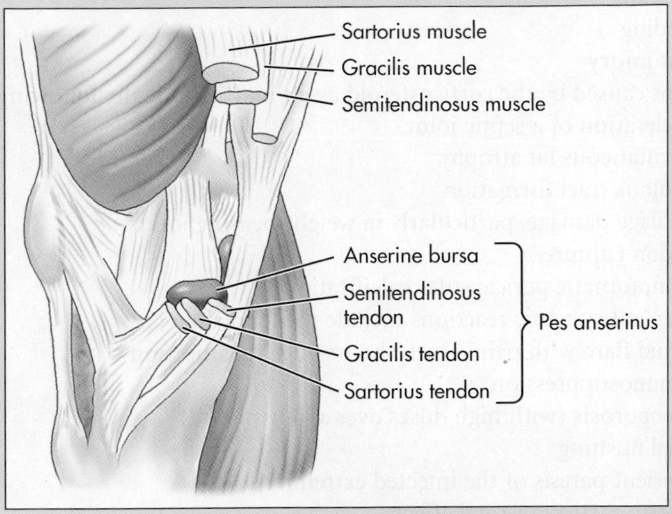

FIGURE 7-18 Pes anserine bursa injection.

- *Injection of pes anserine bursitis:* The pes anserine bursa is located along the medial aspect of the knee joint about 2 cm beneath the medial joint line. With the patient either supine or seated, palpate the point of maximal tenderness, usually 2 cm inferior to the medial joint line at the insertion of the sartorius, gracilis, and semitendinosus muscles. Anesthetize the skin. Then insert the needle slowly until it gently touches the bone. Withdraw the needle 2 to 3 mm, aspirate any fluid, and then change the syringe and needle to inject the corticosteroid (Figure 7-18).

PATIENT EDUCATION POSTPROCEDURE

- Instruct the patient to rest the joint for at least 24 hours and to avoid weight bearing as much as possible.
- Ice may be applied to the area for 20 to 30 minutes as often as every 2 hours as needed until the follow-up visit.
- Instruct the patient to remove the dressing and bandage in 24 hours.
- Warn the patient about the possibility of *steroid flare,* a painful condition that may begin 6 to 12 hours after injection and may last 2 to 3 days. The self-limiting problem may be related to precipitation of crystals within the tissue fluid.
- Instruct the patient to watch for signs of infection (redness, swelling, drainage, foul odor) and return for follow-up if any sign of infection develops.
- Fluid in a joint or bursa may reaccumulate. If so, instruct the patient to return for follow-up.
- Instruct the patient to exercise—to stretch and strengthen the area.

COMPLICATIONS

- Problems caused by the injection process consist of local reactions:
  - Swelling
  - Skin changes, including hypopigmentation

  - Infection
  - Bleeding
  - Joint injury
- Problems caused by the corticosteroid agent may include the following:
  - Acceleration of a septic joint
  - Subcutaneous fat atrophy
  - Fistulous tract formation
  - Cartilage damage, particularly in weight-bearing joints
  - Tendon rupture
  - Asymptomatic pericapsular calcification
- More general systemic reactions include the following:
  - Steroid flare with pain 6 to 12 hours after the injection
  - Immunosuppression
  - Osteoporosis (with high doses over a long period)
  - Facial flushing
  - Transient paresis of the injected extremity
  - Adverse gastrointestinal effects
  - Mood alterations (including euphoria)
  - Fluid retention
  - Menstrual irregularities
  - Allergic or hypersensitivity reactions
  - Glycosemia

PRACTITIONER FOLLOW-UP

Obtain results of culture or other fluid analyses and provide additional follow-up treatment as indicated, depending on the underlying problem.

■ CPT BILLING

Do not bill an E/M code with a joint injection, if the sole purpose for the visit was the joint injection. If the E/M is a significant separate service, the E/M code and the injection are both reportable, with modifier 25 attached to the E/M code.

20600—modifier 25 attached to the E/M code section, small joint or bursa (e.g., fingers, toes); without ultrasound guidance ■ **20605 06**—Arthocentesis, aspiration and/or injection, intermediate joint or bursa (e.g., temporomandibular, acromioclavicular, wrist, elbow or ankle, olecranon bursa); without ultrasound guidance ■ **20610 06**—Arthocentesis, aspiration and/or injection, large joint or bursa (e.g., shoulder, hip, knee, subacromial bursa); without ultrasound guidance

REFERENCES AND RELATED RESOURCES

Bhagra A, Syed H, Reed DA, et al: Efficacy of musculoskeletal injections by primary care providers in the office: a retrospective cohort study, *Internat J Gen Med* 6:237, 2013.

Bellapianta J, Swartz F, Lisella J, et al: Randomized prospective evaluation of injection technique for the treatment of lateral epicondylitis, *Orthopedics* 34:e708, 2011.

Boss SE, Mehta A, Maddow C: Critical orthopedic skills and procedures, *Emerg Med Clin N Am* 31: 261–290, 2013.

Courtney P, Doherty M: Joint aspiration and injection and synovial fluid analysis, *Best Pract Res Clin Rheumatol* 27:37, 2013.

Dean BJ, Lostis E, Oakley T, et al: The risks and benefits of glucocorticoid treatment for tendinopathy: a systematic review of the effects of local glucocorticoid on tendon, *Semin Arthritis Rheum* 43:570, 2014.

Fischer J, Guerts J, Valderrabano V, et al: The risks and benefits of glucocorticoid treatment, *J Clin Rheumatol* 19:373, 2013.

Guerini H, Ayral X, Vuillemin V, et al: Ultrasound-guided injection in osteoarticular pathologies: general principles and precautions, *Diagn Interv Imaging* 93:674, 2012.

Hall MM: The accuracy and efficacy of palpation versus image-guided peripheral injections in sports medicine, *Curr Sports Med Rep* 12:296, 2013.

Hansford BG, Stacy GS: Musculoskeletal aspiration procedures, *Semin Intervent Radiol* 29:270, 2012.

Saikh S, Verma H, Yadav N, et al: Applications of steroid in clinical practice: a review, *ISRN Anesthesiol* 2012:985495, 2012.

Ganglion Cyst Aspiration

Christy L. Crowther-Radulewicz

7

DESCRIPTION

Ganglions of the hand and wrist are common benign lesions. The contents of a ganglion cyst are removed by aspiration. Sometimes steroids are injected into the area to reduce the potential for recurrence.

ANATOMY AND PHYSIOLOGY

Ganglion cysts are outpouchings of bursae, ligament, or tendon sheaths, with no clear etiology and no relation to nerve ganglia. The cyst is an encapsulated and frequently semimobile mass of tissue found near a joint or tendon sheath. Some occur after trauma to the affected area. The cyst fills with thick, gelatinous synovial fluid. This fluid regenerates in the cyst more than 50% of the time after either simple aspiration, aspiration and injection, or surgical excision. Some ganglion cysts spontaneously resolve.

INDICATIONS

- Although some patients seek evaluation of a ganglion because of pain, research shows that most patients are more concerned about the cosmetic appearance of the ganglion, and a large number are also concerned about the possibility of malignancy.
- Aspiration of a ganglion cyst may be considered if the cyst causes pain, decreases joint mobility, or impinges on nearby tissue such as a joint, blood vessels, or nerves. Activities that place stress on the wrist (gymnastics or occupations that require repetitive wrist motion) may also aggravate the cyst and cause it to grow in size, necessitating removal. Ganglion cysts often decrease in size after the area is rested.
- The origin of the majority of surgically treated ganglia is the scaphotrapeziotrapezoid or radiocarpal joints. Because of a large number of recurrences after nonoperative treatment, surgical excision is recommended as the primary definitive treatment for volar wrist ganglia.

CONTRAINDICATIONS

- Anticoagulant therapy or presence of a clotting disorder
- Sepsis
- Recent joint fractures

PRECAUTIONS

- Conduct a thorough history and physical examination of the affected extremity to ascertain that everything else is normal.
- The primary care clinician may defer performing this procedure and refer the patient to a surgeon if there has been a lack of response to previous attempts to drain or inject the cyst.

ASSESSMENT

- Carefully evaluate the site of the cyst, noting its size and its relation to other structures. Ganglia are commonly located on either the dorsum or volar aspect of the wrist. Ask the patient to flex (for a volar cyst) or extend (for a dorsal cyst) the fingers or wrist; this may accentuate the movement of the cyst. Pain can occur with compression of the cystic mass.
- Ganglion cysts often occur in patients who have underlying arthritic conditions.
- Radiographs are of no value unless there is some question of bony pathology.

PATIENT PREPARATION

- Explain that this fluid-filled cyst poses no particular danger. Make certain that the patient understands the high potential for recurrence.
- Obtain written informed consent after discussing the different treatment options with the patient and giving the patient a chance to make a treatment decision.
- The procedure causes mild discomfort.

TREATMENT ALTERNATIVES

- The three major treatment options are observation, aspiration, and surgical excision. *Observation* is acceptable in most instances.
- *Manual reduction* of the cyst by applying finger or thumb pressure is often possible in cysts that have been present for less than 3 months. If this is possible, a padded button or coin can be firmly secured to the area with an elastic bandage for a 3-week period to prevent reaccumulation of the cyst material.
- Indications for more aggressive treatment include pain, obvious interference with activity, evidence of nerve compression, and, rarely, imminent ulceration (in the case of some mucous cysts). The recurrence rate after cyst *aspiration* is high: more than 50% for cysts in most locations.
- *Surgical excision* of the cyst is effective in reducing symptoms if care is taken to completely excise the stalk of the cyst along with a small portion of the joint capsule. A recurrence rate of only 5% is seen with surgical excision. Ganglion surgery is usually performed in either a hospital or an outpatient surgical center because it requires anesthesia and careful technique to decrease the chance of damage to adjacent structures and to reduce the likelihood of recurrence.
- For ganglion cysts that have more well-defined capsules, the following are options:
  - Drain the cyst with an 18-gauge needle.
  - Drain the cyst with an 18-gauge needle, and then inject a corticosteroid into the cyst.
  - Refer the patient to a surgeon for surgical excision of the cyst.
  - Do nothing and hope for a spontaneous remission.

EQUIPMENT

- Skin cleansing solution (alcohol pads; povidone-iodine solution)
- 4 × 4 gauze pads
- Sterile gloves
- Sterile drapes
- 1% lidocaine (from single-dose vials without epinephrine or preservatives)
- One or two 3-ml syringes with a 25-gauge needle
- 5-ml syringe with a 18-gauge needle
- Culture tube (optional)
- Corticosteroid if injection is planned (see Table 7-2)
- Gauze pad, compression dressing, tape

Procedure

1. Scrub skin with alcohol and cleansing solution using gauze pads.
2. Don sterile gloves.
3. Drape the area with sterile drapes.
4. Using an 18-gauge needle and 5-ml syringe, aspirate the mucinoid material within the cyst. Use your fingers to compress the cyst, forcing additional material into the syringe. If blood is aspirated, remove the needle and dress the wound (Figure 7-19).
5. Send aspirate for culture if it is cloudy or if there is any question about the contents.
6. Use extreme caution if the ganglion is near a nerve or an artery.
7. Using the 25-gauge needle and 3-ml syringe, draw up 0.5 ml of 1% lidocaine and 0.5 ml of the corticosteroid. Mix well by gently rotating the syringe back and forth.
8. Inject the medication steadily into the cyst area, and then withdraw the needle.
9. Apply a compression dressing.

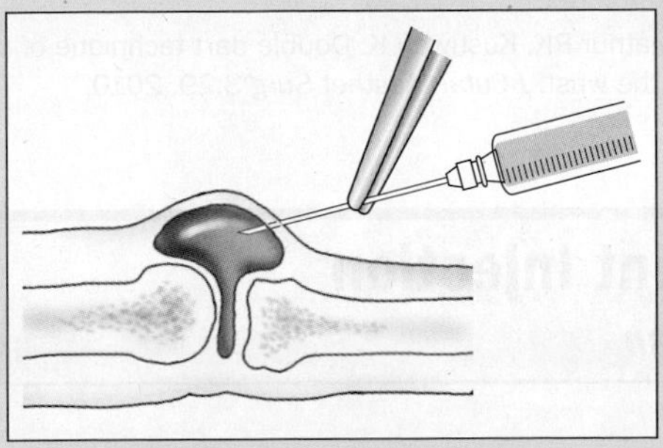

FIGURE 7-19 Ganglion cyst aspiration.

PATIENT EDUCATION POSTPROCEDURE

- Instruct the patient to keep the compression dressing in place for at least 3 hours and the area covered for 3 days.
- Instruct the patient to rest the joint for 24 hours. Keep it elevated for at least 24 hours. Keep weight-bearing to a minimum for a week.

- Some redness, swelling, and heat are normal. Instruct the patient to watch for signs of infection, such as purulent drainage or a foul odor.
- Instruct the patient to take acetaminophen (Tylenol) or ibuprofen every 4 to 6 hours as needed to control mild pain.
- Instruct the patient to return for follow-up in 1 week.

COMPLICATIONS

- Reoccurrence of cyst
- Rare infection of cyst

PRACTITIONER FOLLOW-UP

- Other than checking the aspiration area, usually no follow-up is necessary.
- If a culture specimen is obtained, provide needed follow-up or treatment if required.

■ CPT BILLING

20600—Arthocentesis, aspiration and/or injection, small joint or bursa (e.g., fingers, toes); without ultrasound guidance ■ **20605**—Arthocentesis, aspiration and/or injection, intermediate joint or bursa (e.g., temporomandibular, acromioclavicular, wrist, elbow or ankle, olecranon bursa); without ultrasound guidance

REFERENCES AND RELATED RESOURCES

Dermon A, Kapetanakis S, Fiska A, Alpantaki K, Kazakos K: Ganglionectomy without repairing the bursal defect: long-term results in a series of 124 wrist ganglia, *Clin Orthop Surg* 3:152, 2011.

Gude W, Morelli V: Ganglion cysts of the wrist: pathophysiology, clinical picture, and management, *Curr Rev Musculoskelet Med* 1(3–4):205, 2008.

Hawkes R, O'Connor P, Campbell D: The prevalence, variety and impact of wrist problems in elite professional golfers on the European Tour, *Br J Sports Med* 47:1075, 2013.

Hochberg MC, Altman RD, April KT, Benkhalti M, Guyatt G, McGowan J, Towheed T, Welch V, Wels G, Tugwell P; American College of Rheumatology: American College of Rheumatology 2012 recommendations for the use of nonpharmacologic and pharmacologic therapies in osteoarthritis of the hand, hip, and knee, *Arthritis Care Res*, 64:465, 2012.

Meena S, Gupta A: Dorsal wrist ganglion: current review of the literature, *J Clin Orthop Trauma* 5:59, 2014.

Paramhans D, Navak D, Mathur RK, Kushwah K: Double dart technique of instillation of triamcinolone in ganglion over the wrist, *J Cutan Aesthet Surg* 3:29, 2010.

Trigger Point Injection

Jared Spackman

DESCRIPTION

Although there is no strong clinical evidence for utilizing them, trigger point injections are a method for treating myofascial pain syndrome (MPS) by injecting specific trigger points with an anesthetic agent, such as 1% lidocaine or isotonic saline. Botulinum toxin A injections have shown promise in relieving trigger point pain and certain headaches, but trigger point injections should be considered as only a part of a multifaceted treatment for MPS.

ANATOMY AND PHYSIOLOGY

Myofascial pain syndrome is a common muscle disorder in which trigger points may develop. The etiology remains obscure, but some researchers think that pain might be caused by localized tissue ischemia and acidic accumulation of acids and other inflammatory molecules from prolonged muscle contraction. Other proposed mechanisms involved in the development of trigger points include the thought that within the area, muscle nociceptors respond to sustained noxious stimulation, initiating motor and sensory changes in both the peripheral and central nervous systems. These changes create sensitization in a localized area, and pain and dysfunction are characteristic of this condition. Trigger points produce localized pain with movement and pressure, contributing to a decreased ability to carry out activities of daily living.

There is no consensus on the exact mechanism of inactivation that occurs with injection. Disruption of abnormal muscle fibers and/or nerve endings, local release of intracellular potassium, and interruption of nerve function with a local anesthetic are proposed to be of benefit and bring the symptom relief as reported in the medical literature.

INDICATIONS

- Symptoms and examination consistent with an active trigger point
- Trigger points should be relatively few in number
- Trigger point may either demonstrate a taut band with a local twitch response or have a positive "jump sign" when the patient winces or attempts to pull away from the pressure upon moderate palpation of the muscle

CONTRAINDICATIONS

- Local or systemic infection
- Patient history of bleeding disorders
- Patient pregnancy
- Local muscle trauma

PRECAUTIONS

- Relative contraindications are patients with a high risk for infection (i.e., diabetes), patients who are debilitated, and patients who are on chronic steroid therapy or have compromised immune function.
- Relative contraindication in those who have allergies to anesthetics, though isotonic saline may be used.

ASSESSMENT

- An appropriate history should be collected. Often there is a history of acute trauma or repetitive microtrauma. Lack of conditioning, poor biomechanics, sleep disturbances, and joint problems are known contributors. Acute sports injuries are often implicated as well.
- An appropriate and targeted physical examination should be performed to identify trigger points that would be appropriate for treatment. Latent trigger points without acute symptoms should not be injected. For patients who have other etiologies, such as fibromyalgia, complex regional pain syndrome should not be treated with this modality. Patients presenting with comorbid psychological

concerns, such as major depression or anxiety, should be treated only when clear indications exist.
- Trigger points may occur in any location where skeletal muscle is present. Trigger points often are found within the muscles of the neck, shoulders, and pelvic girdle.

PATIENT PREPARATION

- Explain procedure to the patient and obtain a written consent from the patient.
- Explain to the patient that the procedure may cause discomfort. If the practitioner is using an anesthetic, explain that there may be some soreness or discomfort when the anesthetic effect wanes.

TREATMENT ALTERNATIVES

- Conservative treatment for myofascial pain includes activity modification, physiotherapy, RICE (see "Splinting: Ankle Sprains, Equipment"), massage, transcutaneous electrical stimulation (TENS), and nonsteroidal antiinflammatories.
- Referral should be considered in patients who do not respond to two or three attempts at an area. Referral to a physical medicine specialist or rheumatologist should be considered if there is evidence of comorbid conditions complicating the myofascial pain or evidence of an underlying rheumatologic process.

EQUIPMENT

- Alcohol or povidone-iodine preps
- Syringes of variable sizes, typically a 5 cc syringe will suffice
- 22- to 25-gauge needle for injection
- Sterile gauze pads
- Gloves (either sterile or nonsterile)
- Lidocaine without epinephrine
- Isotonic saline
- Vapocoolant spray (optional)
- Adhesive bandages

Procedure

TRIGGER POINT INJECTION

Note: The skin does not have to be anesthetized before the procedure with a topical anesthetic spray, although doing so may provide a less painful needle entry.

- Draw up the appropriate amount of local anesthetic or isotonic saline utilizing sterile technique.
- Switch the needle to either a 22- or 25-gauge sterile needle.
- Position the patient in a comfortable, relaxed position under adequate lighting.
- Identify the trigger point(s) by palpating the taut band or cord of muscle fibers that may be up to a half centimeter in diameter. Identify the point of maximal tenderness that is the center of the trigger point.
- Don gloves.
- Cleanse the skin overlying the trigger point with alcohol and povidone-iodine.
- Isolate the trigger point between the thumb and index finger to trap the muscle fibers and to prevent displacement by the advancing needle.

- Inject a small amount of anesthetic into each trigger point, fanning out the medication into the trigger point until the muscle relaxes or the local twitch response stops.
- Apply pressure over the injection site.
- Apply a clean bandage.

PATIENT EDUCATION POSTPROCEDURE

- Stretching after the injection is key. The patient, with assistance from the clinician, should stretch the muscle to full length, if possible.
- Active range of motion should continue to resolve stiffness and determine the efficacy of the injection.
- Physiotherapy or active exercises should be performed postinjection.

COMPLICATIONS

Complications could include local infection at the injection site, hematoma, minor bleeding, and myositis ossificans.

PRACTITIONER FOLLOW-UP

Reevaluation of the injection sites may be indicated if symptoms return. Reinjection is not indicated until muscle soreness resolves, which is usually within a week.

■ CPT BILLING

20552—Injection(s); single or multiple trigger point(s), 1 or 2 muscles ■ **20553**—Injection(s); single or multiple trigger point(s), 3 or more muscles

REFERENCES AND RELATED RESOURCES

Jaeger B: Myofascial trigger point pain, *Alpha Omegan* 106(1-2):14-22, 2013.

Kishner S, Schraga ED: Trigger point injection, *Medscape.* Available at http://emedicine.medscape.com. Last updated May 11, 2015. Accessed September 16, 2015.

Shin SJ, Kang SS: Myositis ossificans of the elbow after a trigger point injection, *Clin Orthop Surg* 3(1):81-85, 2011.

Wong CS, Wong SH: A new look at trigger point injections, *Anesthesiol Res Pract,* 2012:492452, 2012.

Zhou JY, Wang D: An update on Botulinum toxin A injections of trigger points for myofascial pain, *Curr Pain Headache Rep* 18(1):386, 2014.

Dislocation Reduction: Finger (DIP and PIP Joints)

Jared Spackman

DESCRIPTION

Reduction is a technique by which two joint surfaces that have lost complete continuity are brought back in approximation to each other with manual force. The force used depends on whether the distal portion of the digit is volar, dorsal, or lateral.

ANATOMY AND PHYSIOLOGY

The second through fifth digits are comprised of three bones that are associated with a single metacarpal proximally. Dislocation of a joint typically occurs when a force is sufficient to create complete loss of continuity between the joint surfaces. This is different from a subluxation, in which only partial loss of continuity occurs. A fracture may or may not appear in conjunction with any finger dislocation, and it is important to determine whether a fracture has occurred or whether any articular surfaces are involved.

Prevention of routine dislocation is the role of the ligaments, fibrocartilage plates, joint capsules, and the bicondylar arrangement of the bones. Many forces can cause dislocation, including hyperextension, hyperflexion, ulnar or radial stress, or straight axial loading. Although less common, a direct crush injury may cause dislocation.

Dorsal dislocations of the proximal interphalangeal (PIP) joint are most common and are often sports related. Volar PIP joint dislocations are the least common and almost always involve an injury to the central slip of the extensor tendon of the joint.

INDICATIONS

- Symptoms and examination consistent with a dislocation of the distal interphalangeal (DIP) or PIP joint of a digit
- Radiograph demonstrates complete joint space discontinuity
- No open wound is present

CONTRAINDICATIONS

- Injury to the nerve or blood supply of the digit
- Fracture of the phalanx, particularly an articular fracture
- Open wound
- Obvious volar plate or ligamentous rupture
- Inability to reduce the fracture with simple manipulation

PRECAUTIONS

- Relative contraindication in those who have prior deformity or other musculoskeletal problems, such as rheumatoid arthritis.
- A hand surgeon should be promptly consulted if any contraindications exist.

ASSESSMENT

- A proper history should be taken. This should include mechanism of injury, timing, and associated symptoms. In finger dislocations, time is of the essence because dislocations are more easily reduced early in the course of events.
- Hand dominance, previous injury history, and any allergies to anesthetics should be asked. Common physical signs include deformity, swelling, erythema, and tenderness to palpation. The patient will often complain of significant pain. The other digits and joints should be examined for injury. Ligamentous and tendon function should be intact. Neurovascular status and joint movement should be assessed.
- A three-view radiograph of the finger (anterior-posterior, lateral, and oblique) should be obtained to confirm dislocation and to assess for a complicating factor, such as a fracture.

PATIENT PREPARATION

- Explain the procedure to the patient and obtain written consent from the patient.
- Explain that the procedure may cause discomfort. If the practitioner is using an anesthetic, explain that there may be some soreness or discomfort when the anesthetic effect wanes.

TREATMENT ALTERNATIVES

- There are no reasonable treatment alternatives to reduce a simple uncomplicated dislocation.
- Referral should be considered in patients if an attempt at reduction is unsuccessful, there is an open dislocation, or when a contraindication is present.
- If a fracture or tendinous injury, such as a mallet finger deformity, is present, referral is indicated.

EQUIPMENT

- Alcohol and povidone-iodine preps
- Syringes of variable sizes, typically a 3- or 5-cc syringe will suffice
- 20-gauge needle for anesthetic solution or isotonic saline withdrawal
- 27-gauge needle for injection
- Sterile gauze pads
- Gloves (either sterile or nonsterile)
- Lidocaine without epinephrine
- Vapocoolant spray (optional)
- Adhesive bandages
- Tape
- Scissors
- Aluminum digital splints

Procedure

DIP OR PIP JOINT REDUCTION

Note: The skin does not have to be anesthetized with a topical anesthetic spray before a nerve block, although doing so may provide a less painful needle entry.

- Using the 20-gauge needle, draw up the appropriate amount of local anesthetic, using sterile technique.
- Switch the needle to a 27-gauge sterile needle.
- Position the patient in a comfortable, relaxed position under adequate lighting.
- Identify the dorsal aspects of both the radial and ulnar aspects of the digit.
- There are several techniques for administering local anesthesia before reducing a finger dislocation. One technique is described here:
  - Don gloves.
  - Cleanse the skin overlying the injection site with alcohol and povidone-iodine.
  - Inject the dorsal skin over the dorsal nerve branches, leaving a small wheal. Direct the needle ulnar and radial in the volar direction toward, but not into the digital nerves, utilizing approximately 1 to 2 ml on each side.
  - Reduction of a dorsal PIP dislocation should be attempted by applying gentle, but continuous distal traction and volar pressure on the middle phalanx at the

PIP joint. Successful relocation will typically provide immediate relief and the appearance of a normal, albeit sometimes swollen joint.

- Reduction of a volar PIP dislocation is performed by placing traction on the middle phalanx, flexing the distal finger, and placing dorsal pressure at the PIP joint.
- Reduction of a DIP joint is performed in similar fashion to the PIP joint.
- Postreduction radiograph should be obtained to confirm a successful procedure.
- Splint the joint in extension and refer the patient to a hand specialist for follow-up.

PATIENT EDUCATION POSTPROCEDURE

- Active range of motion should continue to resolve stiffness.
- Physiotherapy or active exercises should be performed postinjection.

COMPLICATIONS

Complications could include inadequate or delayed reduction, fracture with aggressive reduction, avulsion fracture of a phalangeal condyle, tendon injury, possible soft tissue interposition in the joint, chronic swelling, redislocation, contracture, or infection (if open fracture is present)

PRACTITIONER FOLLOW-UP

- Reevaluation of the joint is indicated within 2 to 3 weeks of reduction.
- Postreduction, referral to a hand therapist is beneficial for regaining range of motion, reducing swelling, and maintaining function.
- Prompt referral to a hand specialist is indicated if there are any signs of neurovascular compromise or if contraindications for reduction exist.

■ CPT BILLING

26700—Closed treatment of metacarpophalangeal dislocation, single, with manipulation, without anesthesia. ■ **26770**—Closed treatment of interphalangeal joint dislocation, single, with manipulation, without anesthesia.

REFERENCES AND RELATED RESOURCES

Borchers JR, Best TM: Common finger fractures and dislocations, *Am Fam Physician* 85(8):805–810, 2012.

Mangelson JJ, Stern P, Abzug JM, et al: Complications following dislocations of the proximal interphalangeal joint, *J Bone Joint Surg Am* 95(14):1326, 2013.

Polansky R, Schraga ED: *Finger dislocation joint reduction,* updated December 3, 2013. http://www.medscape.com.

Wilhelmi BJ, Molnar JA: *Hand anesthesia*, updated October 31, 2013. www.medscape.com.

Wolfson D, Raghavendra M: Anesthesia, regional, digital block, *Medscape reference: drugs, diseases, procedures*. http://www.medscape.com. updated September 23, 2014. Accessed December 10, 2014.

8

Genitourinary Procedures

Jared Spackman and Marilyn Winterton Edmunds

There are a few procedures, mostly involving the urinary tract, commonly performed in primary care practice. Most primary care practices provide numerous opportunities for the new graduate to develop expertise in these procedures.

ANATOMY AND PHYSIOLOGY

The renal and urinary systems are examples of internal organ systems that usually require radiographic or other significant examinations to assess for function. Their general status of health is measured by examining the urine that is produced. The evaluation of abnormalities in these structures is complicated by the reproductive system, whose organs are intertwined with the urinary tract. Thus a clear picture of the different organ systems and their location and function is essential in performing procedures.

The two oval kidneys lie in a retroperitoneal position, against the posterior wall of the abdomen. The left kidney is often slightly larger than the right. The ureter of each kidney conducts urine inferiorly from the kidney to the urinary bladder below. The entry to the bladder is guarded by a valve-like narrow region that prevents backflow from the bladder toward the kidneys.

The urinary bladder is located directly behind the symphysis pubis and is composed of smooth muscle tissue. The muscle layer is formed by a network of crisscrossing bundles of smooth muscle fibers, called the detrusor muscle, which runs in all directions. The bladder empties into the urethra.

In women, the urethra extends down and forward from the bladder for a distance of about 3 cm, ending at the urinary meatus. In contrast, the male urethra extends for about 20 cm, passing through the center of the prostate gland just after leaving the bladder. Two ejaculatory ducts that deliver fluid containing sperm join the urethra in the prostate. After leaving the prostate, the urethra angles down, forward, and then up to enter the penis, ending as a urinary meatus at the tip of the penis (Figure 8-1).

Bladder Scanning with Ultrasound

Jared Spackman

DESCRIPTION

Bladder scanning is a noninvasive procedure that measures urinary bladder volume. It should be performed as part of a routine continence assessment when urinary retention is suspected.

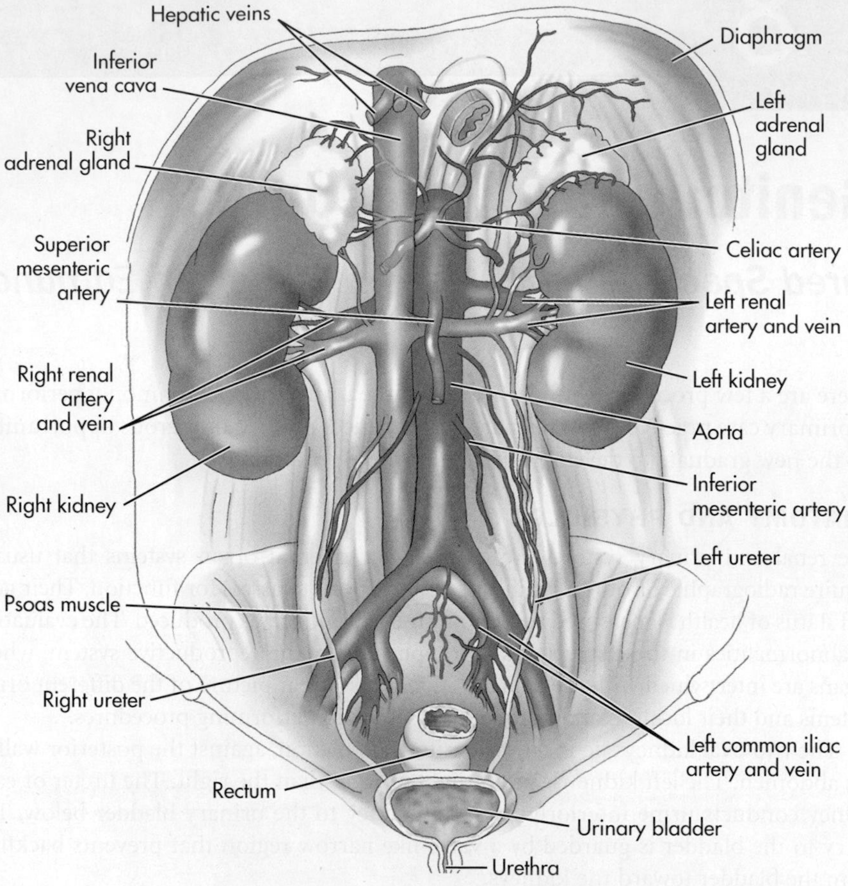

FIGURE 8-1 Location of urinary system organs.

ANATOMY AND PHYSIOLOGY

A bladder scanner is a portable, handheld ultrasound device, which can perform a quick, easy, and noninvasive scan of the bladder. The scanner has an ultrasound probe and transducer to reflect sound waves from the patient's bladder to the scanner. Information is then transmitted into a computer in the handheld unit to automatically calculate the bladder volume.

INDICATIONS

- Assess for urinary retention
- Suspected voiding dysfunction
- Monitor for residual urine in patients who have neurologic conditions
- Assess the ability to void following a trial without a catheter
- Recurrent urinary tract infections

CONTRAINDICATIONS

- If patient has a wound where the scanner probe would normally be placed
- If the patient is pregnant
- If the patient does not give consent

PRECAUTIONS

Precautions for this procedure include standard caution associated with ensuring the patient has given consent and is the correct person being scanned.

ASSESSMENT

The earlier stated "indications for bladder scanning" will determine the need to scan the bladder. The amount (in milliliters) of the results will determine the next step. Evidence-based protocols have varied from inserting a catheter and draining the bladder when a minimum of 100 ml, 200 ml, or 300 ml are determined on scanning. It is important to always evaluate the patient clinically to determine the need to insert a catheter at the current time versus "watchful waiting."

Patients who have contraindications or patients who are combative should be carefully assessed before an attempt to catheterize. In addition, the need for an indwelling catheter versus obtaining a sample with a straight catheter should be determined.

PATIENT PREPARATION

- Explain the procedure to the patient and obtain verbal consent from the patient before the procedure.
- Explain that the procedure may cause only mild discomfort.

TREATMENT ALTERNATIVES

Bladder volume can be determined by other means, including urinary catheterization, but that is not the preferred method because it is an invasive procedure.

EQUIPMENT

- Bladder scanner with head connection
- Ultrasound transmission gel
- Cleaning wipe
- Paper towels (single use only)
- Single-use, disposable apron if required
- Single-use, disposable, nonsterile gloves, if required
- A charged battery

Procedure

BLADDER SCANNING

1. Confirm the identity of the patient in an appropriate fashion.
2. Ensure verbal consent has been obtained from the patient before the procedure.
3. Explain to the patient the risks and benefits of the procedure.
4. The patient should be in a comfortable supine or semiprone position.
5. Prepare the equipment and clean the scan head with antiseptic.
6. Wash hands before the procedure.
7. If indicated, apply nonsterile gloves.
8. Expose the area above the pubic bone; strive to keep exposure to a minimum.
9. Clean the skin overlying the bladder.
10. Set the scanner to the proper gender, if applicable.

11. Apply a small amount of gel on the scanner head or on the suprapubic region.
12. Press the scan head in this area at a downward angle toward the bladder, ensuring the scan head is in the correct position (according to manufacturer specifications). For live scanners, both transverse and sagittal readings are required.
13. Press the button on the scan head and wait for the reading to display.
14. Repeat the procedure three or four times with minor adjustments to ensure accuracy.
15. Use a paper towel or similar wipe to remove excess gel.

PATIENT EDUCATION POSTPROCEDURE

The results and appropriate interventions should be reviewed with the patient and follow-up should be planned.

COMPLICATIONS

There are none.

PRACTITIONER FOLLOW-UP

Practitioner follow-up will be guided by the scan results.

■ CPT BILLING

51798—Measurement of post-void residual urine and/or bladder capacity by ultrasound, non-imaging

8

REFERENCES AND RELATED RESOURCES

Newman D: BladderScan BVI-9400 Diane Newman video for male patients, *BladderScanDevice* July 13, 2012. http://www.youtube.com/watch?v=Z6ASnzmBXwE. Accessed February 22, 2015.

Quality and Governance Service: *Clinical procedure for bladder scanning*, July 2012. http://www.wirralct.nhs.uk/attachments/article/19/CP58SOPCPBladder. Accessed February 22, 2015.

Rigby D, Housami FA: Using bladder ultrasound to detect urinary retention in patients, *Nursing Times* 105:21, 2009.

Male/Female Catheterization

Jared Spackman

DESCRIPTION

Catheterization is a routine medical procedure by which urine can be obtained from the male or female bladder directly. The basic principles regarding catheterization are gender neutral, although specifics related to each gender exist, which will be discussed.

ANATOMY AND PHYSIOLOGY

In males who have a normal lower urinary tract, there are two points of potential obstruction when passing a catheter, the first is the acute upward angulation between the bulbous and membranous urethra. The second is at the bladder neck where a congenital stenosis or prostatic enlargement can narrow this area. The urethral meatus is easy to identify in a male, being located at the distal portion of the glans.

In female patients, age increases the angle between the urethra and the bladder neck. In younger patients, the urethra is angled toward the umbilicus; in older patients, the urethra is angled toward the sacrum. The urethra in females is located just superior to the vaginal introitus and is best visualized in an infant when the child is placed in the frog-leg position (Figure 8-2).

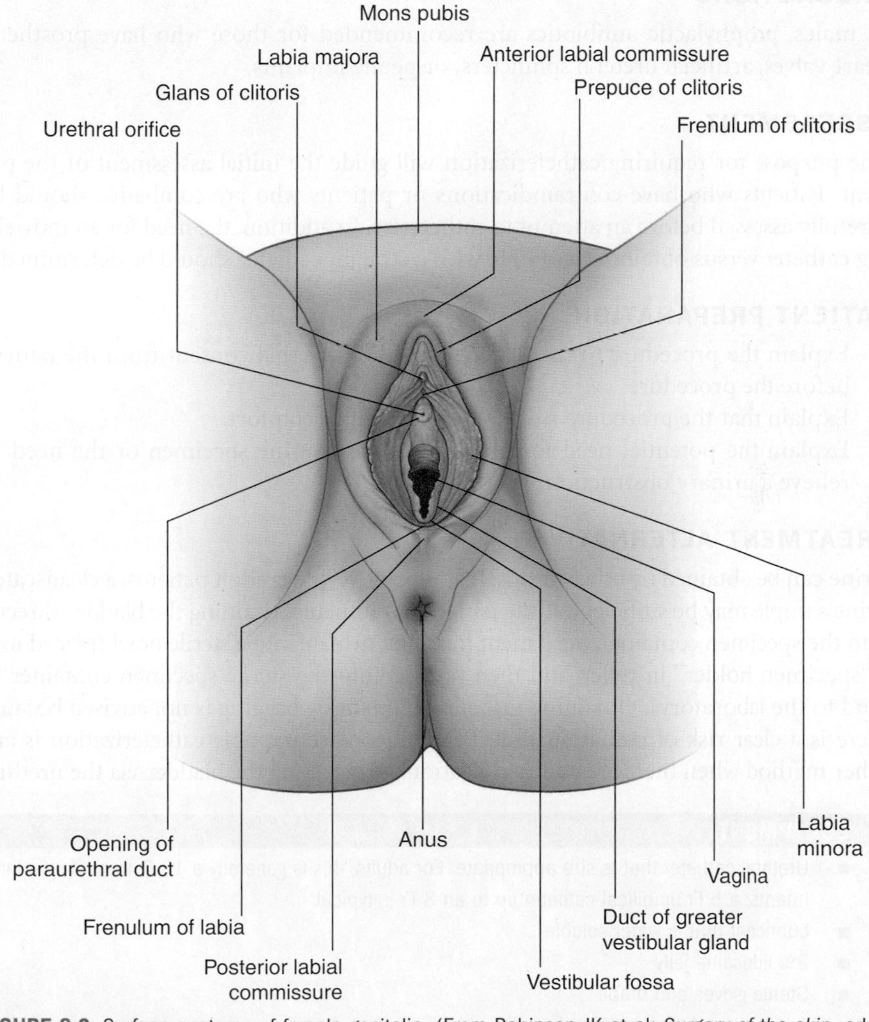

FIGURE 8-2 Surface anatomy of female genitalia. (From Robinson JK et al: *Surgery of the skin,* ed 2, London, 2010, Elsevier.)

INDICATIONS

- Need for an uncontaminated urine specimen
- Monitoring of urine output
- Acute urinary retention
- Chronic urinary obstruction
- Decompression of a neurogenic bladder
- Need to obtain a urine sample from an infant

CONTRAINDICATIONS

- Traumatic injury of the lower urinary tract
- Unclear or uncertain anatomic landmarks
- Lack of antibiotic prophylaxis in at risk patients

PRECAUTIONS

In males, prophylactic antibiotics are recommended for those who have prosthetic heart valves, artificial ureteral sphincters, or penile implants.

ASSESSMENT

The purpose for requiring catheterization will guide the initial assessment of the patient. Patients who have contraindications or patients who are combative should be carefully assessed before an attempt to catheterize. In addition, the need for an indwelling catheter versus obtaining a sample with a straight catheter should be determined.

PATIENT PREPARATION

- Explain the procedure to the patient and obtain verbal consent from the patient before the procedure.
- Explain that the procedure may cause minimal discomfort.
- Explain the potential need for obtaining a clean urine specimen or the need to relieve a urinary obstruction.

TREATMENT ALTERNATIVES

Urine can be obtained by other means. In cooperative, older adult patients, a clean-catch urine sample may be sufficient. If the patient has difficulty draining the bladder directly into the specimen container, the patient may first urinate into a sterile bowl (placed into a "specimen holder" in toilet, and then poured into the sterile specimen container to send to the laboratory). Obtaining urine in an infant by bagging is not advised because there is a clear risk of contamination. Percutaneous suprapubic catheterization is another method when there are contraindications to accessing the bladder via the urethra.

EQUIPMENT

- Urethral catheter that is size appropriate. For adults, this is generally a 16 Fr to an 18 Fr. In infants, a 5 Fr umbilical catheter up to an 8 Fr is typical.
- Lubricant that is water soluble
- 2% lidocaine jelly
- Sterile gloves and drape
- Antiseptic solution, such as betadine
- Closed urinary drainage system or sterile container

Procedure

URINARY CATHETERIZATION

1. The female patient should be placed in the lithotomy or supine position with the legs abducted (frog-leg position). The male may likewise be supine with legs slightly abducted or straight.
2. In an infant, an assistant is helpful to stabilize the legs in an abducted position and to limit movement.
3. Perform proper hand hygiene.
4. Open the catheter pack and have all supplies easily accessible.
5. Don sterile gloves.
6. Cleanse the urethral meatus and surrounding area with antiseptic solution and properly drape the patient.
7. In adults, utilizing lidocaine jelly is helpful if it is known that the patient had a painful/uncomfortable experience in the past or in a first-time catheterization that is expected to be difficult. Inject this into the urethra and leave in place for several minutes before proceeding.
8. In females, separate the labia with one hand to expose the urethral meatus. In males, lift the penis and gently retract the foreskin, if present.
9. Insert the catheter. In adult females, angle upward approximately 30 degrees; in female infants, angle toward the umbilicus. In males, hold the penis perpendicular to the body as the catheter is initially inserted into the urethra, and then move the penis parallel to the body with the distal penis toward the feet. In either case, advance the catheter until urine flow is seen.
10. Gentle pressure of the bladder may assist in urine flow.
11. If the catheter is indwelling, slowly inflate the balloon.
12. Gently withdraw the catheter until resistance is felt, and then hook up the system to the drainage reservoir.
13. Remove gloves and dispose of them and any remaining biohazards appropriately.

PATIENT EDUCATION POSTPROCEDURE

Catheter care should be discussed if the catheter is to remain in place for any period of time. Infection surveillance should be performed and the catheter should be removed as soon as it is no longer needed.

COMPLICATIONS

- Urinary tract infection.
- Transient hematuria.
- Creation of a false passage if too small of a catheter is used, too much force is used, or if there is a significant obstruction or stricture.
- Paraphimosis due to failure to return the foreskin to a normal position after the procedure.

PRACTITIONER FOLLOW-UP

Urgent evaluation of the patient should be performed if any complications occur or if there is concern about urethral injury or false passage.

■ CPT BILLING

51701—Insertion of non-indwelling bladder catheter (e.g., straight catherization for residual urine) ■ **51702**—Insertion of temporary indwelling bladder catheter, simple (e.g., Foley)

REFERENCES AND RELATED RESOURCES

Hollingsworth JM, Rogers MA, Krein SL, et al: Determining the noninfectious complications of indwelling urethral catheters: a systematic review and meta-analysis, *Ann Intern Med* 159(6):401–410, 2013.

Pfenninger JL, Fowler GC: *Procedures for primary care*, ed 3, Philadelphia, 2011, Mosby.

Schumm K, Lam TB: Types of urethral catheters for management of short-term voiding problems in hospitalized adults, *Cochrane Database Syst Rev* 2:CD004013, 2008.

Selius BA, Subedi R: Urinary retention in adults: diagnosis and initial management, *Am Fam Physician* 77(5):643–650, 2008.

Shlamovitz GZ: Urethral catheterization in men, *EMedicine* Updated December 4, 2013. http://emedicine.medscape.com/article/80716-overview. Accessed February 22, 2015.

Urinalysis

Marilyn Winterton Edmunds

8

DESCRIPTION

Urinalysis is an examination of the urine that consists of three parts: the *physical* examination of the urine (e.g., color, turbidity), the *chemical* examination of the urine (e.g., pH, glucose, ketones), and the *microscopic* examination of the urine.

INDICATIONS

- Need to obtain information for screening, diagnosis, and monitoring of disease states.
- It is an inexpensive way to test large numbers of people for renal disease, urinary bladder disease, and asymptomatic development of conditions, such as diabetes mellitus and liver disease.
- During pregnancy, urinalysis is used frequently to screen for metabolic disorders such as diabetes and the proteinuria associated with preeclampsia.

CONTRAINDICATIONS

The collection of urine and performance of urinalysis is a safe procedure with no risk to the patient.

PRECAUTIONS

The practitioner must be aware of conditions, chemicals, and drugs that may interfere with the accuracy of the analysis.

ASSESSMENT

- Take a careful history of symptoms of urgency, frequency, dysuria, dribbling, nocturia, oliguria, pyuria, hematuria, and polyuria.
- Assess for fever and suprapubic or renal flank tenderness.

PATIENT PREPARATION

- In outpatient settings, the patient usually collects the specimen, but a nurse or laboratory technician may assist. Explanation of the correct procedure is vital because the accuracy of the laboratory analysis depends on the quality of the specimen.
- If a female patient is menstruating or has a heavy vaginal discharge, she should insert a vaginal tampon before collecting the specimen.

EQUIPMENT

- Clear, disposable, 6- to 10-oz plastic container (should be chemically clean for urinalysis only and sterile if a culture may be indicated)
- Two or three perineal wipes
- Equipment for hand washing
- Written patient instructions for specimen collection
- Label for the container

ADDITIONAL EQUIPMENT FOR PHYSICAL EXAMINATION

- White background against which to observe urine
- Urinometer or refractometer for specific gravity (spG) or chemical spG tapes

ADDITIONAL EQUIPMENT FOR CHEMICAL EXAMINATION

- Reagent strip
- Manufacturer color chart

ADDITIONAL EQUIPMENT FOR MICROSCOPIC EXAMINATION

- Centrifuge
- Centrifuge tube
- Dropper/pipette
- Glass slide and cover slide
- Microscope
- Nonsterile gloves

8

Procedure

1. In the outpatient setting, a "midstream" voided specimen is the most practical way to obtain urine. Instruct the patient to do the following:
   a. Wash hands.
   b. Open the specimen container, placing the lid sterile side up on the counter.
   c. Female: Stand over toilet, use one hand to separate the labia, and wipe the area of the meatus two or three times, wiping front to back once with each wipe.
   d. Male: Stand over toilet, hold penis with one hand, and wipe two or three times around the urinary meatus, once with each wipe.

e. Urinate first into the toilet, then into the specimen cup, and finish urinating into the toilet. The container does not need to be full, but it should contain at least ¼ cup to allow for adequate testing.
f. Do not touch the inside of the container; touch only the outside of the lid.
g. Screw the lid tightly on the container; label with the patient's name and the date, and deliver it to the collection area or person.

2. The specimen should be examined within 1 hour after collection.

(After 1 hour, multiple changes occur in urine, rendering the analysis inaccurate.) A specimen that cannot be examined within 1 hour may be refrigerated for up to 24 hours; the specimen should be allowed to return to room temperature before the examination.

PHYSICAL EXAMINATION

Note: It is best to pour the urine into the centrifuge tube before the urinalysis is performed; then the urine left in the specimen container may be used for culture if necessary.

1. *Determine appearance:* Hold the urine up to the light, against a white background, to examine for the presence of turbidity and to note the color. Terms used to describe turbidity include "clear," "hazy," "slightly cloudy," "cloudy," "turbid," and "milky."
2. *Specific gravity:* For refractometer, place 1 or 2 drops of urine on the prism, focus the instrument with a good light source, and take the reading directly from the spG scale.

8

CHEMICAL EXAMINATION

1. Mix the specimen well, and then dip the reagent strip completely, but briefly, into the specimen.
2. Remove excess urine when you withdraw the strip from the specimen by tapping the strip against the inside of the container.
3. Hold the strip horizontal when comparing it with the color chart to prevent mixing of reagents.
4. Follow manufacturer directions for each type of reagent to determine the number of seconds required for measurement. Compare the strip against the color chart on the container. When precise timing cannot be performed, most manufacturers suggest reading at 60 seconds, but never later than 120 seconds.

MICROSCOPIC EXAMINATION

1. Examine the urine while it is fresh.
2. Centrifuge 10 ml of urine for 5 minutes at a centrifugal force of -400 g in a specially identified specimen tube.
3. Using a pipette, remove 9 ml of the supernatant (clear fluid) and resuspend the sediment in the remaining 1 ml.
4. Take 1 drop of the resuspended sediment and transfer it to a microscope slide; put a coverslip over the slide.
5. Examine the slide first under low power, reading at least 10 low-power fields (lpf), scanning to evaluate what is on the slide and counting and averaging the number of casts, if any, that are found.
6. Examine 10 high-power fields (hpf) and count the cells; report the average number per field.

Note: Reporting may vary among laboratories. Red blood cells, white blood cells, epithelial cells, and crystals are usually reported as "number per hpf." Casts are listed as "number per lpf." Other elements are listed as "rare," "few," "many," and "packed." The term "too numerous to count" (TNTC) may be used when markedly increased numbers of cells and crystals are seen. Casts, epithelial cells, and crystals must also be identified as to their type.

PATIENT EDUCATION POSTPROCEDURE

Explanations to the patient after the procedure depend primarily on the purpose of the urinalysis (screening; diagnostic; monitoring), the results, and the plan of care.

COMPLICATIONS

There are none.

PRACTITIONER FOLLOW-UP

Additional tests may need to be ordered to clarify the diagnosis if abnormalities are found. Findings should be documented.

■ CPT BILLING

81000–Urinalysis, by dip stick or tablet reagent for bilirubin, glucose, hemoglobin, ketones, leukocytes, nitrite, pH, protein, specific gravity, urobilinogen, any number of these constituents, non-automated, with microscopy ■ **81001**–Urinalysis, by dip stick or tablet reagent for bilirubin, glucose, hemoglobin, ketones, leukocytes, nitrite, pH, protein, specific gravity, urobilinogen, any number of these constituents, automated, with microscopy ■ **81002**–Urinalysis, by dip stick or tablet reagent for bilirubin, glucose, hemoglobin, ketones, leukocytes, nitrite, pH, protein, specific gravity, urobilinogen, any number of these constituents, non-automated, without microscopy ■ **81003**–Urinalysis, by dip stick or tablet reagent for bilirubin, glucose, hemoglobin, ketones, leukocytes, nitrite, pH, protein, specific gravity, urobilinogen, any number of these constituents, automated, without microscopy ■ **81015**–Urinalysis, microscopic only

REFERENCES AND RELATED RESOURCES

Cowling T: *The correct way to perform a medical urinalysis*, 2015. www.brighthub.com/science/medical/articles/71520.aspx. Accessed February 26, 2015.

Nabli SN: *Urinalysis tests and procedures.* www.emedicinehealth.com/urinalysis/page3_em.htm. Accessed February 20, 2015.

Urine Culture

Marilyn Winterton Edmunds

DESCRIPTION

Urine is collected under sterile conditions to assess for the presence of bacteria.

ANATOMY AND PHYSIOLOGY

Urinary tract infections (UTIs) are common among the primary care patient population. Traditional diagnosis and treatment regimens for acute cystitis have been

8

estimated to cost $140 to $200 per episode. Untreated, an uncomplicated UTI can progress to more complicated problems, including kidney infections. Thus the early diagnosis and treatment of UTIs can reduce the morbidity and cost associated with these infections.

UTIs are frequently divided into lower UTIs, or cystitis, and upper UTIs, or acute pyelonephritis.

INDICATIONS

- One of the cardinal symptoms of any UTI is dysuria. Other symptoms include frequency, urgency, burning, nocturia, incontinence, and suprapubic or pelvic pain.
- The differential diagnosis of a UTI must include other inflammatory or infectious problems, such as sexually transmitted diseases, vaginitis, or obstructive disorders.

CONTRAINDICATIONS

Catheterization of a patient who has acute cystitis may predispose susceptible individuals to bacteremia and subsequent endocarditis. The risk of such serious complications is fortunately very small and thus may be only a relative contraindication to the procedure.

PRECAUTIONS

A major problem in collecting urine for cultures arises when there is contamination with vaginal or labial bacteria. Catheterization is one way to solve this problem; however, in most primary care settings, this may not be feasible.

Catheterization also carries the risk of introducing organisms that may cause a UTI.

ASSESSMENT (Table 8-1)

- Obtain patient history of urinary frequency, dysuria, hematuria, nocturia, or fever. Assess for past history of UTIs.
- Assess patient for temperature elevation and renal flank or suprapubic tenderness.

PATIENT PREPARATION

- Explain urine collection procedures to the patient.
- Emphasize the importance of not contaminating the specimen with skin flora from the patient's fingers, labia, or foreskin.

EQUIPMENT

- Sterile specimen container with tight-fitting (screw-on) lid
- Cleansing novelettes
- Soap and water

TABLE 8-1 Differential Diagnosis of Dysuria Syndromes

	HISTORY								PHYSICAL EXAMINATION			LABORATORY				
	DYSURIA		ONSET													
	INTERNAL	EXTERNAL	ACUTE	SUBACUTE	VAGINAL DISCHARGE OR ODOR, PRURITUS, EXTERNAL LESIONS	NEW SP, MULTIPLE SPs, SP WITH STD	FREQUENCY, URGENCY, HEMATURIA, SUPRAPUBIC PAIN, DIAPHRAGM USE	FEVER, CHILLS, SWEATS, NAUSEA, VOMITING	VAGINAL OR CERVICAL DISCHARGE, VULVAR LESIONS	SUPRAPUBIC TENDERNESS	FLANK TENDERNESS, FEVER	ABNORMAL VAGINAL FLUID OR CERVICAL SMEAR	CULTURE OF GENITAL LESIONS, CERVIX, OR URETHRA POSITIVE FOR CT, CC, HSV	PYURIA	MICROSCOPIC HEMATURIA OR BACTERIURIA	URINE CULTURE (>10^2 CFU/ML)
Acute pyelonephritis	+/-	-	+	-	-	-	+/-	+	-	+/-	+	-	-	+	+	+
Acute cystitis	+	-	+	-	-	-	+	-	-	+/-	-	-	-	+	+/-	+
Urethritis caused by STD																
HSV	+	+/-	-	+	+	+	+/-	-	+	-	-	+/-	+	+	-	-
GC	+	-	+	-	+	+	+/-	-	+	-	-	+	+	+	-	-
CT	+	-	-	+	+	+	+/-	-	+	-	-	+	+	+	-	-
Vulvovaginitis (bacterial vaginosis, trichomoniasis, yeast, genital HSV)	-	+	-	+	+	+	-	-	+	-	-	+	+/-	-	-	-
Noninflammatory dysuria (trauma, irritant, allergy)	?	?	?	?	-	?	-	-	-	-	-	-	-	-	-	-

From Johnson JR, Stamm WE: Diagnosis and treatment of acute urinary tract infections, *Infect Dis Clin North Am* 1:776, 1987.

CFU, Colony-forming units; *CT, Chlamydia trachomatis; GC, Neisseria gonorrhoeae; HSV,* herpes simplex; *SP,* sex partner; *STD,* sexually transmitted disease.

8

Procedure

1. In the outpatient setting, a "midstream" voided specimen is the most practical way to obtain urine. Instruct the patient to do the following:
   a. Wash hands and open the container.
   b. *Female:* Using the index and middle fingers of the nondominant hand, spread the labia and wipe the perineal area from front to back. Without allowing the labia to meet, repeat the wiping two more times. If vaginal discharge or menses are present, a tampon should be inserted first.
   c. *Male:* Retract the foreskin and, using the cleansing swab or novelette, clean the end of the penis using a circular motion moving from the meatus outward.
   d. Initiate the urine stream.
   e. After a single stream is achieved, pass the specimen container into the stream and obtain the sample.
   f. Remove the container before the flow of urine stops and before releasing the labia or penis. This decreases the risk of contaminating the specimen with skin flora.
   g. Replace the cap on the container and wipe off the outside of the container.
   h. Wash hands again.
2. Label the specimen container with the patient's name, the date, and the time of collection.
3. The specimen should reach the laboratory within 30 minutes of collection or be refrigerated.

8

INTERPRETATION OF RESULTS

- Evaluate urine cultures in conjunction with other documentation that confirms infection. The presence of bacteria alone does not make a diagnosis of UTI. Many older adult women have asymptomatic bacteriuria.
- Urine cultures that are positive for more than 100,000 colony-forming units (cfu) may be interpreted as being positive for infection, but if there are no white blood cells and the culture is negative for leukocyte esterase, the culture results are more likely to represent colonization than infection.
- Testing for the presence of leukocyte esterase by dipstick is a relatively reliable method for determining the presence of white blood cells in the urine. The sensitivity of dipstick tests diminishes when bacterial counts of less than 10,000 colonies per milliliter are present.

PATIENT EDUCATION POSTPROCEDURE

- Inform the patient that urine culture results will be available within 24 to 48 hours.
- Advise the patient that empiric antibiotic therapy will be initiated before final culture results are available. Should the culture reveal resistant organisms, antibiotic therapy will be adjusted.
- Instruct the patient to immediately report new onset of fever, shaking, chills, headache, nausea, or vomiting.

COMPLICATIONS

Complications of UTI can be serious. Inflammation of the renal parenchyma and pelvis may lead to acute pyelonephritis and possibly to bacteremia.

PRACTITIONER FOLLOW-UP

Posttherapy cultures should be obtained only in those patients who have a history of frequent UTIs, drug-resistant organisms, or persistent symptoms. In these instances, posttreatment cultures should be obtained 7 to 14 days after therapy.

■ CPT BILLING

87086—Culture, bacterial, quantitative colony count, urine ■ **87088**—Culture, bacterial, quantitative colony count, with isolation and presumptive identification of each isolate, urine

REFERENCES AND RELATED RESOURCES

Ban KM, Easter JS: Selected urologic problems. In Marx JA, Hockberger RS, Walls RM, et al, editors: *Rosen's emergency medicine: concepts and clinical practice*, ed 7, Philadelphia, 2009, Mosby Elsevier (chapter 97).

Dean AJ, Lee DC: Bedside laboratory and microbiologic procedures. In Roberts JR, Hedges JR, editors: *Clinical procedures in emergency medicine*, ed 5, Philadelphia, 2009, Saunders Elsevier (chapter 68).

Hooton TM, Bradley SF, Cardenas DD, et al: Diagnosis, prevention, and treatment of catheter-associated urinary tract infection in adults: 2009 International Clinical Practice Guidelines from the Infectious Diseases Society of America, *Clin Infect Dis* 50(5):625–663, 2010.

University of Nebraska Medical Center, Division of Laboratory Science, Clinical Laboratory Science Program: *Urine cultures – general procedure*. http://webmedia.unmc.edu/alliedhealth/honeycutt/CLS418/UrineCultures.pdf. Accessed February 22, 2015.

Urine culture: *WebMD*. www.webmd.com/a-to-z-guides/urine-culture. Last updated September 9, 2014. Accessed February 22, 2015.

9

Women's Health Procedures

Pegah Dixon Conk

Both routine health maintenance procedures and those designed to alleviate structural problems or to prevent pregnancy are common primary care gynecologic procedures performed in almost every primary care office. Most gynecologic procedures require a good foundational knowledge not only of the anatomic structures, but also of the physiology and pathophysiology involved in these tissues, which are so greatly affected by changing hormones.

ANATOMY AND PHYSIOLOGY

The *vagina* is a tubular organ that lies between the rectum and the urethra and bladder. It extends upward and backward from its external orifice in the vestibule between the labia minor and the vulva to the cervix. The *uterus* is a muscular, hollow organ that is flexed between the body and cervix, with the body lying over the superior surface of the bladder, pointing forward and slightly upward. The *cervix* points downward and backward from the point of flexion, joining the vagina at approximately a right angle. Several ligaments hold the uterus in place, but allow for considerable movement. The *ovaries* are nodular glands that are located with one on each side of the uterus, below and behind the uterine tubes. The ovaries are almond-size structures attached to the posterior surface of the broad ligament by the mesovarian ligament (Figure 9-1).

Papanicolaou (Pap) Smear Test

DESCRIPTION

This procedure explains how to obtain smears from the cervix and vagina (and occasionally from the vulva, endometrium, and breast discharge) for cytological examination. The test *(Pap smear)* is recommended for the diagnosis of precancerous and cancerous conditions, for hormonal assessment, and for the diagnosis of inflammatory diseases. High-risk human papilloma virus (HPV) testing can also be used in conjunction with cervical cytology to strengthen the validity of cervical cancer screening. HPV reflex testing is performed only when there is an abnormal result on cytology, and HPV cotesting is performed regardless of the cytology results.

ANATOMY AND PHYSIOLOGY

The cells of the cervix may be harvested and tested for diagnostic purposes. The area most likely to be the site of infection or malignant cells is the transformation zone

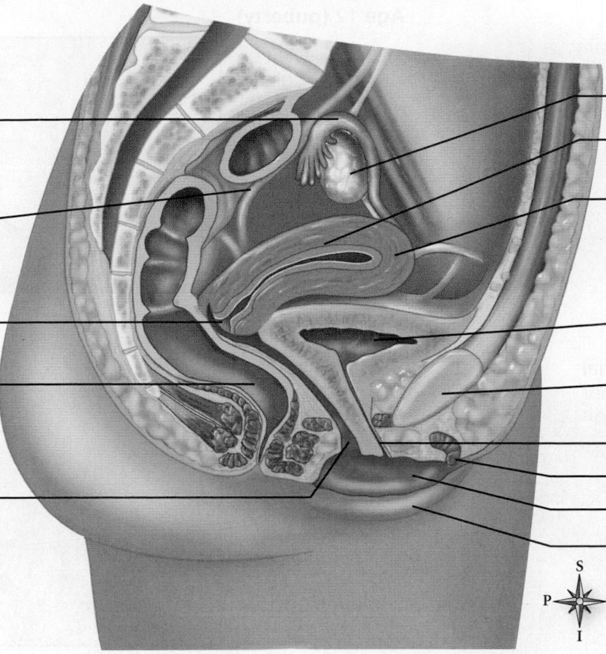

FIGURE 9-1 Female reproductive anatomy. (From Patton KT, Thibodeau GA: *The human body in health & disease,* ed 6, St. Louis, 2014, Mosby.)

(TZ), including the squamocolumnar junction (SCJ). The appearance of the cervix and the location of the transformation zone vary with age (Figure 9-2). The entire TZ must be sampled to maximize the likelihood of effective cell samples. The SCJ migrates inward with aging.

INDICATIONS

- Age 21 to 29 years: Cytology alone every 3 years. Pap smears are NOT recommended for women under the age of 21 regardless of their sexual activity.
- Age 30 to 65 years: Cytology with HPV cotesting every 5 years (preferred) or cytology only with no HPV cotesting every 3 years (acceptable). No testing is needed after the age of 65 with adequate prior negative test results.
- Initial visit for prenatal care or at 6 weeks' postpartum, depending on the history of last Pap test.
- Abnormal vaginal bleeding, postcoital bleeding, or discharge.
- Lower abdominal pain.
- High-risk women may require earlier and more frequent testing. Risk factors include the following:
  - Women who are infected with the HIV virus
  - Women who are immunocompromised (such as women who have had an organ transplant)
  - History of abnormal Pap smear
  - Diethylstilbestrol (DES) exposure while in utero: Refer to gynecologist
  - Women who have undergone a hysterectomy for cervical cancer or cervical dysplasia (CIN 2 or 3) should have cytology testing for 20 years after surgery

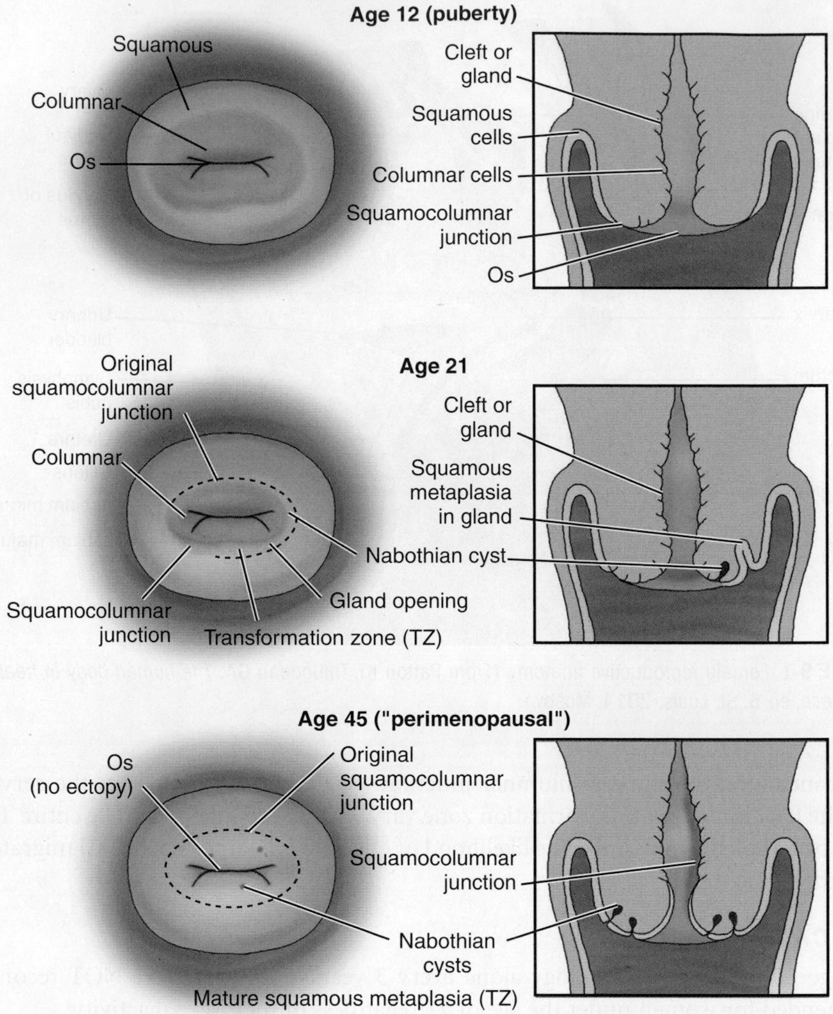

FIGURE 9-2 Appearance of cervix in various age groups.

9

before discontinuing screening. If a woman has undergone a hysterectomy for a reason other than cervical dysplasia or cancer, Pap smears may be discontinued. For women who have had a supracervical hysterectomy, the guidelines for cytology screening are the same as for women who have an intact uterus.

CONTRAINDICATIONS

There are no absolute contraindications to Pap smears. Pap smears to evaluate for cancerous cells are generally deferred in the presence of active vaginitis, active cervicitis, or pelvic inflammatory disease until the acute illness has resolved. For women under 21, the potential harm of Pap screening outweighs the benefits.

PRECAUTIONS

Relative contraindications usually involve situations that may make obtaining or interpreting a Pap difficult:

- Use of lubricating jelly
- Douching, intercourse, or use of vaginal medications within 24 hours of a Pap smear collection
- Active vaginitis or cervicitis
- Pelvic inflammatory disease
- Heavy menstrual flow

This test may be performed at any time when heavy menstrual bleeding is not present. The optimal time to perform the test is in the midcycle for a woman who has not had intercourse for 24 hours and has not placed any substances in her vagina for at least 48 hours, although these conditions are not necessary.

If samples are collected under suboptimal conditions, such as during menses or infection, the results may be reported as unsatisfactory, which always mandates a repeat testing. If the time for taking a Pap smear is not favorable, advise the patient to return at a designated time when the problem is resolved. If the patient insists on having it done despite the advice, warn her about the possibility of an unsatisfactory result and the likelihood of having to repeat the test. If she is unlikely or unable to return, obtain Pap testing despite suboptimal conditions.

ASSESSMENT

- Obtain the patient's general health, obstetrician/gynecologist, and menstrual history.
- Determine whether there are any current problems.
- Answer any questions the patient may have.
- Assess the patient's risk factors for cervical dysplasia and STDs, ask whether she would like *Chlamydia* or gonorrhea testing at the time of the Pap test.

PATIENT PREPARATION

- Advise the patient that she may experience slight discomfort when the cervix is manipulated and the specimen is collected.
- Have the patient empty her bladder before the test.
- Have the patient remove all clothing (except socks and shoes).
- Provide appropriate drapes.

TREATMENT ALTERNATIVES

In women who have never had sexual intercourse and in those with an unusual fear of pelvic examinations, the use of a pediatric or nasal speculum can be useful in visualizing the cervix. In obese women, a wider or longer speculum may be used to better visualize the cervix.

EQUIPMENT

- Examination table suitable for placing patient in lithotomy position
- Well-lighted, warm room with additional "focused" light source
- Cloth or paper drapes
- Two pairs of nonsterile gloves
- Specula of varying sizes

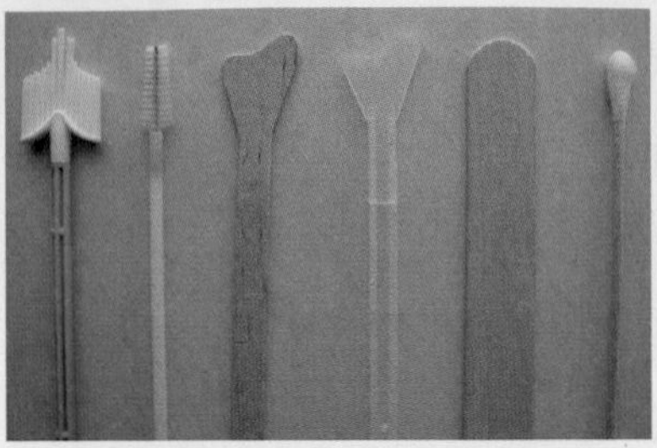

FIGURE 9-3 Sampling devices for a Papanicolaou (Pap) smear (left to right): Cervex-Brush, Cytobrush, wooden spatula, plastic spatula, tongue blade, and cotton swab. Use of the swab and tongue blade is discouraged. (From Pfenninger JL, Fowler GC: *Pfenninger and Fowler's procedures for primary care physicians*, ed 3, Philadelphia, 2011, Mosby.)

- Method for warming speculum if a metal one is used
- Cytobrush or other collection sampling devices (Figure 9-3)
- Cotton-tipped applicators
- Wood or plastic spatula for slides and broom for liquid-based cytology
- Glass slide (frosted on one end) or liquid in a bottle
- Appropriate patient identification and history forms
- Lead pencil for the slide and ink pen for the bottle
- Fixative for the slide (fixative is present in prepackaged bottles)
- Culture or transport medium and Dacron swabs to collect specimens to test for *Chlamydia* or gonorrhea (can be added to a liquid-based Pap test) or herpes, and cotton or Dacron swabs to collect specimens to test for fungal and KOH (potassium hydroxide)/wet mount specimens
- Ring forceps, cervical tenaculum, or cervical hook (rarely needed)

Procedure

1. Complete other parts of the examination (breast and general physical examinations), leaving the pelvic examination for last.
2. Label the frosted end of the glass slide, or the specimen bottle with the patient's name and other identifying data; ensure that all appropriate paperwork is complete and that other culture specimen tubes are present and labeled as needed.
3. Adjust the lighting.
4. Assist patient into the lithotomy position and drape so that only the perineal area is exposed.
5. Wearing a double set of gloves, begin the external examination. Inspect the vulva, examining the hair pattern and anatomy and assessing for estrogen effect, discharge, lesions, and Bartholin and Skene glands.
6. Lubricate the speculum with warm water and insert it into the vagina with a gentle posterior pressure, exposing the cervix. Adjust the speculum to obtain adequate visualization of the cervix, and tighten the screw or lock the speculum in the open position.
7. Encourage the patient to relax by taking deep breaths through her mouth. In case of difficulty with visualization, change the patient's position to high Fowler's and ask the patient to perform the Valsalva maneuver. Having the patient move

further down the table or inserting a smaller or larger/wider speculum can also help in better visualizing the cervix. Inspect the cervix, looking for inflammation or infection. In case of copious discharge, gently blot without rubbing or traumatizing the cervix.

8. Identify cervical landmarks, including the os, TZ, and SCJ. Note the nature of the cervical mucus or discharge. Check for unusual odor, color, and consistency. Examine for any gross lesions (i.e., erosions, leukoplakia, and condylomata). Note the presence of Nabothian cysts.
9. For the slide prep, first obtain an endocervical scraping by rotating a cytobrush in the endocervical canal. Then gently rotate the wooden or plastic spatula 360 degrees in a circular motion over the entire transformation zone. For liquid prep Paps, rotate the broom 360 degrees over the entire transformation zone. Sampling the vaginal pool is of little benefit unless the patient has had a hysterectomy; in this case, be sure to sample the vaginal cuff (Figure 9-4).
10. For slide prep, smear the wooden or plastic spatula sample on the glass slide first, and then quickly apply the cytobrush sample either on the top of the sample or separately on the same slide. Spray a fixative or place the slide in a glass container with ethyl alcohol (ETOH) immediately (within 5 seconds). (The

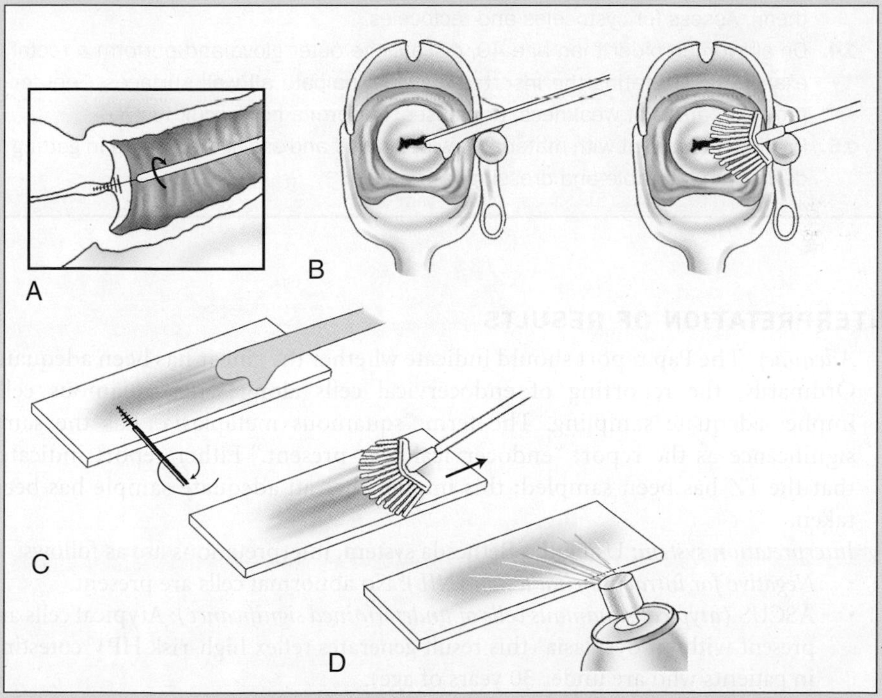

FIGURE 9-4 Procedure for obtaining a slide sample Pap smear. **A,** Obtain endocervical sample with cytobrush. **B,** Use a wooden or plastic spatula to sample the ectocervix. **C,** Spread the spatula sample onto the slide, then "unroll" the brush sample over the first sample. **D,** Immediately spray the slide with fixative.

method you use is often dictated by the laboratory that will be examining the specimen.) If a liquid-based technique is used, swirl broom in the liquid at least 10 times, and shake off the liquid on the inside of the bottle. Some labs and liquid media require the end of the broom left in the sample, and some require that it be removed. If the cervix is friable, indicate it on the laboratory test form and investigate the cause (do a wet mount and/or obtain *Chlamydia*/gonorrhea cultures, if appropriate).

11. Obtain appropriate cervical cultures for STDs after cytologic sampling has been completed. Use the swabs, media, and procedures as dictated by the laboratory that will be performing the testing. If using a liquid-based method, be sure to mark any additional testing desired on the laboratory form so that the testing can be performed on the sample.
12. Slowly withdraw the speculum, examining the vaginal walls as the speculum is removed. Note any abnormalities.
13. Using lubricating gel on the fingers, complete the remainder of the bimanual examination by inserting the fingers of one hand into the vaginal vault and palpating the cervix and uterus (push down on the abdomen with one hand while lifting up with the inserted hand). Assess the uterus for size, position, and irregularity (for presence of fibroids and other masses). Attempt to palpate the ovaries (again, use the hand on top to palpate the ovarian area while pushing toward each ovary with the inserted fingers to "capture" the ovary between them). Assess for cystoceles and rectoceles.
14. On all women older than age 40, discard the outer glove and perform a rectal examination, rotating the inserted finger to palpate all wall surfaces. Feel for prolapse, areas of weakness, or masses. Perform a hemoccult test.
15. Provide the patient with material to wipe herself and assist the patient in getting down from the table and dressing, as needed.

INTERPRETATION OF RESULTS

- *Adequacy:* The Pap report should indicate whether the smear has been adequate. Ordinarily, the reporting of endocervical cells along with squamous cells implies adequate sampling. The term "squamous metaplasia" has the same significance as the report "endocervical cells present." Either report indicates that the TZ has been sampled; this implies that an adequate sample has been taken.
- *Interpretation system:* Using the Bethesda system, interpretations are as follows:
  - *Negative for intraepithelial lesion (NIL):* No abnormal cells are present.
  - ASCUS *(atypical squamous cells of undetermined significance):* Atypical cells are present without dysplasia (this result generates reflex high-risk HPV cotesting in patients who are under 30 years of age).
  - ASC-H *(atypical cells, cannot rule out high-grade lesion):* Atypical cells are present and the pathologist cannot rule out a high-grade lesion.
  - *Low-grade squamous intraepithelial lesion (LSIL) (human papilloma virus [HPV] changes and cervical intraepithelial neoplasia [CIN] I):* Smear contains abnormal precancerous squamous cells consistent with low-grade dysplasia.

- *High-grade squamous intraepithelial lesion (HSIL) (CIN II, CIN III, carcinoma in situ [CIS]):* Smear contains precancerous/preinvasive cancerous squamous cells.
- *Invasive carcinoma:* Smear contains abnormal cells consistent with carcinoma of squamous origin that broke through the basement membrane.

- Vaginal infections, such as bacterial vaginosis and yeast, also appear on Pap results without any specific request for testing. Permission to test for *Chlamydia* and gonorrhea must be requested before the test is performed and can only be added to liquid-prep Paps.

INDICATIONS FOR COLPOSCOPY

- Any of the following Pap smear results:
  - ASCUS with HPV positive cotesting over the age of 24 (under 24 years of age, no colposcopy is needed; repeat Pap test in 1 year)
  - LSIL dysplasia over the age of 24 (under 24 years of age, no colposcopy is needed; repeat Pap test in 1 year)
  - Pap smear with HSIL or ASC-H result, any age
  - Evidence of glandular atypia (AGUS)
  - Two consecutive Pap smears with normal cytology and positive HPV cotesting, or one Pap with normal cytology and type 16 or 18 HPV
  - Cervix with visible lesions or unusual shape

PATIENT EDUCATION POSTPROCEDURE

- Always advise patients that spotting for 24 hours after the procedure is normal.
- Explain clearly how the patient will be informed about the test results (via telephone or mail).
- Recommend that the patient return for well woman examinations annually, and a repeat Pap test as indicated.

COMPLICATIONS

Occasionally, bleeding lasts for several days if the cervix is friable.

PRACTITIONER FOLLOW-UP

- Providers need to be knowledgeable regarding interpretation of the reported results. In the case of ASCUS and LGSIL, patients should be reassured that having cervical cancer is unlikely. In the case of HGSIL, the patient has to be informed that there is a possibility of cancer or that cancer may develop in the future.
- Patients who have ASCUS with positive HPV, LGSIL, or HGSIL should be discussed with and/or referred to a specialist for colposcopy or loop electrosurgical excision procedure (LEEP).
- Pap smear and colposcopy guidelines change frequently. Make sure to stay up-to-date on these guidelines by consulting the ASCCP (American Society for Colposcopy and Cervical Pathology) algorithms. These are continually updated and available on their website, www.asccp.org.

RED FLAG

- Any mass or suspicious lesion on the cervix, in the vagina, or on the vulva should be immediately referred to an OB/GYN.

■ CPT BILLING

There is no additional code for collecting a Pap smear. It is included in the E/M code for the visit. Medicare, however, has a separate code.

Q0091—Screening Papanicolaou smear; obtaining, preparing and conveyance of cervical or vaginal smear to laboratory.

REFERENCES AND RELATED RESOURCES

American College of Obstetricians and Gynecologists: ACOG Practice Bulletin. Clinical Management Guidelines for Obstetrician-Gynecologists. Number 131, November 2012. Cervical cancer screening, *Obstet Gynecol* 120:1222–1238, 2012.

American College of Obstetricians and Gynecologists: ACOG Practice Bulletin. Clinical Management Guidelines for Obstetrician-Gynecologists. Number 140, December 2013. Management of abnormal cervical cancer screening test results and cervical cancer precursors, *Obstet Gynecol* 122:1338–1367, 2012.

Arbyn M, Bergeron C, Klinkhamer P, et al: Liquid compared with conventional cervical cytology: a systematic review and meta-analysis, *Obstet Gynecol* 111:167, 2008.

Hans N, Cave AJ, Szafran O, et al: Papanicolaou smears: to swab or not to swab, *Can Fam Physician* 53:1328, 2007.

Hatcher RA, et al: *Contraceptive technology*, ed 20, New York, 2011, Ardent.

Henley SJ, King JB, German RR, et al: Surveillance of screening-detected cancers (colon and rectum, breast, and cervix) - United States, 2004–2006, *MMWR Surveill Summ* 59:1.64, 2010.

Khan MJ, Castle PE, Lorincz AT, et al: The elevated 10-year risk of cervical precancer and cancer in women with human papillomavirus (HPV) type 16 or 18 and the possible utility of type-specific HPV testing in clinical practice, *J Natl Cancer Inst* 97:1072, 2005.

Kjær SK, Frederiksen K, Munk C, Iftner T: Long-term absolute risk of cervical intraepithelial neoplasia grade 3 or worse following human papillomavirus infection: role of persistence, *J Natl Cancer Inst* 102:1478, 2010.

Massad LS, Einstein MH, Huh WK, et al: 2012 updated consensus guidelines for the management of abnormal cervical cancer screening tests and cancer precursors, *J Low Genit Tract Dis* 17:S1, 2013.

Moyer VA: U.S. Preventive Services Task Force. Screening for cervical cancer: U.S. Preventive Services Task Force recommendation statement, *Ann Intern Med* 156:880, 2012.

Partridge EE, Abu-Rustum NR, Campos SM, et al: Cervical cancer screening, *J Natl Compr Canc Netw* 8:1358, 2010.

Peirson L, Fitzpatrick-Lewis D, Ciliska D, Warren R: Screening for cervical cancer: a systematic review and meta-analysis, *Syst Rev* 2:35, 2013.

Rebolj M, van Ballegooijen M, Lynge E, et al: Incidence of cervical cancer after several negative smear results by age 50: prospective observational study, *BMJ* 338:b1354, 2009.

Rustagi AS, Kamineni A, Weinmann S, et al: Cervical screening and cervical cancer death among older women: a population-based, case-control study, *Am J Epidemiol* 179:1107, 2014.

Whitlock EP, Vesco KK, Eder M, et al: Liquid-based cytology and human papillomavirus testing to screen for cervical cancer: a systematic review for the U.S. Preventive Services Task Force, *Ann Intern Med* 155:687, 2011.

The Wet Mount

DESCRIPTION

The *wet mount,* a simple microscopic procedure, is the most useful technique available for the diagnosis of certain vaginal infections. It should be performed on all patients who have vaginal symptoms, even if the diagnosis seems obvious. This is an accessory tool to the history, the inspection of the vulvar and vaginal mucosa, and the determination of the appearance and pH of the vaginal secretions. Maximum sensitivity is about 80%. The quality of the sample and the skill of the viewer determine the sensitivity of the slide.

INDICATIONS

- Vaginal discharge
- Vulvar or vaginal pruritus
- Vulvar or vaginal pain
- Malodorous vaginal secretions

CONTRAINDICATIONS

There are no absolute contraindications to wet mounts.

PRECAUTIONS

Relative contraindications include recent douching, intravaginal medications, or menses.

ASSESSMENT

Evaluate for signs of infection, pruritus, redness, discharge, and unusual odor.

PATIENT PREPARATION

- Explain the purpose and procedure of the examination to the patient, and answer any questions.
- Patient should empty her bladder before the test.
- Patient should remove her clothing from the waist down.
- Assist the patient into the lithotomy position and drape her with a sheet.

TREATMENT ALTERNATIVES

This is a diagnostic test.

EQUIPMENT

- Examination table suitable for placing the patient in the lithotomy position
- Well-lighted, warm room with additional "focused" light source
- Cloth or paper drapes
- Two pairs of nonsterile gloves
- Specula of varying sizes
- Method for warming speculum, if a metal one is used
- Cotton-tipped applicators
- Glass slides and coverslips
- Culture medium or tubes for collecting specimens to test for *Chlamydia* and gonorrhea
- Normal saline solution
- 10% KOH solution
- Microscope
- pH test tape
- Appropriate patient identification and history forms

9

Procedure

1. Gently insert the vaginal speculum (no lubricants, except water, should be used) and visualize the vaginal walls and cervix, noting any lesions, erosions, ulcerations, leukoplakia, or condylomata. Observe the vaginal discharge: Note the amount, the color, and any odor.
2. The pH test tape may be used to screen for specific types of vaginitis. A piece of the test tape may be directly applied to the vaginal wall or the tape can be touched to the speculum after it is removed. The following conditions are indicated at various pH values:
   a. Normal flora: pH <4.0
   b. Candidiasis: pH 4.0-5.0
   c. Bacterial vaginosis: pH 5.0-6.0
   d. Trichomoniasis: pH 6.0-7.0
3. Collect vaginal discharge with a cotton swab and place it directly onto the slide, being sure to cover a large area. Use a dropper to place a drop or two of normal saline over half the specimen. Cover with a cover slip at an angle to minimize distributing air bubbles.
4. Add one drop of KOH to the other half of the specimen and whiff it immediately for the characteristic "fishy" odor of bacterial vaginosis. Cover with a cover slip in the same manner as the normal saline. Be sure to remember which side has KOH and which has NS. Plan to view the plain saline specimen first to allow time for the KOH to lyse cells before looking for *Candida*.
5. Obtain specimens from the cervix for culture of *Chlamydia* and gonorrhea at the same time that the wet smear specimens are obtained. Insert the appropriate applicators directly into the cervical canal until the tip is completely inside the os. Gently twirl the tip several times in the os (leaving it in there for several seconds to absorb organisms). Withdraw the applicator and place in the proper containers.
6. Remove the speculum and conduct a bimanual examination if it is indicated. Save the speculum so that, if for some reason a repeat specimen needs to be obtained, a sample may be obtained from the upper edges for a repeat wet mount, pH testing, and whiff test.
7. With the 10× lens in place, using low-power light, and with the condenser in the lowest position, place the slide on the stage and lower the objective until it is as close to the slide as possible.
8. Adjust the eyepieces until a single round field is seen. Turn the coarse-focus knob until the specimen is focused. Use the fine-focus knob to bring the specimen into sharp focus.
9. Examine the NS side in a systematic manner, until you have a general impression of the number of squamous cells.
10. Switch to high power (40×) and view again; it may be necessary to slightly increase the amount of light.
11. Move to the KOH side. Switch back to low power to scan the slide for *Candida.* If hyphae, spores, or buds are noted, switch to high power to confirm the impression.
12. Be sure to wipe any spilled fluid from the stage. If the objective becomes contaminated, use only special lens paper to clean it.

INTERPRETATION OF RESULTS

- Evaluate the saline slide for *vaginal epithelial cells* (flat with sharp, clear edges), *clue cells* (epithelial cells covered with bacteria, obscuring the edges of the cell and giving the cell a granular "moth-eaten" appearance), *bacteria* (normal vaginal bacteria), *lactobacilli* (large rods), *white blood cells* (a few are normal, but should not exceed the number of epithelial cells), and *Trichomonas* (ovoid, flagellated organisms recognizable by their motility). Even if one organism is identified, continue to scan the slide systematically to evaluate the specimen fully. Vaginitis may have multiple causes.
- Evaluate KOH slide for evidence of *Candida* (branching pseudohyphae).
- Table 9-1 displays interpretation of results for wet mounts.

PATIENT EDUCATION POSTPROCEDURE

- Provide the patient with medication instructions, including side effects and the importance of completing the medication as directed, if they are needed.
- Partner treatment if necessary.
- Discuss appropriate timing for the resumption of sexual activity.

COMPLICATIONS

There are none.

TABLE 9-1 Diagnoses of Vaginal Conditions Under Microscopy

CONDITION	SYMPTOMS	APPEARANCE OF DISCHARGE	pH	AMOUNT LACTOBACILLI	MICROSCOPY
Vulvovaginal yeast, *Candida Albicans*	Severe vulvovaginal erythema, mild to severe itching	Increased, white, thick, clumpy	<4.7	Moderate	Spores and hyphae seen on KOH
Vulvovaginal yeast, organisms other than *C. Albicans*	Mild vulvovaginal erythema, mild to moderate itching or burning	Increased, color unchanged or white	<4.7	Moderate	Spores only seen on KOH, confirm with culture
Bacterial vaginosis	Mild vulvovaginal erythema, absent to mild inflammation, mild to moderate itching	Homogenous discharge, increased, adherent; gray-white appearance; fishy odor, worse after intercourse	>4.5	Rare	Clue cells seen on saline prep, +whiff test with KOH, few to many WBCs
Trichomonas	Vulvar erythema, severe vulvar itching, petechiae of the cervix/vagina	Copious, yellow-green, frothy, odorous	>4.7	Can be increased or decreased	Trichomonads and many WBCs on saline prep
Vulvovaginal atrophy	Vulvar itching and irritation, vaginal dryness, dyspareunia, decreased vaginal ruggae	Scant discharge	>5	Rare	Parabasal cells, few lactobacilli, few to many WBCs seen on saline prep

Data from Carcio H, Secor RM: *Advanced health assessment of women,* ed 3, New York, 2015, Springer; Lenz G, Lobo M, Gershensen D, Katz V: *Comprehensive gynecology,* ed 6, St Louis, 2012, Mosby.

KOH, Potassium hydroxide; *WBC,* white blood cell.

9

PRACTITIONER FOLLOW-UP

- Arrange follow-up appointments with the patient who has an STD as indicated.
- Follow-up for candidiasis is not necessary.
- Call the patient with any positive culture reports.

■ CPT BILLING

87210—Wet mount for infectious agents (e.g., saline, India ink, KOH preps)

REFERENCES AND RELATED RESOURCES

American College of Obstetricians and Gynecologists: ACOG Practice Bulletin. Clinical Management Guidelines for Obstetrician-Gynecologists. Number 72, May 2006–reaffirmed 2013. Vaginitis, *Obstet Gynecol* 107:1195–1206, 2006.

Anderson MR, Klink K, Cohrssen A: Evaluation of vaginal complaints, *JAMA* 291:1368–1379, 2004.

Baron EJ, Miller JM, Weinstein MP, et al: A guide to utilization of the microbiology laboratory for diagnosis of infectious diseases: 2013 recommendations by the Infectious Diseases Society of America (IDSA) and the American Society for Microbiology (ASM)(a), *Clin Infect Dis* 57:e22, 2013.

Carcio H, Secor RM: *Advanced health assessment of women*, ed 3, New York, 2015, Springer.

Gutman RE, Peipert JF, Weitzen S, Blume J: Evaluation of clinical methods for diagnosing bacterial vaginosis, *Obstet Gynecol* 105:551–556, 2005.

Landers DV, Wiesenfeld HC, Heine RP, et al: Predictive value of the clinical diagnosis of lower genital tract infection in women, *Am J Obstet Gynecol* 190:1004, 2004.

Leboffe M, Pierce B: *Microbiology laboratory theory and application*, ed 2, Englewood, CO, 2011, Morton.

Lenz G, Lobo M, Gershensen D, Katz V: *Comprehensive gynecology*, ed 6, St. Louis, 2012, Mosby.

Treatment of Condylomata Acuminata

DESCRIPTION

Anogenital warts, or condyloma acuminata, are the most common sexually transmitted viral disease in the United States today. *Human papilloma virus* (HPV) is the virus responsible for producing genital warts, which are usually located in the dermal layers of the skin. More than 80 types of HPV viruses have been identified, classified into two categories according to their risk (low or high) of causing cancerous lesions. Certain genotypes preferentially infect the genital tract with some having oncologic properties.

ANATOMY AND PHYSIOLOGY

Condylomata acuminatum is an STD that has become alarmingly prevalent in recent years. Because of the close association with anogenital, head, and neck cancers, genital warts are of increasing concern to health care providers. Genital HPV is caused by virus types such as 6, 11, 16, 18, 31, 33, and 35. The HPV types that are considered "high risk" for malignant potential (most commonly 16 and 18) are more often associated in high-grade lesions and in cervical squamous and adenocarcinomas. Most low-risk subtypes (most commonly 6 and 11) are characterized by the formation of visible or invisible warty growths primarily in the anogenital region. The typical incubation period is 3 weeks to 8 months after exposure, and most condyloma acuminata infections clear within 2 years.

INDICATIONS

This procedure is indicated for visible or symptomatic acuminata condylomata: presence of a hypertrophic, exotropic, or cauliflower-type growth, usually on the prepuce, glans, urethra, penile shaft, and scrotum in men and on the vulva, perianal area, vagina, or cervix in women.

CONTRAINDICATIONS

- Known adverse reaction to the selected treatment modality
- Possibility of cancer (these lesions should undergo a biopsy before ablation)
- Pregnancy (only for some treatment options)

PRECAUTIONS

Repeated history of HPV suggests referral to a specialist for removal.

ASSESSMENT

- The patient may present with genital itching, pain, vaginal discharge, bleeding or burning, or a complaint of a bump or growth. If there are a small number of lesions, the patient may be asymptomatic.
- The typical presentation of condylomata acuminata is of soft, sessile, or papillary swellings that are 2 to 3 mm in diameter and 10 to 15 mm in height, and may occur singly or in clusters. Infection of long duration may create a cauliflower-like mass.
- Warts are usually flesh colored or slightly darker in Caucasians, black in dark-skinned patients, and brownish in Asians. Lymphadenopathy is usually absent.
- On moist skin areas, such as the vagina or vaginal introitus, warts may have the appearance of multiple, fine, finger-like projections. On the cervix, they appear as flat-topped papules 1 to 4 mm in size.
- On nonmucosal dry areas, the warts appear as squared-off keratotic papules.
- Giant condylomata acuminata appear as round, large, soft papules or nodules with a pebbly, strawberry appearance.
- HPV may invade both external and internal surfaces, so particular caution needs to be taken to examine the entire lower genital tract for lesions. These lesions may or may not be visible to the naked eye, so if there is any suspicion of an internal condylomata infection, colposcopy of the genital area after the application of acetic acid is very valuable in the diagnosis.
- Condylomata tend to increase in both number and size during pregnancy and in association with immunodeficiency or poor hygiene, but the natural history is unpredictable. The presence of condyloma acuminata does not mandate a cesarean section, but in severe cases when the genital tract is obstructed by the condylomatous lesions, a cesarean section is the only option for delivery of the fetus. Left untreated, they may regress spontaneously or persist and spread. All methods of treating HPV have significant failure and recurrence rates.

PATIENT PREPARATION

- Warn the patient that the application of chemicals will cause a sharp, stinging pain that will last about 5 minutes.
- Assist the female client into the dorsal lithotomy position and drape her appropriately; a mirror can be offered to the patient so that she may learn how to inspect and identify warts.

TREATMENT ALTERNATIVES

Table 9-2 presents the treatment options. Because many of these treatments remain surgical procedures, primary care practitioners commonly limit their treatment to the chemical ablation or immunologic methods described here. The preferred treatment modality is determined by the size and number of lesions present. Despite treatment, condyloma have the potential to recur (30% to 70% within 6 months of treatment)

TABLE 9-2 Treatments for Condylomata Acuminata

THERAPY	CLEARANCE RATES (%)	RECURRENCE RATES (%)	PAIN	NUMBER OF VISITS	ANESTHESIA	USE IN PREGNANCY	COST
Podophyllin	22-77	11-74	Mild to moderate	3	No	No	$183
Podofilox	45-50	21-33	Mild		No	No	
Trichloroacetic acid (TCA)	81	36	Moderate	3	No	Yes	$183
Cryotherapy	63-88	21-40	Moderate	3	No	Yes	$285
Surgery	93	29	Moderate	2	Yes	Yes	$340
Electrodesiccation	94	22	Moderate	2	Yes	Yes	$340
Interferon	19-62	21-25	Moderate	9-18	No	No	$1500
Laser	31-94	3-95	Moderate	1	Yes	Yes	$2650
Aldara	50	30	Mild		No	No	$796
Sinecatechins	57	10	Mild to moderate		No	No	$447

and also have the potential to spontaneously regress within 3 months. In most cases, treatment with chemical ablation can begin in the office until lesions are few and very small, then home therapy can be prescribed for continued treatment. Cryotherapy with liquid nitrogen is also an option for the treatment of condyloma.

Provider applied therapies:

- Podophyllin 25% (podophyllum [Podofin]) is an inexpensive, but neurotoxic solution contraindicated in pregnancy and breastfeeding women. Podophyllin is applied in the office by a skilled provider and is generally used in combination with another treatment method, such as cryotherapy.
- Cryotherapy is performed in the office with a cryotherapy gun, if available, and is safe for women who are pregnant. Treatment can cause pain.
- TCA (trichloroacetic acid) is a very popular preparation, although it causes a burning pain during treatment.

Patient applied therapies:

- Condylox gel (podofilox) is a purified preparation available only with a prescription. It is meant for patient use at home. It is not neurotoxic, unlike podophyllin, and can be applied with the fingers, making it very convenient. Podofilox is a pure compound and does not contain the toxic substances that podophyllin contains, but it is not to be used on the mucous membrane or perianal tissue. The patient should apply podofilox twice a day for 3 consecutive days, using no more than 0.5 ml each day. The patient must wait 4 days before starting the cycle again. This process may continue for a maximum of 6 weeks or until no warts are visible.
- Aldara (Imiquimod 5%), is an immune response modifier. This product is available as a cream that comes in individual packets and is recommended for the treatment of external genital and perianal warts in patients who are older than 18 years of age. It is thinly applied and rubbed in for 3 days per week on alternate days at bedtime and left on skin for 6 to 10 hours. Treatment can continue until lesions have cleared or for a maximum of 16 weeks.
- Sinecatechins (Veregen), a botanical drug, is an ointment intended for patient self-administration. It is applied three times daily for up to 16 weeks.

EQUIPMENT

- Acetic acid 3% to 5% (full-strength white vinegar) if lesions are to be identified
- Several large "scopette" swabs
- Trichloroacetic acid (TCA) 85% or 0.5% podophyllin or podofilox for treating lesions (podophyllin resin is neurotoxic, thus contraindicated for internal use and in pregnancy)
- Several cotton-tipped applicators

9

Procedure

1. If desired, use a large scopette swab dipped in acetic acid to generously swab the external genitalia. Leave on for 3 to 5 minutes. Acetowhitening or blanching of lesions will occur. This can be helpful to identify all areas to treat.
2. While the acetic acid is working on external lesions, gently insert the speculum and inspect the vaginal and cervical surfaces. If there is no history of a recent Pap smear, obtain a Pap and any indicated vaginal or cervical cultures. Inspect the vagina and cervix for condyloma. You can also paint these areas with acetic acid to look for white patches representing HPV.

3. Treatment may be instituted with trichloroacetic acid or podophyllin. Apply petroleum jelly approximately 3 to 5 mm away from the lesion in a circular pattern to protect the normal tissue and reduce irritation caused by dripping or running of the liquid. Do not smear any petroleum jelly on the lesions because treatment effectiveness will be decreased. Lidocaine ointment can be used as well.
4. Using a regular cotton-tipped wooden stick applicator, apply TCA in small amounts directly onto the visible wart surface. Avoid getting the solution on normal skin. For smaller lesions, use the wooden end to apply treatment; for larger lesions, use the cotton-tipped end. Treated warts develop a white appearance several seconds after the application of TCA. Avoid contact of healthy skin against the treated surface. The treated areas should slough in 1 to 2 days. Apply to lesions once a week or more often if well tolerated by the patient for up to 4 weeks. After the procedure, the treated area can be dusted with baking soda to neutralize acid. If there is a spillage on the unprotected skin during the procedure, immediately rinse with saline solution and apply baking soda on it. Podophyllin is applied to a small area of skin, allowed to dry, and then washed off 6 hours after application. Large areas should not be treated in a single application because of pain and neurotoxicity. Do not apply podophyllin to the vagina or cervical tissues. This can be applied in office one to two times per week.

PATIENT EDUCATION POSTPROCEDURE

- Advise the patient to take a sitz bath in 4 hours or sooner if burning continues.
- Teach the patient how to apply topical podofilox solution, aldara, or sinecatechins at home to treat external genital warts.
- Treated areas should be washed and dried gently each day of the healing process.
- Advise the patient to return to the clinic for evaluation and an additional application of TCA, if necessary, in 7 to 10 days.
- Advise the patient to refer her sexual partners for examination and treatment (85% of exposed partners have or will develop genital warts).
- Recurrence is possible without reinfection because treatment does not always eradicate very small warts. It does not eliminate the virus, only diminishes the viral load. Advise the patient to practice safe sex.
- Advise the patient to use condoms during therapy or until a complete cure is obtained.
- If the patient is starting a new relationship, discuss both partners' sexual and medical histories.
- Stress the importance of an annual gynecologic examination with Pap smear as indicated.

9

COMPLICATIONS

Infection can occur. Watch for pain, elevated temperature, redness or swelling, foul odor, and discharge or drainage. The patient can experience pain postprocedure. Ibuprofen or acetaminophen, as well as sitz baths can help to alleviate pain.

PRACTITIONER FOLLOW-UP

- Patient should be asked to return once the therapeutic regimen is completed so that the effectiveness of treatment may be evaluated.
- If the area treated at one visit is too large, extensive necrosis and pain may occur. Reasonably sized areas should be treated over multiple visits. Refer patient to a

gynecologist or a dermatologist for large lesions requiring laser treatment or excision.

- Recurrence or persistence of the lesions is common.

■ CPT BILLING

If the visit is for the procedure only, do not bill an E/M code in addition. If the patient comes in for her annual examination, you may bill both the E/M code for the examination, and the CPT code for the procedure with a 25 modifier.

46900–Destruction of lesion(s), anus; (e.g., condyloma, papilloma, molluscum contagiousum, herpetic vesicle), simple; chemical ■ **46910**–Destruction of lesion(s), anus; (e.g., condyloma, papilloma, molluscum contagiousum, herpetic vesicle), simple; electrodesiccation ■ **46916**–Destruction of lesion(s), anus; (e.g., condyloma, papilloma, molluscum contagiousum, herpetic vesicle), simple; cryosurgery ■ **46917**–Destruction of lesion(s), anus; (e.g., condyloma, papilloma, molluscum contagiousum, herpetic vesicle), simple; laser surgery ■ **46922**–Destruction of lesion(s), anus; (e.g., condyloma, papilloma, molluscum contagiousum, herpetic vesicle), simple; surgical excision ■ **46924**–Destruction of lesion(s), anus; (e.g., condyloma, papilloma, molluscum contagiousum, herpetic vesicle), extensive; (e.g., laser surgery, electrosurgery, cryosurgery, chemosurgery) ■ **56501**–Destruction of lesion(s), vulva; simple (e.g., laser surgery, electrosurgery, cryosurgery, chemosurgery) ■ **56515**–Destruction of lesion(s), vulva; extensive (e.g., laser surgery, electrosurgery, cryosurgery, chemosurgery) ■ **57061**–Destruction of vaginal lesion(s); simple (e.g., laser surgery, electrosurgery, cryosurgery, chemosurgery) ■ **57065**–Destruction of vaginal lesion(s); extensive (e.g., laser surgery, electrosurgery, cryosurgery, chemosurgery)

REFERENCES AND RELATED RESOURCES

Blomberg M, Friis S, Munk C, et al: Genital warts and risk of cancer: a Danish study of nearly 50,000 patients with genital warts, *J Infect Dis* 205:1544, 2012.

Centers for Disease Control: Sexually transmitted disease treatment guidelines, *Genital Warts* 2010. http://www.cdc.gov/std/treatment/2010/genital-warts.htm.

Ciobotaru B, Leiman G, St John T, et al: Prevalence and risk factors for anal cytologic abnormalities and human papillomavirus infection in a rural population of HIV-infected males, *Dis Colon Rectum* 50:1011, 2007.

Hatcher RA et al: *Contraceptive technology*, ed 20, New York, 2011, Ardent.

Lacey CJ, Goodall RL, Tennvall GR, et al: Randomised controlled trial and economic evaluation of podophyllotoxin solution, podophyllotoxin cream, and podophyllin in the treatment of genital warts, *Sex Transm Infect* 79:270, 2003.

Meltzer SM, Monk BJ, Tewari KS: Green tea catechins for treatment of external genital warts, *Am J Obstet Gynecol* 200:233.e1, 2009.

van Seters M, van Beurden M, ten Kate FJ, et al: Treatment of vulvar intraepithelial neoplasia with topical imiquimod, *N Engl J Med* 358:1465, 2008.

Veregen: a botanical for treatment of genital warts, *Med Lett Drugs Ther* 50:15, 2008.

Pessary Use

DESCRIPTION

A *vaginal pessary* is an ancient medical therapy that can be a viable alternative to surgery for those who have pelvic organ prolapse (POP) and stress urinary incontinence (SUI). Today, they are made of rubber or plastic and often include a metal band or spring-type frame. Many different forms of pessaries have been developed over the years, but fewer than a dozen have unique properties or are specifically helpful. Pessaries are used primarily to support the uterus, the cervical cuff, or hernias of the pelvic floor and are effective because they increase the tension of the pelvic floor.

ANATOMY AND PHYSIOLOGY

Any condition that causes loss of turgor to the muscles holding the uterus in place may result in prolapse of the uterus. The degree of prolapse generally progresses over time. Figure 9-5 illustrates the different degrees of prolapse.

INDICATIONS

- Pessaries are used for the treatment of pelvic organ prolapse (uterine, cystocele, or rectocele) in high-risk patients or patients who decline or must postpone surgery.
- Pessaries assist in healing cervical decubitus ulcers associated with uterine prolapse before corrective surgery. Typically, vaginal estrogen is used in combination with the pessary to promote healing.
- A pessary can be used in pregnancy to manage POP and cervical insufficiency.
- Pessaries have been used with increasing frequency to control urinary stress incontinence by exerting pressure beneath the urethra or by improving the posterior urethrovesical angle.

CONTRAINDICATIONS

Pessaries are contraindicated in acute genital tract infections and in adherent retroversion of the uterus. Avoid latex pessaries in those women who are allergic to latex. Pessary use in sexually active women who are unable to remove and insert the pessary themselves is contraindicated as the inability to manage the pessary around intercourse could be discouraging.

PRECAUTIONS

Be certain that the patient will be compliant with follow-up and management before fitting a pessary.

ASSESSMENT

- Before fitting the pessary, perform a Pap smear and pelvic examination to rule out cervical or vaginal infections.
- Perform a bimanual examination, noting the length, shape, and position of the cervix, vagina, and uterus.

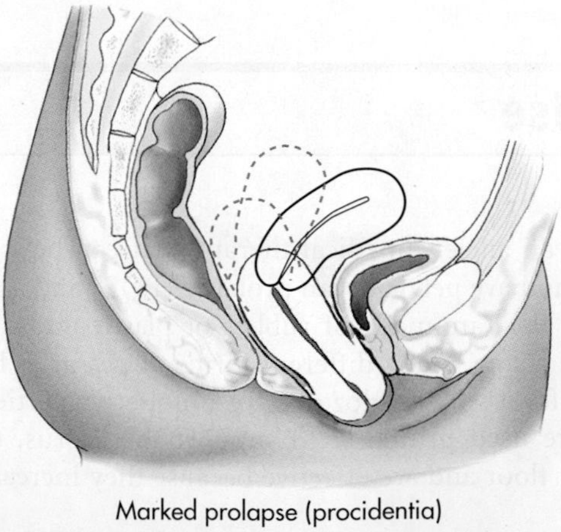

Marked prolapse (procidentia)

FIGURE 9-5 Depiction of prolapse of uterus.

TABLE 9-3 Pessary Devices

TYPES	DESCRIPTION
Support pessaries	Two dimensional and sit in the long axis of the vagina. These are typically more easily removed by the patient, allow for intercourse while in place, and are more comfortable.
Ring	Used to treat uterine prolapse and cystocele. Most commonly used pessary; available with and without support.
Lever (Smith, Hodge, Risser)	Useful in uterine prolapse and cystocele; no longer commonly used.
Gehrung	Used to treat cystocele and rectocele.
Shaatz	Rigid ring pessary; same as Gellhorn, but without the stem.
Space-filling pessaries	Three dimensional and have a large base that supports the cervix or cuff. Used in women who have severe POP, especially posthysterectomy. They are not effective as a treatment for SUI. Difficult for patient to remove, and intercourse is not possible with pessary in place.
Gellhorn	Used to treat POP. Most women can be managed with the 2.5-, 2.75-, and 3-inch sizes. Can be difficult to remove manually.
Donut	Used to treat POP. Similar sizes to Gellhorn.
Cube	Prevents prolapse using suction. Highly effective, but associated with malodorous discharge and vaginal erosions. Recommended to remove and wash the device nightly.
Inflatable (inflatoball)	Designed to be easier for patient management. The bulb is attached to a port to inflate and deflate device. The stem can protrude from vagina. Made of latex.
Incontinence pessaries	Used for treatment of SUI only. Causes an increase in urethral resistance associated with SUI by compressing the urethra against the upper posterior portion of the symphysis pubis.
Incontinence ring and dish	Both used to treat SUI; the dish is more rigid, but has minimal added benefit compared with the incontinence ring.
Bell-shaped incontinence	Bell-shaped design for easy removal and insertion. Used for treatment of SUI.
Cylindrical intra-vaginal device	Tampon-shaped design for ease of use. Treats SUI. Can only be ordered from Australia and New Zealand.
Continence ring	A balloon obstructs the flow of urine during rest and when patient has an urge or at scheduled time for voiding, the balloon is deflated to allow urine to pass.
Disposable intra-vaginal device	Inserted with an applicator; similar to a tampon. Used to treat SUI.

PATIENT PREPARATION

- Explain to the patient that pessaries do NOT cure uterine prolapse, but that they may be used for months or years for relief of symptoms under proper supervision.
- Have the patient get into the lithotomy position. Offer her a mirror so that she may watch the fitting process and explain the insertion process step-by-step as you go through the pessary fitting.

TREATMENT ALTERNATIVES

- Pelvic muscle exercises with the aid of biofeedback can be used instead of and in conjunction with a pessary.

EQUIPMENT

- Well-lighted, warm room with additional "focused" light source
- Lubricant
- Nonsterile gloves
- Examination table
- Table 9-3 describes various pessary devices, which are pictured in Figure 9-6.

9

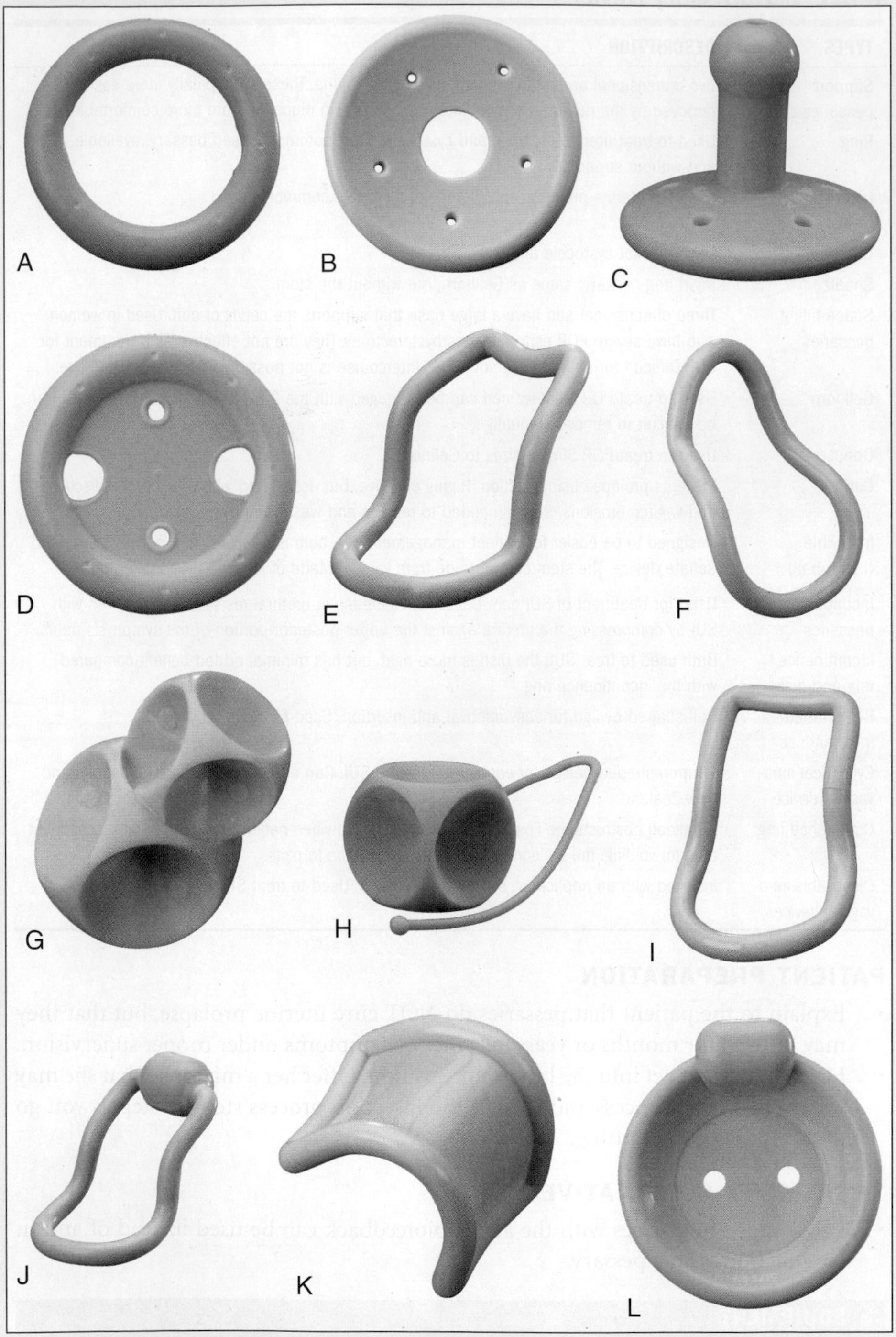

FIGURE 9-6 Various types of pessaries: **A,** Ring. **B,** Shaatz. **C,** Gellhorn. **D,** Ring with support. **E,** Hodge. **F,** Smith. **G,** Tandem cube. **H,** Cube. **I,** Hodge with knob. **J,** Hodge. **K,** Gehrung. **L,** Incontinence dish with support. (Images provided by CooperSurgical, Inc.)

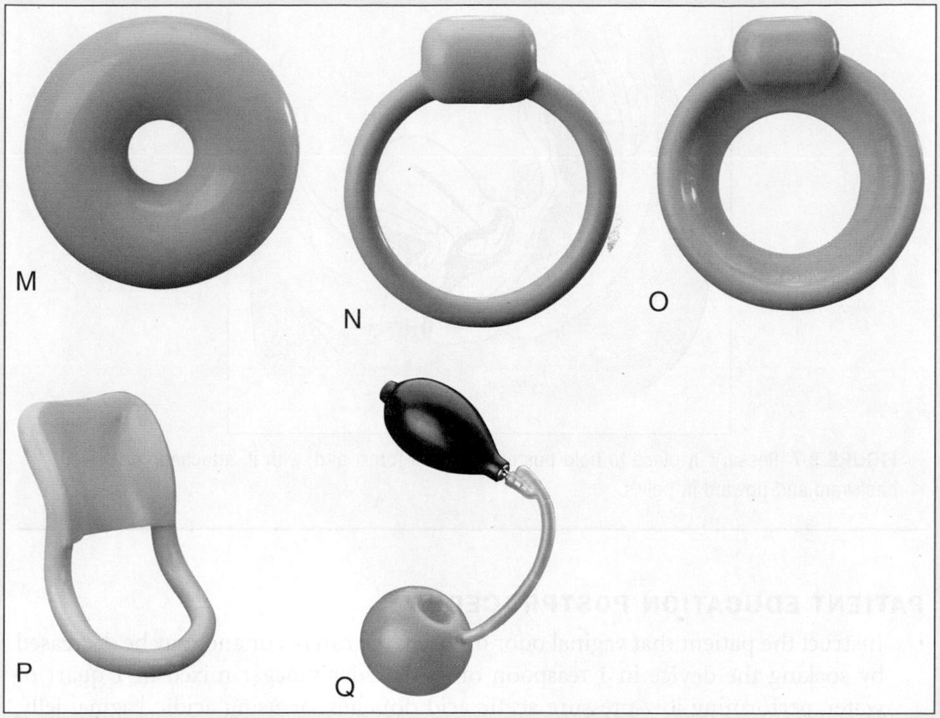

FIGURE 9-6, cont'd **M,** Donut. **N,** Incontinence ring. **O,** Incontinence ring. **P,** Hodge. **Q,** Inflatoball (latex). (Images provided by CooperSurgical, Inc.)

Procedure

1. Choose a pessary designed to alleviate the symptoms this particular woman is having (see Table 9-3). Each pessary has specific instructions for placement and removal.
2. Correct fit is somewhat subjective, but very important: Too large a pessary can cause irritation and ulceration, and one that is too small may not stay in place or may protrude. There should be room for one finger width on all sides of the pessary frame and the vaginal wall, but no part of the pessary should be visible at the introitus (Figure 9-7).
3. Instruct the woman on pessary insertion and removal, allowing plenty of time for practice. She should be asked to stand, walk, and squat to determine (1) whether pain occurs, (2) whether the pessary becomes displaced, or (3) whether the uterus remains in the desired position.

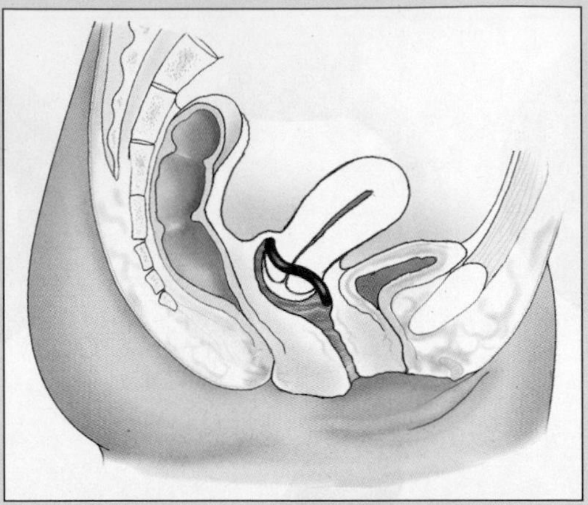

FIGURE 9-7 Pessary in place to hold posterior vaginal fornix and, with it, attached cervix wall backward and upward in pelvis.

PATIENT EDUCATION POSTPROCEDURE

- Instruct the patient that vaginal odor or discharge can occur and may be decreased by soaking the device in 1 teaspoon of apple cider vinegar mixed in 1 quart of water, performing low-pressure acetic acid douches, or using acidic vaginal jelly, such as Trimo-San (Milex Inc.).
- All pessaries should be removed and cleaned at least monthly, and some forms need to be removed nightly (cube and inflatable) for cleaning and to protect vaginal mucosa from the effects of constant pressure.
- Instruct the patient to wash the pessary with warm soap and water and to not use any talcum powder or perfumed powders.
- If vaginal infection occurs, the patient should soak the pessary in rubbing alcohol for 20 minutes before reuse.
- Instruct the patient to bring the device with her to her annual gynecologic examination to evaluate its fit.
- Pessaries should be reevaluated for appropriate fit after pregnancy, miscarriage, or abortion.

9

COMPLICATIONS

- Toxic shock is a theoretical, but unreported, complication.
- Vaginal lacerations or abrasions can occur if the pessary is improperly fitted or left in place without periodic cleaning.

PRACTITIONER FOLLOW-UP

- Practitioners should be available to answer any questions, especially in the first 2 to 3 months of initial pessary use.
- Practitioner should schedule a 2-week follow-up examination to check fit and placement.
- Practitioners and patients should consider annual pessary replacements to avoid problems with rubber or plastic deterioration.

CPT BILLING

You should not bill a E/M code if the visit is for the fitting and insertion of the pessary only. If the visit was for a discussion of treatment options for stress urinary incontinence, and the pessary was inserted at that visit, then an E/M code can be billed, as well.
57160—Fitting and insertion of pessary or other intravaginal support device

REFERENCES AND RELATED RESOURCES

Cundiff GW, Amundsen CL, Bent AE, et al: The PESSRI study: symptom relief outcomes of a randomized crossover trial of the ring and Gellhorn pessaries, *Am J Obstet Gynecol* 196:405.e1, 2007.

Fernando RJ, Thakar R, Sultan AH, et al: Effect of vaginal pessaries on symptoms associated with pelvic organ prolapse, *Obstet Gynecol* 108:93, 2006.

Friedman S, Sandhu KS, Wang C, et al: Factors influencing long-term pessary use, *Int Urogynecol J* 21:673, 2010.

Gorti M, Hudelist G, Simons A: Evaluation of vaginal pessary management: a UK-based survey, *J Obstet Gynaecol* 29:129, 2009.

Lenz G, Lobo M, Gershensen D, Katz V: *Comprehensive gynecology*, ed 6, St. Louis, 2012, Mosby.

Lone F, Thakar R, Sultan AH, Karamalis G: A 5-year prospective study of vaginal pessary use for pelvic organ prolapse, *Int J Gynaecol Obstet* 114:56, 2011.

Nager CW, Richter HE, Nygaard I, et al: Incontinence pessaries: size, POPQ measures, and successful fitting, *Int Urogynecol J Pelvic Floor Dysfunct* 20:1023, 2009.

Powers K, Lazarou G, Wang A, et al: Pessary use in advanced pelvic organ prolapse, *Int Urogynecol J Pelvic Floor Dysfunct* 17:160, 2006.

Diaphragm Fitting

DESCRIPTION

The *diaphragm* is one type of *barrier* contraceptive method. Barrier contraceptives are possibly the oldest contraceptive devices. The diaphragm was introduced in the United States in the early 1900s and rapidly became "the" modern contraceptive device. It has essentially remained unchanged since then with the addition of spermicide and the development of a "wide-seal" style the only alterations.

ANATOMY AND PHYSIOLOGY

Diaphragms work by mechanically blocking sperm from entering the cervix. When used with a spermicidal jelly, the annual failure rate of the diaphragm is 6% with perfect use and 12% with typical use.

INDICATIONS

- Rapidly reversible contraception without hormonal influences
- Inability or unwillingness to use other contraceptive methods
- Provide some aid in protection against certain STDs in addition to hormonal contraceptive uses

CONTRAINDICATIONS

- Abnormalities in vaginal or pelvic anatomy that interfere with proper fit or stable placement
- A history of toxic shock syndrome
- Fitting sooner than 6 weeks' postpartum or before completed involution
- A large cystocele or rectocele

- Uterine prolapse
- Recurrent urinary tract infections

PRECAUTIONS

- Lack of motivation
- Uncomfortable with touching vagina
- Inability to learn insertion technique because of problems with dexterity

ASSESSMENT

- Determine when the last Pap smear was performed. If indicated, repeat the Pap and pelvic examination to rule out cervical or vaginal infections.

PATIENT PREPARATION

- Discuss in detail with the patient all available contraceptive choices, including the advantages and disadvantages of each.
- Explain the fitting procedure and proper diaphragm use, including statistics related to contraceptive effectiveness, and answer any questions. Show video on diaphragm fitting, if available.
- Explain the procedure to the patient; have her get into the lithotomy position. Offer her a mirror so that she may watch the fitting process and explain the insertion process step-by-step as you go through the diaphragm fitting.

TREATMENT ALTERNATIVES

Other forms of contraception

DIAPHRAGM TYPES (Figure 9-8)

- *Arching spring:* Forms an arc when compressed. Good for women with relaxed pelvic support, cystocele, or rectocele. The firmer rim makes insertion easier. This is the most popular diaphragm in the United States.

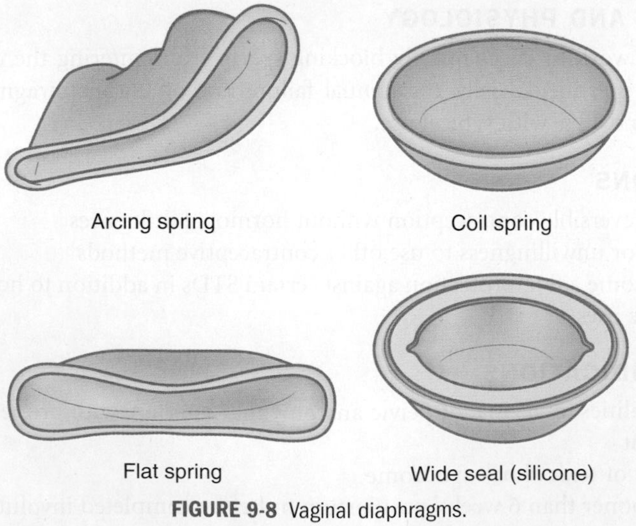

FIGURE 9-8 Vaginal diaphragms.

- *Coil spring:* Firm spring strength; best for women with average vaginal tone and average pubic arch depth.
- *Flat spring:* Gentle spring strength; comfortable for women with very firm vaginal tone. Recommended for smaller women with narrow or shallow pubic arches. Excellent choice for nulliparous women.
- *Wide seal:* Wide outer flange made of silicone, rather than a rim. May provide a better barrier than other rims. Available with an arching or coil spring.

EQUIPMENT

- Diaphragm fitting kit (contains diaphragms varying in size from 55 to 95 mm in circumference, in 5-mm increments)
- Lubricant
- Examination gloves
- Lithotomy table
- Well-lighted, warm room with additional "focused" light source
- Mirror

Procedure (Figure 9-9)

1. To *determine an approximate diaphragm size,* insert your index and middle fingers into the patient's vagina until your middle finger reaches the posterior wall of the vagina.
2. Use the tip of your thumb to mark the point at which your index finger touches the pubic bone. The diaphragm is sized correctly if its opposite rim lies in front of your thumb when you place the diaphragm rim on the tip of your middle finger. (Some providers use an empirical approach and begin with a 75-mm diaphragm because most women wear a 70- to 80-mm diaphragm.)
3. Insert a sample diaphragm in the chosen size by bending the diaphragm in half with the concave side facing the ceiling and sliding it down the posterior wall of the vagina. Aim the entering part of the diaphragm high in the vagina up behind the cervix to lie in the posterior fornix.
4. Check the diaphragm fit by moving your finger around the entire rim of the diaphragm, making sure that it lies in the posterior fornix and snugly behind the pubic bone. Feel for the cervix.
5. The patient should find a properly sized diaphragm comfortable. She should not feel the diaphragm when walking, standing, sitting, or voiding. Have her try each diaphragm in all these positions.
6. It is wise to try a diaphragm one size larger and one size smaller. Choose the largest size diaphragm that is comfortable for the patient and fits snugly in the vagina.
7. To remove the diaphragm, hook one finger under the rim of the diaphragm, and it will fold over on itself. Another method is to slide a finger over the rim to break

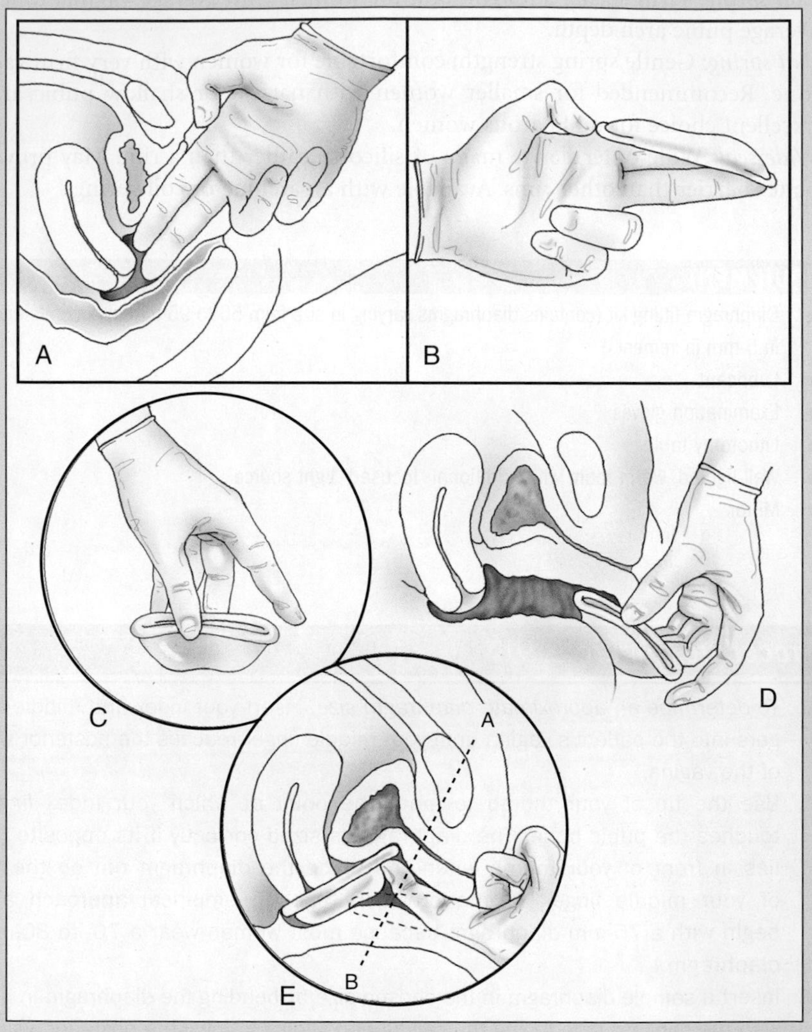

FIGURE 9-9 Procedure for inserting diaphragm. **A** and **B,** Clinical examination to measure for appropriate diaphragm size. **C,** Fold the diaphragm for insertion. **D,** Insert the diaphragm. **E,** Proper positioning of the diaphragm: Cervix is palpable behind the diaphragm *(A)* and rim fits snug, but without discomfort behind the symphysis pubis *(B)*.

9

the suction (this is the method women who have longer fingernails will want to use) (Figure 9-10).

8. Have the patient practice and demonstrate insertion and removal. Women may facilitate insertion by placing one leg up on a stool, by squatting, or by lying on their backs with knees bent. The patient should make sure the diaphragm is in the proper position after insertion.

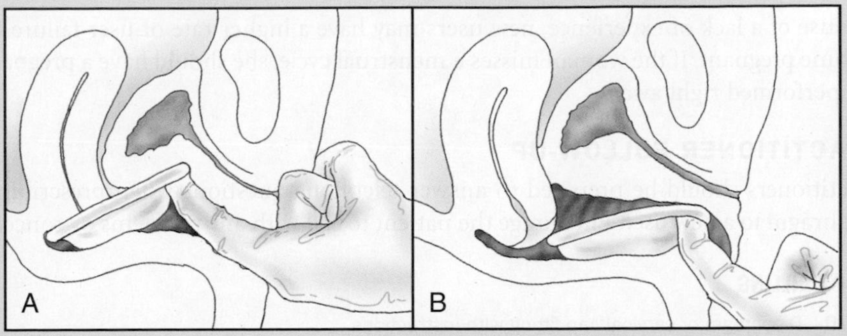

FIGURE 9-10 Procedure for removal of diaphragm. **A,** Hook finger under rim. **B,** Pull diaphragm out through the introitus.

PATIENT EDUCATION POSTPROCEDURE

- Teach the patient the *anatomy* of the vagina. Using a model, assist the patient in learning and identifying landmarks. She should check the position of the diaphragm by inserting her fingers into the vagina. If she cannot reach the posterior fornix, she can feel to make sure that the cervix (which feels like the tip of the nose) is covered by the latex dome of the diaphragm and that the anterior rim is under the symphysis pubis.
- Check the diaphragm for *leaks* before each use by holding it up to a light or by seeing whether it will hold water.
- Place approximately 1 teaspoon of *contraceptive jelly* in the dome of the diaphragm and spread a small amount around the rim. The jelly should come in contact with the cervix. If the wide-seal diaphragm is used, place the jelly also under the rim to provide extra protection.
- The diaphragm must stay in place for 6 hours after intercourse. If intercourse is repeated while the diaphragm is in place, additional spermicidal jelly, vaginal contraceptive film, or foam should be inserted into the vagina. It is recommended that the diaphragm not stay in place for more than 24 hours.
- Only contraceptive jelly or water-based lubricants should be used. Oil-based products will destroy the latex.
- Wash the diaphragm with mild soap and warm water, and blot it dry. It should be stored in the container provided with the diaphragm in a cool place. Talcum powder and other preparations should not be applied to the diaphragm.
- A diaphragm should be replaced every 2 years or should be refitted in the event of weight gain or loss of 10 pounds or greater, after the delivery of a child, or in the event of pelvic surgery. Silicone diaphragms have a longer shelf life; therefore, they can be replaced less frequently.
- Make the patient aware of the signs and symptoms of *toxic shock syndrome:* sudden high fever, vomiting, diarrhea, dizziness, faintness, weakness, sore throat, aching muscles and joints, and rash.
- Discuss *urinary tract infections* related to diaphragm use. Instruct the patient to call promptly if she begins to develop symptoms of a urinary tract infection.

COMPLICATIONS

Because of a lack of experience, new users may have a higher rate of user failure and become pregnant. If the woman misses a menstrual cycle, she should have a pregnancy test performed right away.

PRACTITIONER FOLLOW-UP

Practitioners should be prepared to answer telephone questions when prescribing a diaphragm to a new user. Encourage the patient to call with any problems or concerns.

CPT BILLING

57170—Diaphragm or cervical cap fitting with instructions

REFERENCES AND RELATED RESOURCES

Carcio H, Secor RM: *Advanced health assessment of women*, ed 3, New York, 2015, Springer.

Cook L, Nanda K, Grimes D: Diaphragm versus diaphragm with spermicides for contraception, *Cochrane Database Syst Rev* 1: CD002031, 2009.

Hatcher RA, et al: *Contraceptive technology*, ed 20, New York, 2011, Ardent.

Lenz G, Lobo M, Gershensen D, Katz V: *Comprehensive gynecology*, ed 6, St. Louis, 2012, Mosby.

Cervical Cap Placement

DESCRIPTION

The *cervical cap* is another barrier method of contraception; it acts similarly to the diaphragm in that it prevents sperm from entering the cervix. A small amount of spermicide is usually placed in the dome to aid in effectiveness, although no studies have been done to document the necessity of this step. The cervical cap is a small, cup-like, polyurethane device that fits over the cervix and is held in place by suction. Three types of caps are made, but the most popular and widely available in the United States is the cavity rim cap, which is made of rubber and looks much like a thimble (Figure 9-11). This cap is available in four sizes, 22, 25, 28, and 31 mm, with the cap depth increasing as the rim size increases.

ANATOMY AND PHYSIOLOGY

The cervix varies in appearance and size for every woman. Therefore the limited number of cervical cap sizes precludes 6% to 10% of women in the United States from having a properly fitting cap. With perfect use, nulliparous women have a 9% failure rate versus 26% for parous women.

INDICATIONS

- Prevention of pregnancy
- Desire for rapidly reversible contraception without hormonal influences
- Inability or unwillingness to use other contraceptive methods
- STD protection in addition to hormonal contraceptive use

CONTRAINDICATIONS

- Cervical caps should not be used in the following situations:
  - Lack of motivation
  - Patient who is uncomfortable touching her vagina
  - Inability to learn proper insertion technique

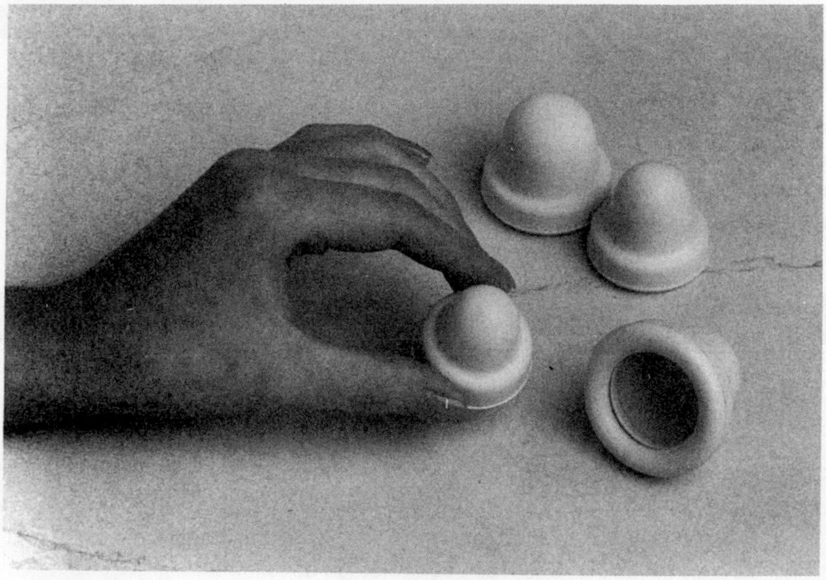

FIGURE 9-11 Cervical cap.

- Abnormalities in cervical or vaginal anatomy that interfere with fit or stable placement (e.g., cervical polyps)
- Unresolved or abnormal Pap smear result
- Current vaginal or cervical infection
- Latex allergy
- History of toxic shock syndrome
- Uterine prolapse

- Fitting should not be done sooner than 6 weeks' postpartum or before completed involution.

PRECAUTIONS

Discuss the fact that this is the least reliable barrier method available, despite perfect use.

ASSESSMENT

Before fitting the cervical cap, perform a Pap smear and pelvic examination to rule out cervical or vaginal infections.

PATIENT PREPARATION

- Discuss in detail with the patient all other available contraceptive choices and their advantages and disadvantages.
- Explain and discuss the fitting procedure and proper cervical cap use, including failure rates.
- Have patient get into the lithotomy position. Offer her a mirror, so that she may watch the fitting process, and explain the insertion process step-by-step as you go through the cervical cap fitting.

TREATMENT ALTERNATIVES

Consider another form of contraception, particularly if women are hesitant to try to insert the cervical cap.

EQUIPMENT

- Cervical cap fitting set that includes one of each of the four sizes of cervical caps (22, 25, 28, and 31 mm)
- Lubricant
- Nonsterile gloves
- Well-lighted, warm room with additional "focused" light source
- Examination table

Procedure

1. Perform a bimanual examination, noting the length, shape, and position of the cervix, and any irregularities in the shape of its circumference. Estimate the appropriate cap size.
2. Fold the rim and compress the cap dome to insert it, dome outward, into the vagina. Place it over the cervix. On unfolding the dome, a desirable suction will be created between the cervix and the rim of the cap. Achieving a correct fit is somewhat subjective, and it can be evaluated as follows:
   a. The cap covers the entire cervix; no cervix is felt.
   b. No space exists between rim and cervix (check the ENTIRE circumference for gaps with your index finger).
   c. Suction is adequate 2 minutes after insertion. Pinching the cap dome and gentle tugging will not dislodge the cap, the dome remains collapsed, suction is equal on both sides, and it takes some effort to dislodge the cap.
   d. Rotation of the cap is not significant; if it does rotate, it should not tilt from the cervix. (If it does not rotate at all, it is too tight and a larger cap is needed; if it rotates too easily, it is too large, and a smaller size is recommended.)
   e. The dome is midline and faces the introitus (so that penile thrusts will not hit the cap at an angle and dislodge it).
   f. The cap is not close to the introitus.
   g. Try one size larger and one smaller to confirm the fit of the chosen cap. If two sizes seem appropriate, choose the smaller cap.
3. Instruct the patient on cap insertion and removal, allowing plenty of time for practice. The cap is removed by inserting one or two fingers between the rim and cervix and pulling down and out. Removal is easier if the suction is broken over the posterior rim. When the patient is comfortable with insertion and removal, place the cap on several times, both correctly and incorrectly, and have the patient identify the cap placement and adjust it as necessary.
4. A second visit is advisable for follow-up of proper placement. Advise the patient that her partner can be taught insertion and removal as well.

PATIENT EDUCATION POSTPROCEDURE

- Instruct the patient to practice insertion and removal before using the cervical cap for contraception the first time. Patients should wear it for 8 hours and check the fit and comfort level.
- Before insertion, the patient should fill the dome one third full with spermicidal jelly; she should not apply it to the inner rim.

- Instruct the patient to insert a cervical cap at least 30 minutes before intercourse to increase suction.
- Instruct the patient to use a condom along with the cap for the first month of use or for the first eight acts of intercourse, checking the cap after each use. Patients and their partners should use different sexual positions to see whether the cap will dislodge. If it is dislodged more than once, a smaller size may be necessary or certain sexual positions become unsafe.
- The patient should allow the cap to remain in place for at least 8 hours after intercourse.
- The patient should not allow the cap to remain in place for longer than 48 hours at a time.
- The cap should be washed with warm soap and water, and blotted dry. Talcum powder or other powders are not recommended to use.
- Instruct the patient to check for tears or holes by holding the cap up to the light or filling it with water.
- If vaginal infection occurs, the patient should soak the cap in rubbing alcohol for 20 minutes before reuse.
- The patient should bring the cap to her annual gynecologic examination to evaluate its fit.
- The patient should not use a cervical cap during menses.
- Cervical caps should be refitted after pregnancy, miscarriage, or abortion and should not be worn in the first 6 weeks' postpartum.

COMPLICATIONS

- Toxic shock is a theoretical, but unreported, complication.
- Vaginal lacerations or abrasions can occur if the cap is left in place for too long.

PRACTITIONER FOLLOW-UP

- Practitioners should be available to answer any questions, especially in the first 2 to 3 months of initial cap use.
- The practitioner should schedule a 2-week follow-up examination to check the fit and placement.
- The Food and Drug Administration mandates a follow-up Pap smear 3 months after the first fitting, after which the routine annual Pap smear is required.
- Patients should consider cap replacements annually to avoid problems with deterioration.
- Vaginal odor or discharge occurs in 5% to 27% of cap users and may be decreased by soaking the cap in 1 teaspoon apple cider vinegar mixed in 1 quart water or placing a drop of chlorophyll in the dome before insertion. Too frequent soaking can more rapidly deteriorate rubber, however.

■ CPT BILLING

57170—Diaphragm or cervical cap fitting with instructions

REFERENCES AND RELATED RESOURCES

Carcio H, Secor RM: *Advanced health assessment of women*, ed 3, New York, 2015, Springer.
Hatcher RA, et al: *Contraceptive technology*, ed 20, New York, 2011, Ardent.
Lenz G, Lobo M, Gershensen D, Katz V: *Comprehensive gynecology*, ed 6, St. Louis, 2012, Mosby.

Endometrial Biopsy

DESCRIPTION

Endometrial sampling by office-based endometrial biopsy provides a minimally invasive option for the diagnosis of endometrial hyperplasia, pathology, or cancer. The endometrial biopsy has generally replaced diagnostic surgical dilation and curettage.

There are several benefits of endometrial biopsy versus dilation and curettage. The procedure is performed in the office rather than the hospital setting, there is minimal cervical dilation, there is a decreased risk of uterine perforation, and it is less expensive. Endometrial biopsy can be used in conjunction with a pelvic or transvaginal ultrasound to evaluate postmenopausal bleeding, pre- or perimenopausal abnormal uterine bleeding, or atypical glandular cells (AGC) Pap. Endometrial biopsy can also be used for the ongoing monitoring of women who have prior endometrial hyperplasia or carcinoma and who have not had a hysterectomy.

An endometrial biopsy should only be performed by providers who have received special training in biopsy technique.

ANATOMY AND PHYSIOLOGY

The endometrial biopsy samples the endometrium, or uterine lining, with either a suction device or an endometrial brush. The device enters the cervix through the os and typically takes only a small amount of cervical dilation with a sound. The low and high pressure devices use suction to sample the endometrium. The low pressure devices are thin, flexible plastic tubes that use suction to sample the endometrium. These are the most commonly used devices. The high pressure devices are used less frequently because they are more rigid and thus more uncomfortable for the patient. The endometrial brush is similar to the endocervical brush and can provide good results in postmenopausal women, especially when used in conjunction with a low pressure device.

INDICATIONS

- Abnormal uterine bleeding (AUB):
  - Under 45 years old: Persistent AUB that occurs with unopposed estrogen (obesity; anovulation), failed medical management of bleeding, or women at high risk for endometrial cancer (tamoxifen therapy; Cowden and Lynch syndromes).
  - Age 45 years to menopause: Any persistent AUB such as frequent menses (interval between onset of menses is less than 21 days), prolonged bleeding (over 7 days), or heavy bleeding (total volume of over 80 ml or entirely saturating through a large pad every hour).
  - Postmenopausal: Any uterine bleeding and/or endometrial stripe of over 4 mm on ultrasound.
- Abnormal cervical cytology results:
  - Presence of endometrial cells in a woman 40 years or older who also has AUB or risk factors for endometrial cancer
  - Presence of AGC, endometrial
  - AGC: All categories other than endometrial if 35 years or older; or at risk for endometrial cancer
- Other indications:
  - Screening of women who are at increased risk of endometrial cancer

9

- Monitoring of women who have prior endometrial pathology, such as endometrial hyperplasia

CONTRAINDICATIONS

- Known or suspected pregnancy
- Acute cervical, vaginal, or pelvic infection
- An obstructing cervical lesion (as in women who have cervical cancer)
- Uncontrolled bleeding disorders

PRECAUTIONS

- If patient is bleeding heavily, the endometrial biopsy may be insufficient and need to be repeated.
- Vagal response may occur with endometrial biopsy.

ASSESSMENT

Obtain patient history. Determine risk of pregnancy, risk of STDs, bleeding disorders, current state of vaginal bleeding, last Pap smear, and abnormal vaginal discharge. Obtain a Pap smear and any cultures if indicated. A negative urine beta-human chorionic gonadotropin (BHCG) should also be obtained before the procedure. A bimanual examination should be performed to evaluate the orientation and size of the uterus.

PATIENT PREPARATION

Review the indication for the endometrial biopsy with the patient and describe the procedure to the patient. Explain that the procedure will likely cause cramping. If possible, 600 to 800 mg of ibuprofen taken preprocedure can help reduce this effect. Answer all questions and obtain consent before the biopsy.

TREATMENT ALTERNATIVES

Dilation and curettage and hysteroscopy can provide endometrial sampling, but are more invasive.

EQUIPMENT

- Gloves
- Speculum
- Well-lighted, warm room with additional "focused" light source
- Povidone-iodine (Betadine) swabs (if allergic to iodine, use chlorhexidine [Hibiclens])
- Uterine sound
- Cotton swabs
- Single-tooth tenaculum
- Ring forceps
- Local anesthetic agent (e.g., 1% chloroprocaine), and 0.5 mg atropine for vasovagal response, and a 10-ml syringe with a 25-gauge, 3-inch needle, if a paracervical block is indicated
- Endometrial biopsy sampling device

Procedure

1. Assist patient in the dorsal lithotomy position and drape as needed, perform bimanual examination, and insert warm speculum.
2. Cleanse the cervix with an antiseptic solution, such as providone-iodine.
3. If needed, grasp the cervix with a tenaculum or ring forceps to hold the cervix in place and provide traction, especially when the position of the uterus is retroflexed

9

or anteflexed or if the device will not pass through the cervical os. The tenaculum or ring forceps are not always needed if the sampling tool is able to be passed through the cervix without complication and the uterus is close to midline. This can decrease the patient's discomfort. If using these devices, consider a paracervical block or topical anesthetic.

4. Using moderate, steady pressure, insert the sampling device through the cervical os and advance to the uterine fundus (Figure 9-12, A). When resistance is

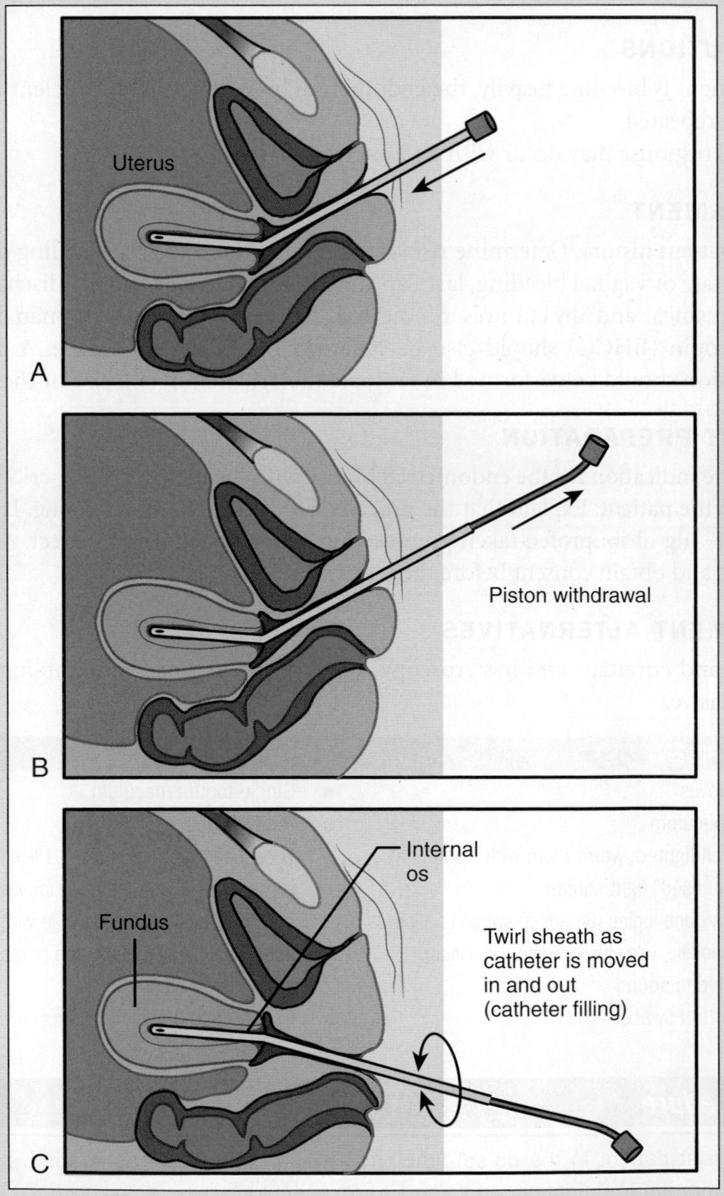

FIGURE 9-12 Procedure of endometrial biopsy. **A,** Insert the sampling device through the cervical os and advance to the uterine fundus. **B,** Stabilize the sheath with one hand while pulling the piston out to create suction. **C,** Slowly twist the piston while pulling it out in a corkscrew motion to obtain sample. (Redrawn with permission from Renee L. Cannon.)

met, stop advancement. Many sampling devices are marked in centimeters to measure uterine depth.

5. If the device will not pass through the cervix, use a uterine sound or small dilator to gently dilate the os.
6. Stabilize the sheath with one hand while pulling the piston out as far as it will go to create suction (Figure 9-12, B). Move the end of the sampling device to sample different areas of the uterus. With the commonly used, low-suction device (i.e., Pipelle), slowly twist the piston while pulling it out in a corkscrew motion (Figure 9-12, C).
7. Advance the piston and dispense the contents of the sampling device into a formalin container. More than one pass may be needed to ensure an adequate sample is obtained.
8. Remove the tenaculum, if present. Bleeding can generally be controlled with a cotton swab and pressure, but, if needed, Monsel's solution or silver nitrate can provide hemostasis.

PATIENT EDUCATION POSTPROCEDURE

- Have patient remain in a recumbent position for a few minutes postprocedure to reduce the chance of a vasovagal response. She will likely experience some cramping after the procedure, which can be managed with analgesics such as nonsteroidal antiinflammatories (NSAIDs), aspirin, or acetaminophen.
- Advise the patient to call if she experiences any fever, increasing pain, foul-smelling vaginal discharge, continuous cramping for 48 hours or more, or bleeding that is heavier than a normal period.

COMPLICATIONS

- Cramping
- Vasovagal reaction
- Light vaginal bleeding or spotting for several days
- Excessive uterine bleeding (rare)
- Uterine perforation (rare)
- Pelvic infection (rare)
- Bacteremia (rare)

PRACTITIONER FOLLOW-UP

Patients may come back into the office for a follow-up appointment in 2 weeks to discuss pathology and any treatment plan.

■ CPT BILLING

If the visit is for the procedure only, no additional E/M code should be charged.
58100–Endometrial sampling (biopsy) with or without endocervical sampling (biopsy), without cervical dilation, any method (separate procedure)

REFERENCES AND RELATED RESOURCES

American College of Obstetricians and Gynecologists: ACOG Practice Bulletin. Clinical Management Guidelines for Obstetrician-Gynecologists. Number 120, July 2012. Diagnosis of abnormal uterine bleeding in reproductive aged women, *Obstet Gynecol* 120:197–206, 2012.

American College of Obstetricians and Gynecologists: ACOG Practice Bulletin. Clinical Management Guidelines for Obstetrician-Gynecologists. Number 136, July 2013. Management of abnormal uterine bleeding associated with ovulatory dysfunction, *Obstet Gynecol* 120:197–206, 2012.

9

Carcio H, Secor RM: *Advanced health assessment of women*, ed 3, New York, 2015, Springer.
Lenz G, Lobo M, Gershensen D, Katz V: *Comprehensive gynecology*, ed 6, St. Louis, 2012, Mosby.
Polena V, Mergui JL, Zerat L, Sananes S: The role of Pipelle Mark II sampling in endometrial disease diagnosis, *Eur J Obstet Gynecol Reprod Biol* 134:233, 2007.
Sierecki AR, Gudipudi DK, Montemarano N, Del Priore G: Comparison of endometrial aspiration biopsy techniques: specimen adequacy, *J Reprod Med* 53:760, 2008.
Trimble CL, Method M, Leitao M, et al: Management of endometrial precancers, *Obstet Gynecol* 120:1160, 2012.

Contraceptive Implant Insertion and Removal

DESCRIPTION

The etonogestrel implant is a reversible contraceptive that provides long-term protection from pregnancy (3 years). It is appropriate for use in selected patients. It was first marketed as Implanon, but was subsequently modified to be radio-opaque and marketed as Nexplanon. Nexplanon and Implanon are otherwise bioequivalent.

With this implantable system, a rod containing the contraceptive hormone etonogestrel is implanted just under the skin in the gap between the biceps and triceps muscles, and the hormone is slowly released into the blood supply. Removal of the implant immediately restores fertility.

This is a procedure that should be learned in a hands-on class with supervision, giving the practitioner an opportunity to practice the different manipulative skills required on a rubber model before the procedure is attempted on a patient. Directions are provided here to help the clinician review the steps of the procedure before performing it. The procedure should NOT be attempted without first attending a training class and obtaining certification.

ANATOMY AND PHYSIOLOGY

The implant is a rod (40 mm long and 2 mm wide) made of semirigid plastic, containing 68 mg of the progestin etonogestrel. The etonogestrel is slowly released over 3 years, at first 68 to 70 mcg/day, then decreasing to 35 to 46 mcg/day after the first year, to 30 to 40 mcg/day at the end of the second year, and then to 25 to 30 mcg/day at the end of the third year. The etonogestrel implant is over 99% effective. There are three explanations for the mechanism of action:

- Hypothalamic and pituitary suppression of the luteinizing hormone surge (ovulation prevention)
- Thickening of the cervical mucus, which serves as a barrier to sperm penetration
- Suppression of cyclic maturation of the endometrium, leading to an atrophic endometrial lining unfit for implantation of the fertilized egg

9

INDICATIONS

Used to prevent pregnancy, the etonogestrel implant is particularly useful in patients who have a poor history of compliance with other forms of birth control or are advised against taking estrogen-containing birth control methods.

CONTRAINDICATIONS

- Hypersensitivity to any component of the method
- Current or past history of thrombosis or thromboembolic disorders (this is according to the package labeling, though the WHO [World Health Organization]

and CDC [Centers for Disease Control and Prevention] have indicated that progestin-only contraceptives represent a reasonable contraceptive choice for these women)
- Undiagnosed abnormal genital bleeding
- Known or suspected breast cancer or history of breast cancer with progestin-sensitive tumor
- Known or suspected pregnancy
- Hepatic tumor or active liver disease
- Positive or unknown antiphospholipid antibodies

PRECAUTIONS

- Immediately before insertion, ascertain that the patient has used effective contraception. Corroborate this with a negative pregnancy test.
- The implant can be inserted at any time in the menstrual cycle as long as the provider is reasonably sure that the patient is not pregnant. If pregnancy cannot be ruled out, the insertion could be delayed until there is another pregnancy test that proves that the patient is not pregnant; however, there is no evidence that the etonogestrel implant causes abnormal fetal development.

ASSESSMENT

Assess for pregnancy by reviewing the woman's sexual, menstrual, and contraceptive history, and obtain a urine pregnancy test. Also assess for any possible contraindications to the etonogestrel implant before placement.

PATIENT PREPARATION

- Describe the advantages of the etonogestrel implant, and describe the insertion and removal procedures.
- Discuss the possibility of potential side effects, such as bleeding irregularities, headache, acne, weight gain, abdominal pain, breast tenderness, vaginitis, depression, and local site reactions.
- Obtain informed written consent.

TREATMENT ALTERNATIVES

Other long-term methods of birth control, such as intrauterine devices or Depo Provera, could be an alternative to the implantable device.

EQUIPMENT

INSERTION OF THE ETONOGESTREL CONTRACEPTIVE IMPLANT
(Figure 9-13)

- A sterile drape
- Antiseptic skin cleanser
- A 2- to 5-ml syringe and a 25-gauge needle (1.5 inches in length)
- 1% lidocaine or chloroprocaine
- Steri-Strips, gauze sponges, stretch bandage
- Pairs of sterile gloves (for procedure)
- Preloaded insertion device, sterile
- Well-lighted, warm room with additional "focused" light source

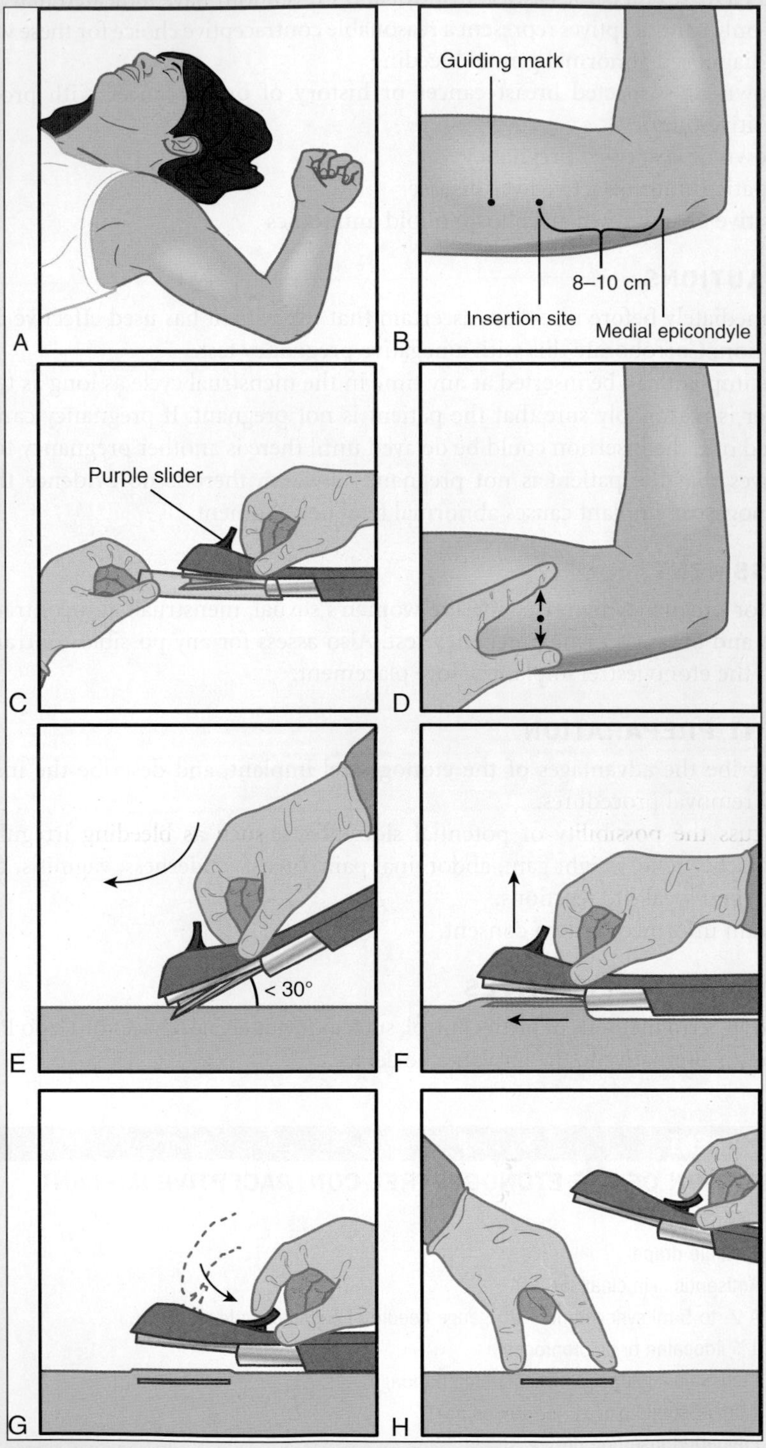

FIGURE 9-13 Insertion of etonogestrel implant. (NEXPLANON® materials/image reproduced with permission of Merck Sharp & Dohme B.V., a subsidiary of Merck & Co., Inc., Kenilworth, New Jersey, U.S.A. All rights reserved.)

9

Procedure

1. The nondominant arm should be used for insertion of the implant. The patient should be comfortably positioned on her back near the edge of the table with her arm flexed at the elbow and externally rotated. The arm will rest on a thick paper drape.
2. Identify a spot for insertion approximately four fingerbreadths superior and lateral to the medial epicondyle of the humerus. The site should be between 6 and 10 cm from the medial epicondyle. The site will depend on anatomic features individual to each patient, such as the area at which the crease between the biceps and triceps muscle is clearest. The device should be inserted in this crease.
3. Prepare the skin with the antiseptic scrub solution.
4. Fill syringe with 1% lidocaine or chloroprocaine and inject 1 to 2 ml into the incision site to make a raised wheal along the planned insertion tract. Test for anesthesia with the needle.
5. Open the sterile etonogestrel system. Hold the applicator above the needle cap on the textured surface between the thumb and forefinger, and remove the clear plastic needle cover. Place the needle against the insertion site at a less than 30-degree angle to the skin. While applying traction to the skin, puncture the skin with the tip of the needle. The needle is sharp enough that a separate incision is not needed. Lower the applicator so that it is parallel to the skin and advance the needle into the subdermal connective tissue. While doing this, make sure to "tent" or lift the skin with the tip of the needle to ensure that the implant is not inserted too deeply. Advance the needle fully, and press the slider downward until the needle retracts. You can then remove the applicator. Hold the gauze over the site for hemostasis.
6. Verify placement of the device by palpating the skin above the device. Both ends should be palpable. At this time, ask the patient to palpate the implant as well.
7. Place Steri-Strips for closure, then wrap with a pressure bandage.

9

Removal of Etonogestrel Contraceptive Implant *(Figure 9-14)*

- Use all of the anesthetic agent, sterile draping, syringes with needles, antiseptic solution, gloves, 4 × 4 gauze (as many as needed), stretch bandage, and Steri-Strips.
- The following additional supplies are needed for removal:
    - Small, sterile, curved hemostats
    - Number 11 scalpel

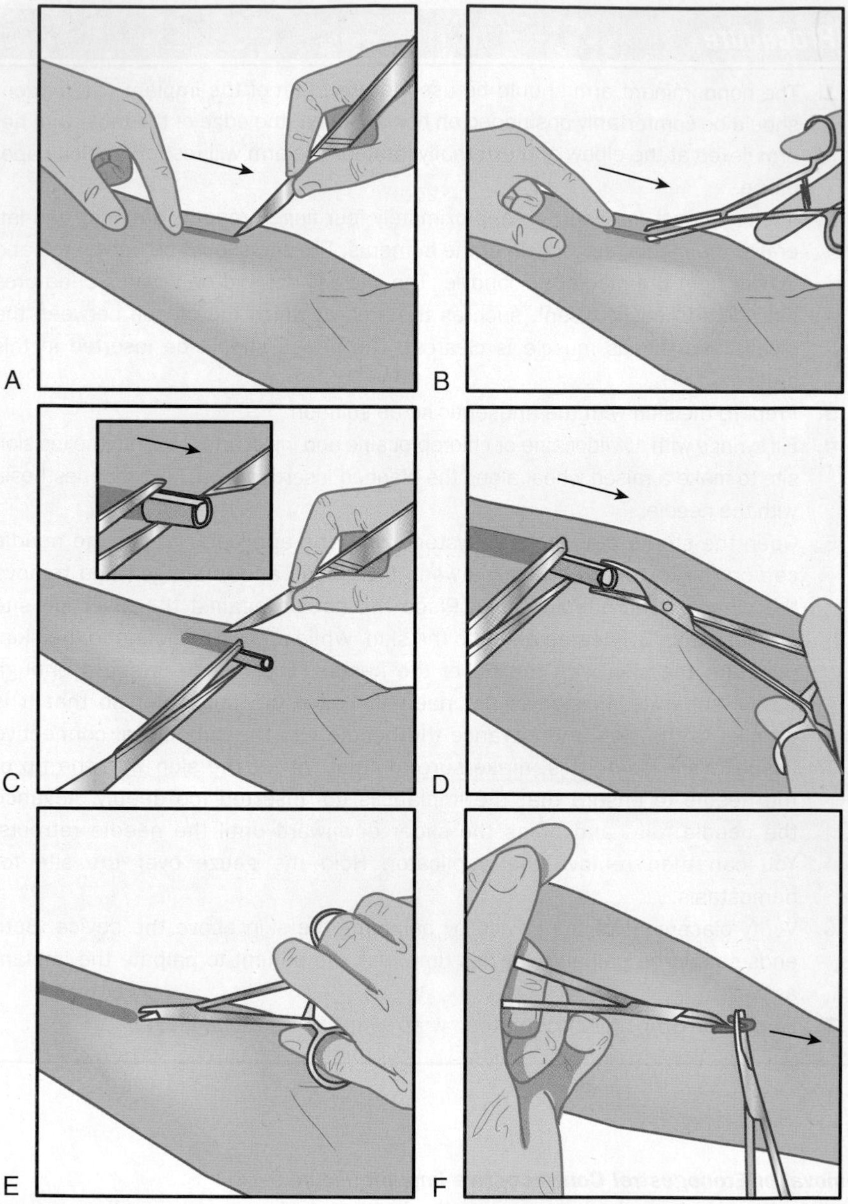

FIGURE 9-14 Removal of etonogestrel implant. (NEXPLANON® materials/image reproduced with permission of Merck Sharp & Dohme B.V., a subsidiary of Merck & Co., Inc., Kenilworth, New Jersey, U.S.A. All rights reserved.)

Procedure

1. Position the patient's arm in the same position as with insertion.
2. Palpate the location of the device. If you are unable to palpate the device, stop the procedure and send for imaging. MRI is needed for Implanon; Nexplanon can be detected by an x-ray.

3. Cleanse the area with antiseptic cleaner.
4. Push down on the end closest to the axilla (distal end), and inject a small wheal (no more than 0.5 ml) of 1% lidocaine under the elevated end of the rod. Too much anesthetic obscures the end of the rod and makes it difficult to remove.
5. Continue to apply pressure to the distal end of the device, and use the scalpel to make a small (2-3 mm) longitudinal incision over the end of the rod. Increase the depth of the incision until you feel the rod. The rod will generally be encased in a fibrous sheath. Continue to dissect away the sheath with the scalpel until the rod comes into view.
6. Using a curved hemostat, gently grasp the end of the rod and pull it free from the skin. If there is resistance, the sheath may need to be further dissected. Use gauze and pressure for hemostasis if needed.
7. Apply Steri-Strips to the incision site, and wrap with a pressure dressing. If the patient wants a new implant inserted after removal of an expired implant, the new rod may be immediately inserted through the same incision used for implant removal.

PATIENT EDUCATION POSTPROCEDURE

Use the same instructions both before insertion and removal:

- The patient should keep the insertion/incision clean and dry.
- The patient could experience some pain at the incision site, but it is not common. This can be relieved with acetaminophen (Tylenol) or ibuprofen (Motrin).
- Some bruising is common at the incision site. The extent of bruising may be decreased by applying an ice bag as needed for the first few hours after insertion/removal, keeping the dressing in place for 1 day.
- Report any signs of infection: redness, swelling, increased pain, foul odor, or purulent discharge. Warn the patient not to try to reinsert a capsule into the arm if it falls out (very rare).

COMPLICATIONS

- Infection
- Hematoma formation
- Local irritation or rash
- Expulsion
- Allergic reaction

PRACTITIONER FOLLOW-UP

- If placing the device more than 5 days after patient's last menstrual period, a backup birth control method is advised for 7 days after placement. Options include condoms, abstinence, or continued use of the former birth control method until the implant is effective.
- Emphasize the importance of using condoms if the patient is at risk for sexually transmitted infections.
- Emphasize the importance of yearly gynecologic examinations.
- Encourage the patient to call if troubled by abnormal bleeding.

■ CPT BILLING

The insertion charge does not include the implant itself. This is an additional charge. If the reason for the visit is the procedure itself, there is no additional E/M code.

11981–Insertion, non-biodegradable drug delivery implant ■ **11982**–Removal, non-biodegradable drug delivery implant ■ **11983**—Removal, with reinsertion, non-biodegradable drug delivery implant ■ **J7307**–Etonogestrel implant system, including implant and supplies

REFERENCES AND RELATED RESOURCES

American College of Obstetricians and Gynecologists: ACOG Practice Bulletin. Clinical Management Guidelines for Obstetrician-Gynecologists. Number 121, July 2011-reaffirmed 2013. Long acting reversible contraception: implants and intrauterine devices, *Obstet Gynecol* 118:184–196, 2011.

Centers for Disease Control and Prevention (CDC): U.S. medical eligibility criteria for contraceptive use, 2010, *MMWR Recomm Rep* 59:1, 2010.

Darney P, Patel A, Rosen K, et al: Safety and efficacy of a single-rod etonogestrel implant (Implanon): results from 11 international clinical trials, *Fertil Steril* 91:1646, 2009.

Finer LB, Jerman J, Kavanaugh ML: Changes in use of long-acting contraceptive methods in the United States, 2007–2009, *Fertil Steril* 98:893, 2012.

Hatcher RA, et al: *Contraceptive technology*, ed 20, New York, 2011, Ardent.

Lidegaard Ø, Løkkegaard E, Jensen A, et al: Thrombotic stroke and myocardial infarction with hormonal contraception, *N Engl J Med* 366:2257, 2012.

Incision and Drainage of a Bartholin Cyst

DESCRIPTION

Bartholin's glands provide lubrication to the vaginal area. Bartholin gland cysts and abscesses are common problems in women of reproductive age. Although the cysts are usually asymptomatic, they may become enlarged or infected and cause significant pain.

ANATOMY AND PHYSIOLOGY

Bartholin's glands are located on either side of the vaginal orifice (Figure 9-15). Bartholin's cyst is a postinflammatory pseudocyst that forms proximally to the obstructed

9

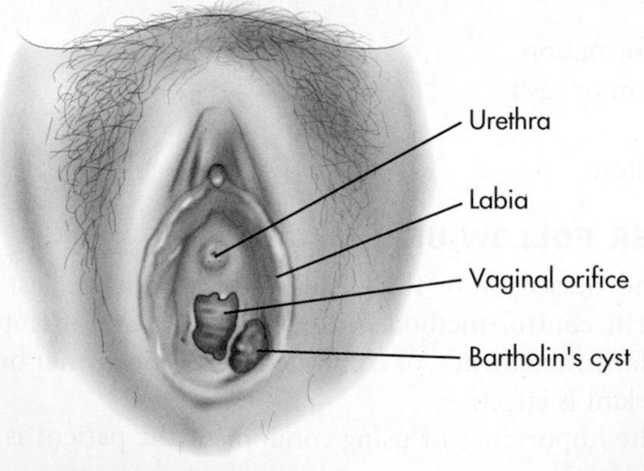

FIGURE 9-15 Bartholin's glands are on either side of the vaginal orifice. A Bartholin's cyst occurs when the gland becomes inflamed or infected.

duct of the Bartholin's gland. The cyst can be unilateral or bilateral when one or both of the glands become inflamed or infected. The affected area becomes swollen and painful from the retention of sterile secretions (mucus plug) or infected exudates. The most frequent cause is congenital narrowing of the gland that causes a backup of natural secretions. The most common pathogens cultured from the abscess are *Gonococcus, Staphylococcus aureus, Streptococcus faecalis, Escherichia coli,* and *Pseudomonas.*

INDICATIONS

If the Bartholin gland has become swollen and painful, incision and drainage may be necessary. Culture of secretions should be taken to help diagnose the cause of swelling and infection so that adequate treatment may be determined.

CONTRAINDICATIONS

Do not attempt if the patient is pregnant; refer patient to an obstetrician.

PRECAUTIONS

- Use universal precautions for blood-borne pathogens; use eye protection.
- Inject the lidocaine slowly, on the top margin of the abscess, to avoid pressure buildup and sudden squirting of exudates from the punctate.

ASSESSMENT

- Assess for previous history of abscesses of Bartholin's glands.
- Look for swelling, tenderness, and pain of the labia during intercourse and during both walking and sitting.
- Palpate for enlarged inguinal lymph nodes and other palpable masses in the area of the glands.

PATIENT PREPARATION

- Explain the procedure to the patient.
- Obtain informed written consent.
- Have the patient empty her bladder.

TREATMENT ALTERNATIVES

- If the cyst is only mildly painful and appears to be "unripened," Keflex (cephalexin) 500 mg every 12 hours for 10 days coupled with sitz baths four times a day may diminish swelling and resolve infection.
- Often the primary care clinician will choose to lance the cyst or abscess because this technique can be effective for other common abscesses; however, simple lancing of a Bartholin gland cyst or abscess may result in recurrence. If a patient has had a previous history of Bartholin gland cyst or abscess, more definitive treatment methods include use of a Word catheter and marsupialization, both of which can be performed in the office. These methods allow for a new epithelialized tract for drainage of glandular secretions. Marsupialization is more complicated than Word catheter placement, but it causes the patient less discomfort. Generally, marsupialization is reserved for patients who have one or two failed Word catheter placements and is generally performed by a physician. Word catheter placement will be reviewed in this section.

- The management of Bartholin cysts through the insertion of a silver nitrate stick into the cyst cavity immediately postdrainage is another treatment option that is more simple and possibly more effective than Word catheter placement, but there are limited data to support this. The only complication to this method is significant patient discomfort.

EQUIPMENT

- Sterile drapes
- Sterile gloves
- Well-lighted, warm room with additional "focused" light source
- Antiseptic cleaner
- Two 10-ml syringes
- An 18- and 25-gauge needle, 1½ inch
- 250 ml of 0.9% NaCl
- One bottle of 1% lidocaine
- No. 11 scalpel
- Sterile curved hemostat
- Sterile pickup
- Iodoform gauze ½ or ¼ inch wide
- 4 × 4 gauze pads
- Vaginal culture swab
- Sanitary napkins
- Word catheter with saline, needle and syringe for placement (if needed)

Procedure

1. Have the patient lie down in the lithotomy position.
2. Use an antiseptic solution to scrub the perineum.
3. Put on gloves and drape the patient with sterile drapes.
4. Inject 5 to 10 ml of 1% lidocaine along the top margin of the abscess using the 25-gauge needle.
5. Incise the cyst along the top margin of the abscess at or behind the hymenal ring sufficiently to allow for drainage. Collect drainage for culture.
6. Insert the gloved fingers of one hand into the vaginal vault behind the abscess, and press the abscess against gloved fingers of the other hand to help force the exudate from the abscess.
7. Insert a curved, sterile hemostat into the abscess and break up all the soft tissue walls inside the abscess.
8. Irrigate the wound with 0.9% NaCl using the 20-ml syringe with the 18-gauge needle. Continue irrigation until the solution runs clear.
9. Prepare the Word catheter by testing the balloon with a 5-cc syringe filled with normal saline. Insert the tip of the Word catheter into the cavity so that the end is entirely within the space. Inflate the balloon. Take the end of the catheter and place it in the vagina. The Word catheter will remain in place for at least 4 weeks. The patient will need to return to the office for removal, which involves deflating the catheter and removing the catheter.
10. Cover the abscessed area with 4 × 4 gauze pads and attach a sanitary napkin.

PATIENT EDUCATION POSTPROCEDURE

- Instruct the patient to change the 4 × 4 gauze and sanitary napkin every 4 to 6 hours.
- Schedule a return appointment for reevaluation 24 hours after the procedure.

- Patient should have a sitz bath in warm water four times a day for 1 week.
- Instruct the patient to report any signs of infection to the practitioner.
- Instruct the patient to return for follow-up at 1 week.

COMPLICATIONS

Infection

PRACTITIONER FOLLOW-UP

Within 24 hours of the procedure, remove half of the gauze. If the wound appears clear, instruct the patient to remove the remainder of the gauze 24 hours later. According to evidence, there is no benefit in antibiotic therapy for uncomplicated skin abscesses. The provider may want to consider antibiotic therapy in women who have recurrent infection, MRSA, systemic signs of infection, extensive surrounding cellulitis, and immunosuppression.

RED FLAG

- Bartholin's gland masses are more likely to be malignant in postmenopausal women; make immediate referral to OB/GYN rather than performing drainage.

CPT BILLING

56420—Incision and drainage of Bartholin's gland abscess ■ **56740**—Excision of Bartholin's gland or cyst

REFERENCES AND RELATED RESOURCES

Haider Z, Condous G, Kirk E, et al: The simple outpatient management of Bartholin's abscess using the Word catheter: a preliminary study, *Aust N Z J Obstet Gynaecol* 47:137, 2007.

Kessous R, Aricha-Tamir B, Sheizaf B, et al: Clinical and microbiological characteristics of Bartholin gland abscesses, *Obstet Gynecol* 122:794, 2013.

Lenz G, Lobo M, Gershensen D, Katz V: *Comprehensive gynecology*, ed 6, St. Louis, 2012, Mosby.

Marzano DA, Haefner HK: The Bartholin gland cyst: past, present, and future, *J Low Genit Tract Dis* 8:195, 2004.

Thurman AR, Satterfield TM, Soper DE: Methicillin-resistant Staphylococcus aureus as a common cause of vulvar abscesses, *Obstet Gynecol* 112:538, 2008.

Intrauterine Device (IUD)

DESCRIPTION

Devices inserted into the uterus to prevent conception have been inventive and diverse for hundreds of years. A device used in Japan and Europe in the 1930s lost its popularity because of major concerns about the possible association it had with pelvic infections. The IUD had never gained popularity in the United States until the 1960s, when the Population Council made a concerted effort to reintroduce the device.

In the early 1960s, a variety of newly designed IUDs appeared on the market, using different products in the shape of bows, butterflies, loops, rings, and spirals. Because of the adverse outcomes and publicity associated with one of these devices, the Dalkon Shield, interest in this form of contraception was absent for many years. Current devices have been proven to be mostly safe, with a low incidence of adverse events. There are currently three types of IUDs available in the United States: the copper-releasing IUD (for 10 years of use) and two levonorgestrel-releasing IUDs (the Skyla [for 3 years of use] and the Mirena [for 5 years of use]).

Despite lingering misconceptions, such as IUDs being an abortifacient, causing ectopic pregnancy, infertility, and others, IUDs have been proved to be a very effective and safe contraceptive alternative. The copper-T IUD, Skyla, and Mirena are 99.8% effective. The IUD is not contraindicated for the nulliparous woman, but insertion can be more difficult. Some nulliparous patients may benefit from misoprostol before placement to facilitate insertion.

Mechanisms of Action

The copper IUDs prevent fertilization primarily via a spermicidal action. The endometrium reacts biochemically and morphologically to the foreign body with sterile inflammation, which incapacitates viable motile sperms, hence preventing them from reaching the fallopian tubes. Fertilization occurs in less than 1% of menstrual cycles.

The progestin-releasing IUDs (Mirena and Skyla) have several suggested mechanisms of contraceptive action: thickening of the cervical mucus, thus preventing passage of sperm into the uterus; inhibition of sperm capacitation or survival; disruption of tubal motility; partial inhibition of follicular development and ovulation; and alteration and suppression of the endometrium (atrophy).

INDICATIONS

The IUD is indicated for women who are unwilling or cannot take oral contraceptives or are unable to comply regularly with user-dependent methods, such as barrier contraceptives or oral contraceptives. The hormonal IUDs are also used for therapeutic purposes to alleviate severe dysmenorrhea, menorrhagia, endometriosis, adenomyosis, and myoma formation. The copper-T IUD is also indicated for emergency postcoital contraception.

CONTRAINDICATIONS

- This procedure requires the practitioner to have formal training and supervised clinical experience before being implemented. The practitioner should not attempt to insert an IUD without this educational preparation.
- Do not use with pregnancy or suspected pregnancy, incomplete involution after abortion or childbirth, uterine anomaly (congenital abnormalities, such as a bicornuate uterus or a uterus less than 6 or greater than 10 cm on sonogram), fibroid tumors that distort the endometrial cavity, endometrial polyps, history of pelvic inflammatory disease (PID), unless there has been a subsequent intrauterine pregnancy, acute PID, postpartum endometritis or infected abortion in the past 3 months, known or suspected cervical neoplasia, genital bleeding of unknown etiology, lower genital tract infections (acute untreated cervicitis; vaginitis) until infection is controlled, current breast cancer or history of progestin-sensitive breast cancer (pertains to progestin IUDs only), active hepatic disease or hepatic tumors (progestin IUDs only), allergy to copper or diagnosed Wilson's disease (pertains to copper-T IUD only), allergy to silicone and/or polyethylene, previously inserted IUD that has not been removed, strong history of syncope during cervical

manipulation (e.g., Pap smears), and cognitive or physical limitations that prevent the patient from recognizing danger signs and the presence of the string.

- The copper-T IUD is also contraindicated for women who have severe dysmenorrhea and menorrhagia; however, either of the other two progestin IUDs can be a therapeutic solution to this problem (diminished bleeding).

PRECAUTIONS

Because of the possibility of introducing bacteria into the uterus from the existing vaginal flora, strict aseptic technique is mandatory. In case of stenosis of the cervix, do not use excessive force to overcome resistance to sounding the uterine cavity. A vasovagal reaction can occur (e.g., syncope; bradycardia; diaphoresis).

ASSESSMENT

History

- Ask about parity, menstrual history (last and previous menstrual periods), anemia, menorrhagia, metrorrhagia, dysmenorrhea, current mode of contraception, metal and drug allergies, coagulopathies, Wilson disease, liver disease, history of syncope, current medications, ectopic pregnancies, PID, STDs, stability of relationship (monogamy versus promiscuity), vaginal discharge, endometriosis, abnormal Pap smear, breast masses, and progesterone sensitivity.

Physical Examination

- Obtain Pap smear (if indicated based on history), cervical cultures (*Chlamydia*/gonorrhea), and urine pregnancy test. If cervical cultures return positive after IUD is inserted, the STD should be treated and the IUD may be left in. It is recommended to repeat testing in 3 months to ensure that the infection has cleared. If a Pap smear comes back abnormal, the IUD may be left in place until the level of dysplasia is determined via colposcopy.
- Observe for cervical lesions; uterine position, shape, size, and tenderness; and adnexal/uterine tenderness.

PATIENT PREPARATION

- After detailed explanation and discussion, obtain written informed consent.
- Patient needs information on indications versus contraindications, advantages versus disadvantages of the selected IUD, and details of the procedure.
- Reinforce verbal information with a video provided by the manufacturer.
- Ask the patient to take home the package insert along with the consent form to read.
- Discuss efficacy, signs of infection, and the possibility of expulsion or partial expulsion (cramping, vaginal discharge, lengthening of the string, or device protruding from the cervix), as well as the emergent nature of it (patient must see the provider immediately).
- If possible, at the time of scheduling, advise the patient to return when having her menses (if feasible) in a fed state and to take an antiprostaglandin (e.g., 400 to 800 mg of ibuprofen) 1 hour before the procedure. Advise her to avoid intercourse until insertion or to practice strict reliable birth control. IUDs can be placed at any time during the menstrual cycle if pregnancy can be reasonably excluded.

TREATMENT ALTERNATIVES

The decision to use an IUD pivots on the menstrual history, contraindications, and planning a future pregnancy. If the woman is planning a pregnancy in less than 1 year, insertion of an IUD is not economically wise. If the IUD is not a good choice, select another reliable method comparable to the high efficacy of IUDs (e.g., oral contraceptives, Nexplanon, Depo-Provera, or bilateral tubal ligation).

EQUIPMENT

- Sterile gloves
- Speculum
- Well-lighted, warm room with additional "focused" light source
- Povidone-iodine (Betadine) swabs (if allergic to iodine, use chlorhexidine [Hibiclens])
- Uterine sound
- Cotton swabs
- Single-tooth tenaculum
- Scissors
- Ring forceps
- Local anesthetic agent (e.g., 1% chloroprocaine), 0.5 mg atropine for vasovagal response, and a 10-ml syringe with a 25-gauge, 3-inch needle, if paracervical block is indicated
- IUD kit with inserter (Figure 9-16)

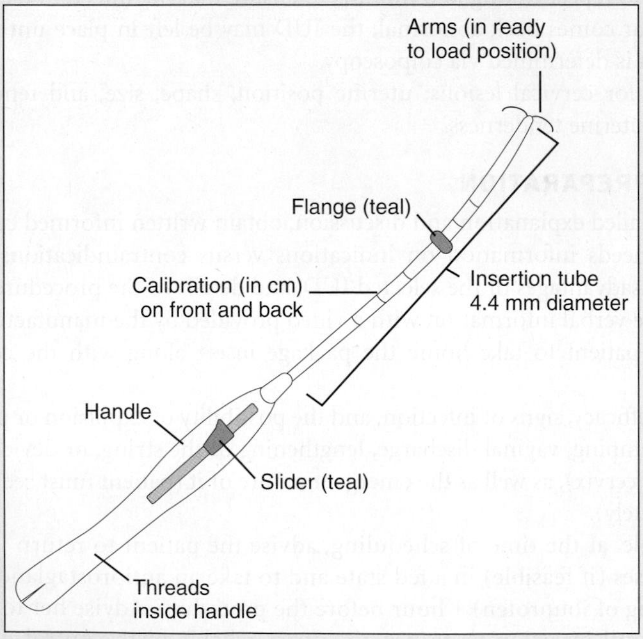

FIGURE 9-16 Example of intrauterine device (IUD).

Procedure

PREPARATION FOR COPPER-T, MIRENA, AND SKYLA IUD INSERTION

1. Drape the patient and place her in the lithotomy position. Perform a careful bimanual examination to rule out vaginal/pelvic infection, and determine again the position of the uterus (unrecognized retroflexion can lead to perforation of the uterine wall).
2. Insert a warm speculum, and inspect the cervix for abnormal discharge or lesions. The procedure has to be performed under aseptic conditions with universal precautions for blood-borne pathogens.
3. Beginning at the os, paint the cervix with an antiseptic solution in concentric circles, spiraling outward on the cervix, and paint vaginal vault. Repeat procedure two more times.
4. If paracervical block is indicated, inject 1 ml of 1% chloroprocaine with 0.4 mg of atropine in the anterior lip of the os (if uterus is anteverted) and in the posterior lip (if retroverted).
5. After 1 minute, grasp the anterior portion of the cervix (if uterus is anteverted and posteriorly if retroverted) with the tenaculum or ring forceps, about 1.5 to 2 cm from the os. Close the tenaculum/ring forceps slowly to the first notch. Reveal the left lateral vaginal fornix by moving the cervix with the tenaculum/ring forceps to the right. Inject 4 ml of anesthetic agent at 3 o'clock into the cervical mucosa 1 to 2 cm from the os. Deflect the cervix to the left and inject the same way at 9 o'clock. As the needle is withdrawn, inject the additional 1 ml left in the barrel under the mucosa. Wait for 1 to 2 minutes before proceeding.
6. Sound the uterus slowly and gently to determine the direction of the cervical canal and the depth of the uterus. If the os gives resistance due to spasm, wait a few minutes and attempt sounding again. Never force entry of the sound or applicators! Place a cotton swab at the cervix when the sound is all the way in. Hold the sound and the swab together and remove them at the same time. The distance between the tip of the sound and the tip of the swab determines the depth of the fundus, so the clinician will know how far the IUD can be inserted.
7. After procedure is completed, remove the tenaculum or ring forceps. If there is bleeding from the tenaculum, place a cotton swab with pressure at the sites. If this does not provide hemostasis, Monsel's solution or silver nitrate sticks may be used.

MIRENA AND SKYLA INSERTION (Figure 9-17)

1. The Mirena and Skyla IUDs packaging contains a partially preassembled IUD and applicator (see Figure 9-16). The applicator is a plastic insertion tube containing the string and IUD. The string is located completely within the tube. There is a flange for indicating the cervical depth and a handle with a slider that is used to release the IUD and retract the insertion tube.
2. Using the sterile technique, move the slider (pink in Skyla and blue in Mirena) all the way forward in the direction of the arrow. This moves the IUD into the

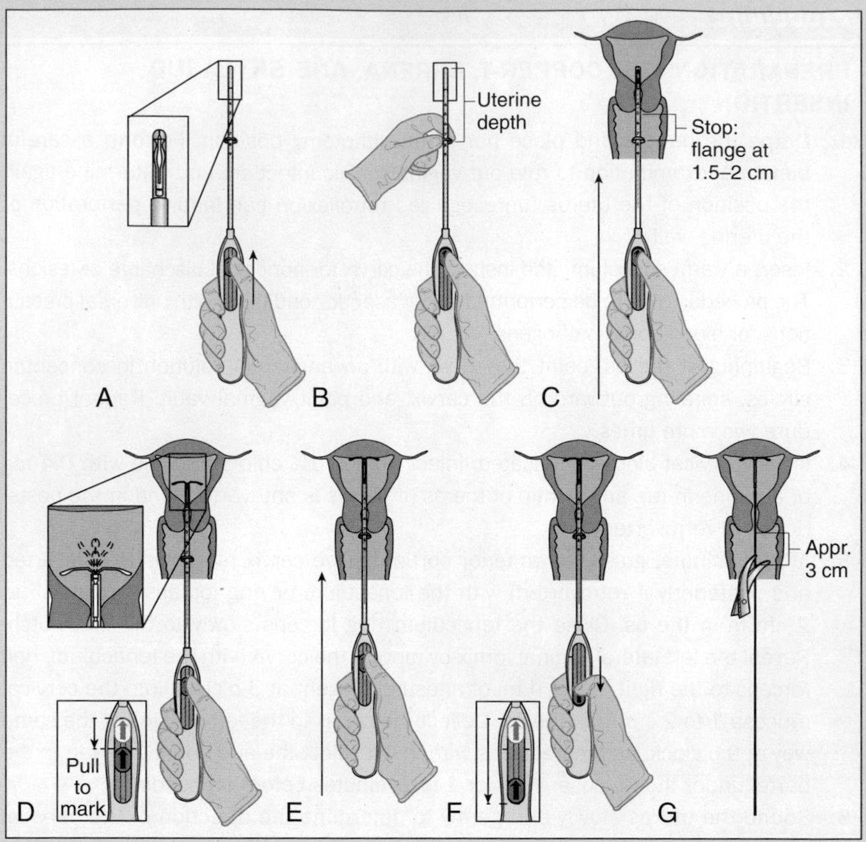

FIGURE 9-17 Technique for inserting levonorgestrel-releasing intrauterine device (LNG IUD). (Redrawn with permission from Bayer HealthCare Pharmaceuticals Inc.)

insertion tube, resulting in the tips of the arms meeting and forming a rounded end that extends slightly beyond the insertion tube. The strings are completely contained within the handle and do not need to be secured.

3. Hold the slider in place with the thumb and, either by using the groove located within the sterile packaging or with a sterile gloved hand, move the flange on the barrel to the desired depth. This will be the depth of the uterus determined by sound.
4. While exerting traction on the tenaculum, advance the inserter through the cervix until the flange is 1.5 to 2 cm from the os, and hold there while moving the slider halfway down. There is a mark there to show where to stop insertion and allow the IUD arms to release, which takes about 10 seconds.
5. Advance the inerter until the flange touches the cervix, which places the IUD at the correct fundal position. Hold the inserter in place and release the IUD by moving the slider all the way back down toward the handle. Remove the inserter and cut the strings about 3 cm from the external os.

COPPER-T IUD INSERTION (Figure 9-18)

1. The package contains the IUD with attached string, insertion tube with elliptical flange, and a solid plastic rod with a ring at one end. Wearing sterile gloves, the provider loads the IUD into the insertion tube by bending the transverse arms of the IUD downward toward the vertical arm and placing the thread and IUD into the tube until the IUD is secure. This tucks the transverse arms into the tube next to the vertical arm. The IUD should not be in the tube more than 5 minutes before insertion or it may not release appropriately. If sterile gloves are not available, it is possible to load the IUD into the insertion tube through the packaging. After loading the IUD into the tube, take the solid rod and pass through the other end of the tube until it barely touches the end of the IUD. Mark the depth of the uterus measured before with the sliding plastic flange.
2. Advance the insertion tube while exerting traction by the tenaculum to align the cervix with the uterine cavity. Insert the tube into the uterus to the correct depth. When the tube reaches the fundus, withdraw the unit a few millimeters. The

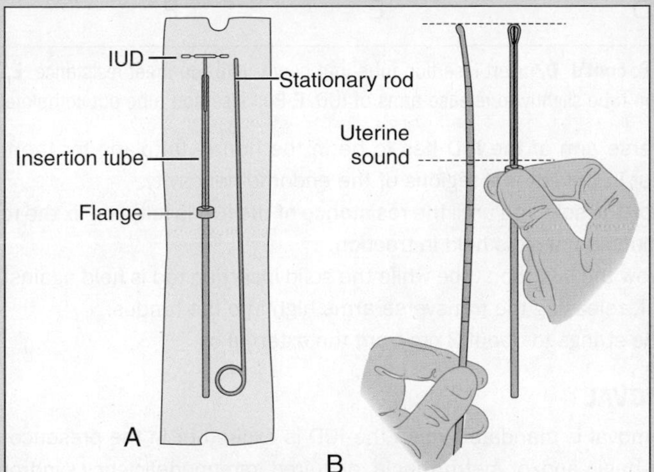

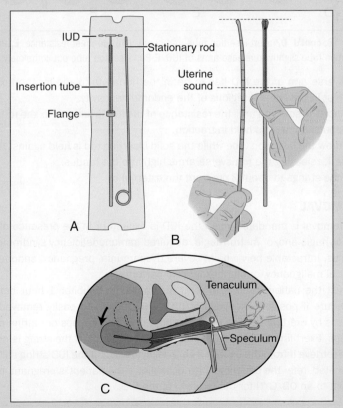

FIGURE 9-18 Technique for inserting copper-T intrauterine device (IUD). **A,** Prepare the IUD by inserting the arms into the insertion tube and introducing the stabilized rod into the tubing. **B,** Place the tenaculum on the cervix and straighten the uterine axis. Sound the uterus to measure depth and check effectiveness of anesthetic. **C,** Set flange to indicate uterine depth. Rotate flange so that the long axis is in the same direction as the IUD arms will open.

9

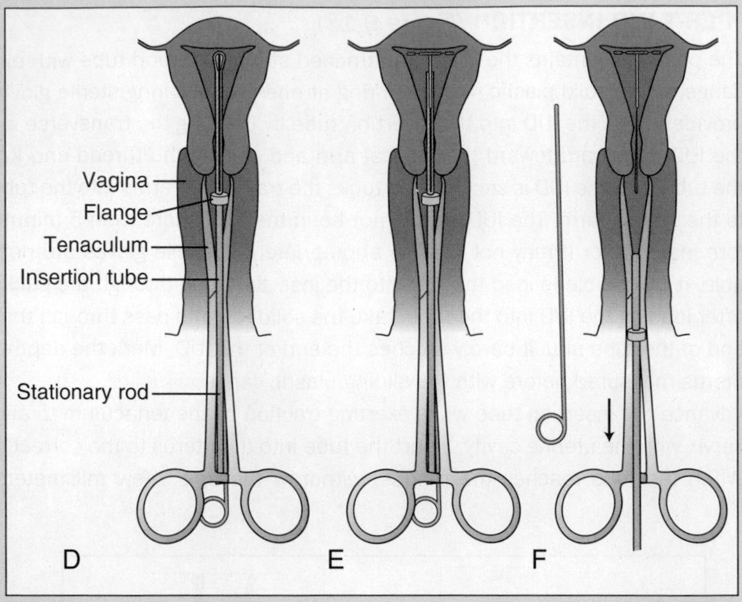

FIGURE 9-18, cont'd **D,** Insert insertion tube into cervix until you meet resistance. **E,** Pull back insertion tube slightly to release arms of IUD. **F,** Pull insertion tube out completely.

transverse arm of the IUD has to be in the horizontal plane for the tips of the T to rest in the cornual regions of the endometrial cavity.

3. Advance the solid rod until the resistance of the IUD is felt, and fix the rod against the tenaculum as it is held in traction.
4. Withdraw the insertion tube while the solid insertion rod is held against the stem of the T, releasing the transverse arms high into the fundus.
5. Trim the strings to about 3 cm from the external os.

IUD REMOVAL

1. IUD removal is mandated when the IUD is expired or in the presence of severe menorrhagia and/or metrorrhagia, acquired immunodeficiency syndrome, endometritis, intractable pelvic pain, severe dyspareunia, pregnancy, endometrial or cervical malignancy, or uterine/cervical perforation.
2. Instruct the patient to take an oral prostaglandin inhibitor 1 hour before the procedure if possible. All types of IUDs can usually be easily removed during menses by exerting traction on the string with a ring forceps or uterine dressing forceps. Exert firm traction on the string close to the os. If the string is not seen, try to retrieve it from the os with a cervical cytobrush. If the IUD string still cannot be located, refer the patient to a gynecologist. If the patient is pregnant, refer the patient to an OB/GYN for the removal of the IUD.

PATIENT EDUCATION POSTPROCEDURE

- Before and after the procedure, emphasize the danger of untreated sexually transmitted diseases, PID, and the risk with IUDs, and encourage regular condom use and testing.

- Explain the efficacy, advantages, side effects (e.g., Mirena diminishes menstrual flow or causes amenorrhea, whereas the copper-T IUD can cause dysmenorrhea and heavy bleeding), possible infection, perforation of cervix or uterus, expulsion (contraceptive effect is lost), and embedment into the myometrium (possible lower efficacy).
- Advise the patient to alert the provider immediately for sudden abnormal discharge, unusual odor, and pelvic pain.
- If frequent heavy bleeding exists beyond a few weeks of insertion, the patient should return for evaluation because it may indicate cervical or endometrial pathology.
- Advise the patient to continue Pap smears and annual examinations.
- Discuss reversibility and resumption of fertility (copper-T IUD: Immediate reversal; Hormonal methods: Rapid reversal, 79.1% cumulative conception rate in 1 year). Emphasize that achieving amenorrhea with hormonal IUD methods is an advantage and not an adverse side effect.
- With hormonal IUD, warn the patient that during the first 3 to 6 months of use, the number of bleeding and spotting days may be increased and can be irregular. The irregular bleeding may linger for more than 6 months, but by 1 year of use, about 20% of users have no bleeding.

COMPLICATIONS

- Expulsion of IUD occurs in 3% to 10% of women with the copper-T IUD and 3% to 6% of women with Mirena and Skyla IUDs. Objective findings of IUD expulsion include the following:
    - The IUD appears in the cervical os or in the vagina.
    - The IUD string is lengthened (partial expulsion).
    - The IUD cannot be located even under ultrasonography or radiography of the abdomen.
    - Excessive bleeding with hormonal IUD may precede partial or complete expulsion.
- Other complications:
    - Menorrhagia/metrorrhagia (copper IUD)
    - Anemia (copper IUD)
    - Abdominal pain and/or dyspareunia/dysmenorrhea
    - Symptomatic or asymptomatic pelvic infection (PID)
    - Pregnancy
    - Ectopic pregnancy
    - Fetal damage
    - Tubal damage
    - Vaginitis/leukorrhea
    - Septicemia
    - Spontaneous abortion
    - Septic abortion
    - Fragmentation of the IUD
    - Perforation of the uterus
    - Embedment in the uterus
    - Jaundice (hormonal IUDs)
    - Infertility resulting from PID, perforation, or other rare catastrophic events
    - Headache, acne, or ovarian cysts (with hormonal IUDs)

PRACTITIONER FOLLOW-UP

- Advise patient to return in 4 to 6 weeks after insertion for a bimanual examination and inspection of the IUD string.
- Reiterate importance of reporting adverse events (signs of infection, menorrhagia, etc.) and to return for yearly examinations.

RED FLAG

- When removing IUDs, if you meet more than minimal resistance, stop removal and refer to an OB/GYN.

CPT BILLING

58300—Insertion of IUD ■ **58301**—Removal of IUD

The CPT procedure codes do not include the cost of the supply. Report the supply separately using a HCPCS code:

J7300—Intrauterine copper contraceptive ■ **J7301**—Levonorgestrel-releasing intrauterine contraceptive system, 13.5 mg ■ **J7302**—Levonorgestrel-releasing intrauterine contraceptive system, 52 mg

If a patient comes in to discuss contraception options during an annual visit, but no procedure is provided at that visit, there is no additional code. The discussion is not reported separately.

If the provider and patient discuss a number of contraceptive options, decide on a method, and then an implant or IUD is inserted during the visit, an E/M service may be reported, depending on the documentation.

If the patient comes into the office, requesting an IUD, followed by a brief discussion of the benefits and risks and the insertion, an E/M service is not reported since the E/M services are minimal.

If the patient comes in for another reason and, during the same visit, a procedure is performed, then both the E/M services code and procedure may be reported.

REFERENCES AND RELATED RESOURCES

Browne H, Manipalviratn S, Armstrong A: Using an intrauterine device in immunocompromised women, *Obstet Gynecol* 112:667, 2008.

Centers for Disease Control and Prevention (CDC): U. S. medical eligibility criteria for contraceptive use, 2010, *MMWR Recomm Rep* 59:1, 2010.

Committee on Adolescent Health Care Long-Acting Reversible Contraception Working Group, The American College of Obstetricians and Gynecologists: Committee opinion no. 539: adolescents and long-acting reversible contraception: implants and intrauterine devices, *Obstet Gynecol* 120:983, 2012.

Fraser IS: Non-contraceptive health benefits of intrauterine hormonal systems, *Contraception* 82:396, 2010.

Hatcher RA, et al: *Contraceptive technology*, ed 20, New York, 2011, Ardent.

Hubacher D, Grimes DA, Gemzell-Danielsson K: Pitfalls of research linking the intrauterine device to pelvic inflammatory disease, *Obstet Gynecol* 121:1091, 2013.

Jensen JT, Nelson AL, Costales AC: Subject and clinician experience with the levonorgestrel-releasing intrauterine system, *Contraception* 77:22, 2008.

Lewis RA, Taylor D, Natavio MF, et al: Effects of the levonorgestrel-releasing intrauterine system on cervical mucus quality and sperm penetrability, *Contraception* 82:491, 2010.

Lyus R, Lohr P, Prager S, Board of the Society of Family Planning: Use of the Mirena LNG-IUS and Paragard CuT380A intrauterine devices in nulliparous women, *Contraception* 81:367, 2010.

Nelson AL: Contraindications to IUD and IUS use, *Contraception* 75:S76, 2007.

Thonneau PF, Almont T: Contraceptive efficacy of intrauterine devices, *Am J Obstet Gynecol* 198:248, 2008.

Wu JP, Pickle S: Extended use of the intrauterine device: a literature review and recommendations for clinical practice, *Contraception* 89:495, 2014.

10

Men's Health Procedures

Jared Spackman

There are a variety of specific procedures for male children or adults related to the external genitalia. These procedures may be performed in primary care settings or in emergency departments if the procedure is an emergency.

Male Circumcision (Gomco Technique)

DESCRIPTION

Male circumcision is the process of removing the skin that covers the distal portion of the glans penis. It typically is performed during infancy.

Note: This procedure description is intended for those who have observed and have been trained to perform the Gomco circumcision technique on infants in states where this is already within the designated scope of practice. This is an advanced procedure requiring supervision and authorization. The procedure outline is intended as a resource for review and refamiliarization of the procedure, not as a guide for those without experience or training.

ANATOMY AND PHYSIOLOGY

Figure 10-1 illustrates the anatomy of the male genitalia and urinary tract system. The skin that forms the foreskin is continuous with the skin of the shaft of the penis and is also connected to the dermis of the lower abdomen. The prepuce, which is a fold of skin that covers the glans, consists of an external keratinized layer and an internal mucosal layer. The prepuce serves the function of covering the glans and is innervated in a complex manner with both somatosensory and autonomic functions.

Infant circumcision has become somewhat controversial over the past decade, with groups advocating for and against circumcision. Evidence-based medicine evaluation has stated that there is a lack of strong enough evidence to recommend routine circumcision of all males and that it is important to counsel parents as to the potential risks and benefits of this procedure.

The potential benefits of circumcision involve a decreased incidence of sexually transmitted diseases, urinary tract infections (UTIs), and penile cancer.

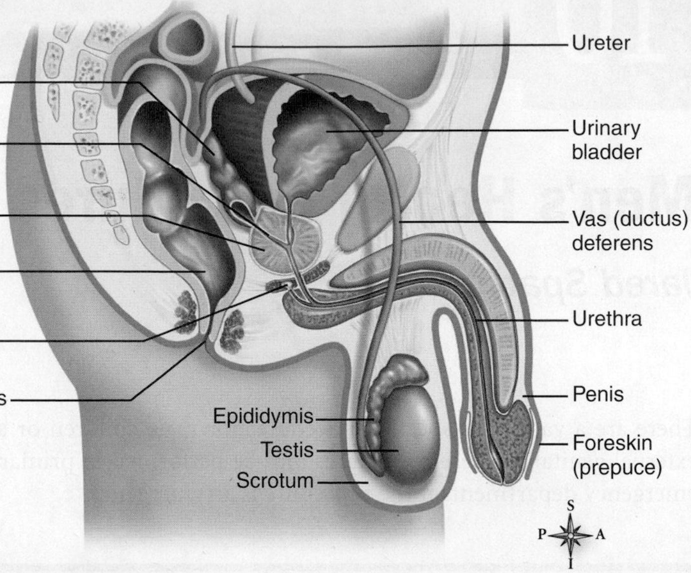

FIGURE 10-1 Anatomy of the male genitourinary system. (From Patton KT, Thibodeau GA: *The human body in health & disease,* ed 6, St. Louis, 2014, Elsevier.)

INDICATIONS

Although many families request circumcision for religious, cultural, or hygienic reasons, there are actually few absolute indications for this procedure.

Indications include phimosis, paraphimosis, balanitis, and posthitis.

Relative indications include male infants who develop UTIs and require recurrent catheterization in conjunction with this.

CONTRAINDICATIONS

- Prematurity of the infant or extremely low birth weight.
- Penile anomalies, such as chordee, hypospadias, epispadias, gonadal hypoplasia, or ambiguous genitalia.

PRECAUTIONS

Abnormalities of clotting are relative contraindications and are discouraged in such individuals.

ASSESSMENT

This procedure describes the Gomco technique, but there are principles that are common to all techniques.

The Gomco clamp technique is an excellent option for infants. In toddlers who are larger, hemostasis can become problematic and a Plastibell should be considered.

10

PATIENT PREPARATION

- Explain the procedure to the parent and obtain written consent from the parent.
- The infant should be properly identified if the procedure is performed other than in an outpatient setting.
- Explain to the parents that the procedure may cause discomfort and bleeding.
- Explain that occasionally the shaft of the penis may be lacerated during the procedure. Small lacerations will typically heal without intervention. Slightly larger lacerations may need absorbable suture.
- If an anesthetic block is to be applied to the penis, explain the risks and benefits of local anesthetic.

TREATMENT ALTERNATIVES

- Treatment alternatives include other methods of circumcision such as the Plastibell, Mogen clamp, or freehand by a trained urologist.
- An additional alternative is to simply not perform the procedure and leave the penis and foreskin intact.

EQUIPMENT

- Examination gloves
- Alcohol swabs
- Infant papoose board
- Sterile gloves of appropriate size
- Hibiclens
- Sterile water
- 2 × 2 gauze sponges
- Sterile drapes
- Syringes
- 25-gauge needles
- 1% lidocaine without epinephrine and buffer solution, if appropriate
- Gomco clamp with all bell sizes available
- Scalpel
- Petroleum jelly
- Curved hemostats (2)
- Straight hemostat
- Skin marker (if desired)
- Absorbable suture

Procedure

MALE CIRCUMCISION USING GOMCO CLAMP

1. The infant should be restrained on a circumcision board in a comfortable and secure manner (Figure 10-2).
2. Examine the penis and identify appropriate landmarks. The corona can be marked with a skin marker because this feature can become less palpable as the procedure continues. Also identify the presence or absence of congenital defects that would create a contraindication for the procedure.
3. Identify the base of the penis and perform a bilateral dorsal penis block with no more than 0.5 ml of anesthetic injected in each side (Figure 10-3).
4. Don sterile gloves.
5. Cleanse the penis with hibiclens and sterile water.
6. Drape the area.

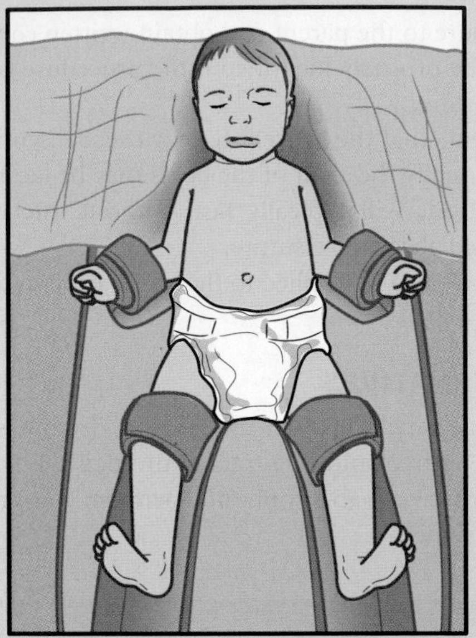

FIGURE 10-2 Infant placed on circumcision board to restrain him during circumcision procedure.

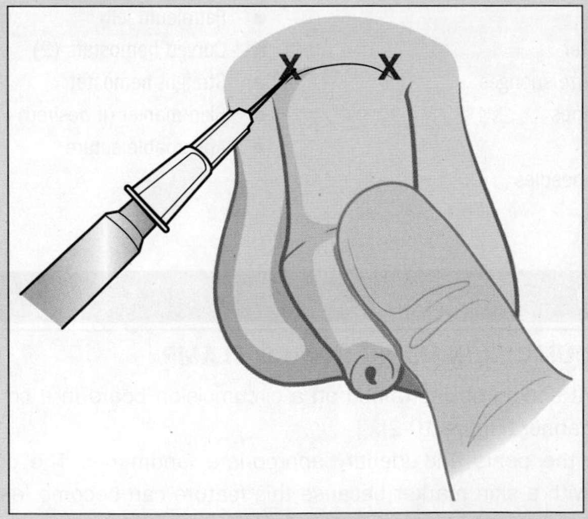

FIGURE 10-3 Bilateral dorsal penis block.

7. Grasp the foreskin on either side with the two curved hemostats, avoiding the urethral meatus and tent up the foreskin from the glans.
8. Use the third hemostat and gently insert this into the preputial ring and sweep right and left, avoiding the ventral frenulum. This should release the adhesions between the inner mucosal layer and the glans.

9. The hemostat is then removed and a straight crush line should be obtained on the dorsal aspect of the foreskin, no closer than 1 cm from the corona.
10. Tent the crush line up with blunt scissors taking care to avoid the glans. This line should then be cut in the center (Figure 10-4, A).
11. Retract the foreskin proximally using the hemostats or a 2 × 2 sponge after everting the foreskin slightly.
12. Any remaining adhesions should be bluntly divided using a probe or gauze sponge until the entire coronal sulcus can be visualized while avoiding the ventral frenulum.

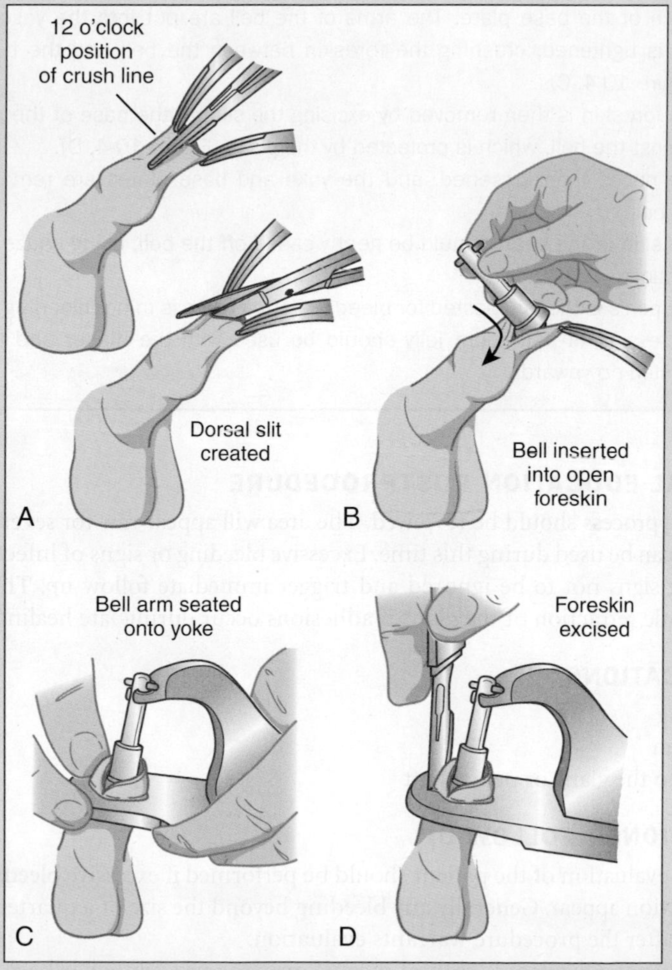

FIGURE 10-4 **A,** Tent the crush line up with blunt scissors taking care to avoid the glans. This line should then be cut in the center. **B,** Foreskin is then brought over the glans and the bell of the Gomco is placed over the glans. **C,** Foreskin pulled through the base plate of the clamp, the rocker arm of the clamp is attached and brought into the notch of the base plate, and the arms of the bell are put into the yoke and the nut is tightened, crushing the foreskin between the bell and the base plate. **D,** Foreskin is then removed by excising the skin at the base of the plate and against the bell.

13. The foreskin is then brought over the glans and the bell of the Gomco is placed over the glans (Figure 10-4, B).
14. The bell should be of appropriate size to ensure uniform length and symmetry of the shaft skin.
15. The foreskin should be carefully pulled through the base plate of the clamp. This can be performed by gently pulling the foreskin up with the two curved clamps, and then clamping the foreskin back together with the third clamp proximal to the curved clamps. Gently release each of the curved clamps once the foreskin is securely through the hold in the base plate.
16. The rocker arm (top plate) of the clamp is then attached and brought into the notch of the base plate. The arms of the bell are put into the yoke and the nut is tightened, crushing the foreskin between the bell and the base plate (Figure 10-4, C).
17. The foreskin is then removed by excising the skin at the base of the plate and against the bell, which is protected by the glans (Figure 10-4, D).
18. The nut is then loosened, and the yoke and base plates are removed from the bell.
19. The skin of the shaft should be gently eased off the bell, using gauze and mild traction.
20. The penis is then inspected for bleeding (often there is minor bleeding present).
21. A dressing of petroleum jelly should be used with the diaper and the penis pointed downward.

PARENTAL EDUCATION POSTPROCEDURE

The healing process should be reviewed. The area will appear raw for several days and petroleum can be used during this time. Excessive bleeding or signs of infection should be warning signs not to be ignored and trigger immediate follow up. The area may require gentle retraction of the glans if adhesions occur during late healing.

COMPLICATIONS

- Bleeding
- Infection
- Injury to the glans or penis shaft

PRACTITIONER FOLLOW-UP

- Urgent evaluation of the patient should be performed if excessive bleeding or signs of infection appear. Generally any bleeding beyond the size of a quarter within the diaper after the procedure warrants evaluation.
- Any signs of a displaced urethral meatus once the procedure has been performed should initiate referral to a pediatric urologist.

■ CPT BILLING

54150—Circumcision, using clamp or other device with regional dorsal penile or ring block ■ **54150-52**—Circumcision, using clamp or other device, without dorsal penile or ring block ■ **54160**—Circumcision, surgical excision other than clamp, device, or dorsal split, neonate (28 days of age or less) ■ **54161**—Circumcision, surgical excision other than clamp, device, or dorsal split, neonate (older than 28 days of age)

REFERENCES AND RELATED RESOURCES

American Academy of Pediatrics: Task Force on Circumcision. Circumcision policy statement, *Pediatrics* 130:585–586, 2012.

Baker M: Doctors back circumcision, *Nature* 488:568, 2012.

Malone P, Steinbrecher H: Medical aspects of male circumcision, *BMJ* 335:1206–1207, 2007.

Peleg D, Steiner A: The Gomco circumcision: common problems and solutions, *Am Fam Physician* 58(4):891–898, 1998.

Wheeler R, Malone P: Male circumcision, *Arch Dis Child* 98(5):321–322, 2013.

Manual Detorsion of the Testes

DESCRIPTION

Manual detorsion of the testes is a procedure in which the provider manually manipulates a torsed testicle in an attempt to restore normal blood supply to the testicular region. Testicular torsion is considered a true urologic emergency and must be differentiated from other complaints on testicular pain because a delay in diagnosis and management can lead to a loss of the testicle.

ANATOMY AND PHYSIOLOGY

The testes are ovoid structures that are typically suspended longitudinally in the scrotum. The tunica vaginalis attaches to the lower portion of the testes, and if this attachment is abnormally high or the soft tissue structures that attach to the spermatic cord are abnormal, torsion can result. Several structures may be impacted by a twisting, or torsion, of the testes. The spermatic cord is the main structure impacted by torsion. It houses several contents, including the ductus deferens, the testicular artery, and a plexus that combines to form the testicular vein and the genital branch of the genitofemoral nerve.

INDICATIONS

- Symptoms and examination consistent with torsed testes
- Sudden onset of unilateral, severe testicular pain, may be accompanied by nausea and vomiting
- Scrotal swelling or redness

CONTRAINDICATIONS

Resolution of the acute pain without detorsion (especially in light of a delay in treatment) raises the possibility of necrosis of the testicle. An urgent surgical consult is advised.

PRECAUTIONS

Other etiologies should be considered. These include orchitis, epididymitis, trauma, or tumor.

ASSESSMENT

Testicular torsion is most typically a condition that affects male children and adolescents. Acute pain and scrotal swelling should be considered as caused by a torsion until proven otherwise.

A testicular torsion is considered a true urologic emergency because the lack of treatment or a delayed treatment can lead to potential necrosis for future testicular development. A torsion can occur during activity, but can also develop during sleep. The cardinal symptoms involve unilateral scrotal pain, swelling, and nausea and/or vomiting.

PATIENT PREPARATION

- Explain the procedure and obtain written consent from the parent, if applicable.
- Explain that the procedure may cause discomfort. Typically, the provider will not use a local or general anesthetic because this can cloud the examination.

TREATMENT ALTERNATIVES

- Treatment alternatives are limited to urologic referral for manual detorsion or surgical exploration.
- Time is of the essence because optimal success requires a detorsion within 6 to 8 hours. A torsion lasting more than 24 hours will usually result in some degree of testicular necrosis.

EQUIPMENT

- Gloves that can be either sterile or unsterile
- A Doppler ultrasound should be available postprocedure to confirm a restoration of blood flow to the testes

Procedure

MANUAL DETORSION OF TESTICLE

Note: The patient can be either standing or supine for the procedure.

1. As the torsion is usually inward (medial), detorsing the testes involves manipulating the testes externally or "opening a book."
2. If the left testicle is the involved side, grasp the testes between the thumb and index finger and turn the testes clockwise 180 degrees. This may need to be repeated more than once because degrees of torsion can exceed 180 degrees. Resolution of symptoms and restoration of normal anatomy should guide the degree of detorsion.
3. If the right testicle is involved, grasp the testicle between the thumb and index finger and turn the testes counterclockwise 180 degrees. As noted earlier, resolution of symptoms and restoration of normal anatomy should guide how many times to repeat the procedure. It may require two to three cycles.
4. Successful treatment will occur in many cases, but not in all. Immediate relief of pain is a good indication of successful treatment (Figure 10-5).

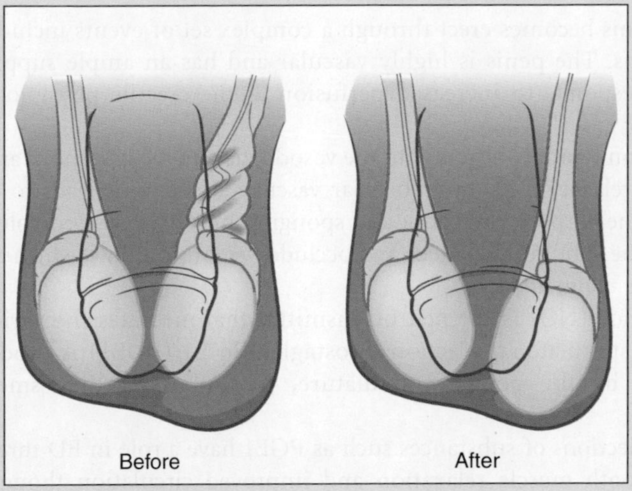

FIGURE 10-5 Successful detorsion of the testes.

PATIENT EDUCATION POSTPROCEDURE

- A Doppler ultrasound is necessary to ensure a return of blood flow to the testicle.
- Surgical exploration is also an important component to treatment because residual torsion or retorsion can threaten the testicle.

COMPLICATIONS

Although the procedure itself is often painful, there is no known complication related to manual detorsion.

PRACTITIONER FOLLOW-UP

Urgent evaluation of the patient should be performed postmanipulation by a urologist.

CPT BILLING

There is no separate CPT code. The charge for the procedure is included in the E/M code

REFERENCES AND RELATED RESOURCES

Ogunyemi OI: *Testicular torsion*. http://emedicine.medscape.com/article/2036003-overview. Updated November 17, 2014. Accessed November 22, 2014.

Saxena AK: *Manual detorsion of the testes*. http://emedicine.medscape.com/article/1413565-overview. Updated July 19, 2013. Accessed November 22, 2014.

Penile Injection Therapy

DESCRIPTION

Penile injection therapy is a nonsurgical method for the treatment of erectile dysfunction (ED).

ANATOMY AND PHYSIOLOGY

The male penis becomes erect through a complex set of events including multiple organ systems. The penis is highly vascular and has an ample supply of erectile tissue that responds to increased perfusion as the erectile physiologic processes progress.

An erection typically begins with the vasodilation of the cavernous artery, which is triggered by relaxation of the trabecular vascular tissue. This leads to engorgement of blood in the corpora cavernosa and spongiosum. The increased volume of blood compresses the subtunical venules and occludes venous outflow, which allows for the erection to be maintained.

Nitric oxide (NO) is the neurotransmitter that mediates the variety of sexual stimuli that stimulate an erection. Prostaglandin E1 (PGE1) is produced during an erection by the penile musculature, leading to further smooth muscle relaxation.

Penile injections of substances such as PGE1 have a role in ED through inducement of smooth muscle relaxation and improved circulation though the penile structures.

INDICATIONS

- Detailed history and physical examination consistent with vasogenic ED.
- Failure of response to first-line treatments, such as lifestyle modification; treatment of underlying conditions that include obesity, hypertension hyperlipidemia, diabetes, metabolic syndrome, and surgeries or injuries that affect the pelvic area or spinal cord; or certain medications.
- Failure of first-line pharmacologic oral agents, such as PDE5 inhibitors.

CONTRAINDICATIONS

- Prior allergic reaction to the medication being administered
- History of a penile implant
- History of priapism

PRECAUTIONS

Relative contraindications include the following:

- History of prior abnormality of the penis, including a curvature or birth defect
- History of coagulopathy
- Penile infection (current)
- Peyronie's disease

ASSESSMENT

The assessment should be complete and thorough. A process of care has been developed by a cadre of specialists including multiple medical specialties. It includes the following:

- Rational approach to diagnosis and treatment
- Emphasis on clinical history taking and focused physical examination
- Specialized tests and referrals based on defined situations
- Stepwise management approach with ranking of treatment options
- Incorporation of patient's and partner's needs and preferences in the decision-making process (goal-directed approach)

In brief, the history needs to be thorough and include medical, sexual, and psychosocial aspects. The organic and psychogenic aspects of ED must be distinguished. There may be a history of comorbid conditions, medications, or substance abuse that would contribute to ED.

The sexual history is useful to separate ED from other sexual function disorders, such as anorgasmia or loss of sexual desire.

The focused physical examination should include the following systems: genitourinary, vascular, and neurologic. Vital signs, including blood pressure and heart rate, should be recorded and evaluated. The patient should be assessed for any signs or hypogonadism.

Comorbid conditions, such as vascular disease, diabetes, hypertension, or depression, should also be ruled out or addressed appropriately.

PATIENT PREPARATION

- Explain the procedure to the patient and/or parent and obtain written consent from the patient and/or parent, if applicable.
- Explain that the procedure may cause discomfort and slight bleeding.

TREATMENT ALTERNATIVES

Treatment alternatives include other options along the spectrum of treating ED. First-line treatment is usually oral agents, such as PDE5 inhibitors that include sildenafil (Viagra). There are other second-line agents, such as transurethral agents, that act in a vasoactive manner, an example being alprostadil (MUSE). Other alternative treatments are vacuum erection assistance devices used in conjunction with a constrictive ring around the base of the penis. Finally, penile implants may be used in those failing all conservative treatments.

EQUIPMENT

- Gloves that can be either sterile or unsterile
- Alcohol swabs
- Syringes
- 25-gauge needles
- Ampules of the agent to be used

Procedure

PENILE INJECTION FOR ERECTILE DYSFUNCTION

Note: The frequency of injection (once the patient is trained) should be no more than once a day and no more than three times a week.

1. The medication must be refrigerated and the patient should be instructed to refrigerate the medication between doses.
2. Use alcohol to cleanse the top of the bottle containing the medication.
3. Draw up the appropriate dose, which is typically 1.0 ml.
4. Switch to a 25-gauge needle.
5. The locations for injection are limited to each lateral aspect of the penis, proximal to the head of the penis. Alternating sites between the left and right and proximal and distal aspects of the shaft is recommended.

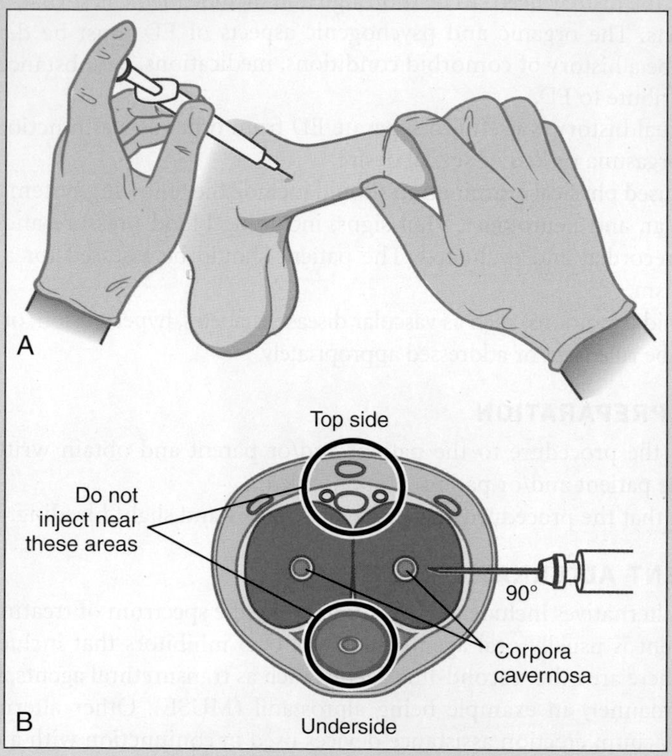

FIGURE 10-6 Penile injection.

6. Grasp the head of the penis between the index finger and thumb. Gently pull the penis away from the body until the skin of the shaft is taut. Avoid any area of the shaft where a vein is located.
7. Wipe the injection site with the alcohol swab.
8. Penetrate the skin with light pressure and at a right angle, push until a distinct "give" is felt; the needle should be located within the erectile tissue of the penis.
9. Inject the medication and remove the needle. Apply pressure with the alcohol swab for 2 to 3 minutes after the injection (Figure 10-6).

PATIENT EDUCATION POSTPROCEDURE

An erection will often occur 5 to 15 minutes after the injection. Many patients will not achieve an erection until sexual foreplay begins. Some patients have noted decreased penile sensation and difficulty with ejaculation, although this is often caused by an underlying pathologic condition.

COMPLICATIONS

- Bleeding from the injection site.
- Prolonged erection (priapism). This is easily managed, but it is critical that the patient contact the health care provider immediately. Immediate contact information or information to seek immediate evaluation should be given to any patient using this treatment.

- Transitory pain. This usually resolves within a few minutes and will often involve the head of the penis.
- Scarring or deformity of the penis (rare, but possible).
- Infection of the penis.

PRACTITIONER FOLLOW-UP

Urgent evaluation of the patient should be performed if priapism occurs. This is typically treated with drainage of the penis and injection of epinephrine. This should be performed by a urologist.

■ CPT BILLING

54235—Injection of corpora cavernosa with pharmacologic agent(s) (e.g., papaverine, phentolamine) ■ **J2440**—Injection, papaverine HCl, up to 60 mg ■ **J2760**—Injection, phentolamine mesylate, up to 5 mg

The frequency with which this can be billed depends on the Medicare carrier or commercial payer. Several Medicare carriers have limited the benefit to once per beneficiary lifetime.

REFERENCES AND RELATED RESOURCES

Brock G, Medscape Multispecialty: *Anatomy and physiology of normal erection and pathophysiology of ED*. http://www.medscape.org/viewarticle/432628_4. Accessed November 13, 2014.

Padma-Nathan H: Diagnostic and treatment strategies for erectile dysfunction: the 'Process of Care' model, *Int J Impot Res* 12(suppl 4):S119–S121, 2000.

University of Utah Department of Urology and Men's Health: *Self injection & erectile dysfunction*. https://uuhsc.utah.edu/menshealth/conditions/ed/injection.php. Accessed November 15, 2014.

WebMD: *Alprostadil to treat erectile dysfunction, reviewed by C. Jennings, MD*, September 12, 2013. http://healthcare.utah.edu/urology/sexual-dysfunction/erectile-dysfunction/self-injection.php. Accessed November 22, 2014.

11

General Principles of Radiograph Interpretation

*Sabrina Jarvis**

DESCRIPTION

Health care providers often have to determine the most appropriate diagnostic radiology imaging to best diagnosis and treat their patients. This includes consideration of possible patient exposure to radiation and contrast dye, and the financial cost to patients who may be either underinsured or who have no insurance. In the primary care setting, it is vital to use evidence-based data to help the provider order the correct imaging test that will provide maximum information with minimal risk to the patient. These imaging studies include computed tomography, magnetic resonance imaging, medical ultrasonography, nuclear medicine scans, mammography, and basic radiographs. It can often be confusing as to what specific radiology test should be ordered for a particular medical condition. One valuable resource is the American College of Radiology (ACR). On their website (www.acr.org), health care professionals can find evidence-based radiology guidelines (ACR Appropriateness Criteria) for various common medical conditions. Under each medical condition topic is a list of rated diagnostic radiology imaging tests, with included variants, followed by a concise narrative discussion. These discussions include evidence-based research and describe the advantages and limitations of the radiology imaging in terms of the particular clinical condition (http://www.acr.org/Quality-Safety/Appropriateness-Criteria).

One common procedure performed in many clinics today is basic radiography to help confirm clinical impressions. This chapter contains a basic introduction on skeletal and abdominal radiographic interpretation with a focus on chest radiography. Depending on the power setting, x-rays penetrate body tissues to varying degrees. As such, they are one of the simplest, most cost-effective tools for evaluating some internal soft tissues and bones. Although the primary care practitioner should have a basic knowledge of radiograph film interpretation, a definitive reading must be performed by a qualified physician.

ANATOMY AND PHYSIOLOGY

It is essential for the primary care clinician to have a good understanding of the skeletal anatomy as a prelude to viewing any radiograph. The bones of the chest are especially important to be able to identify (Figure 11-1).

---

*Christy L. Crowther-Radulewicz offered content support to this chapter.

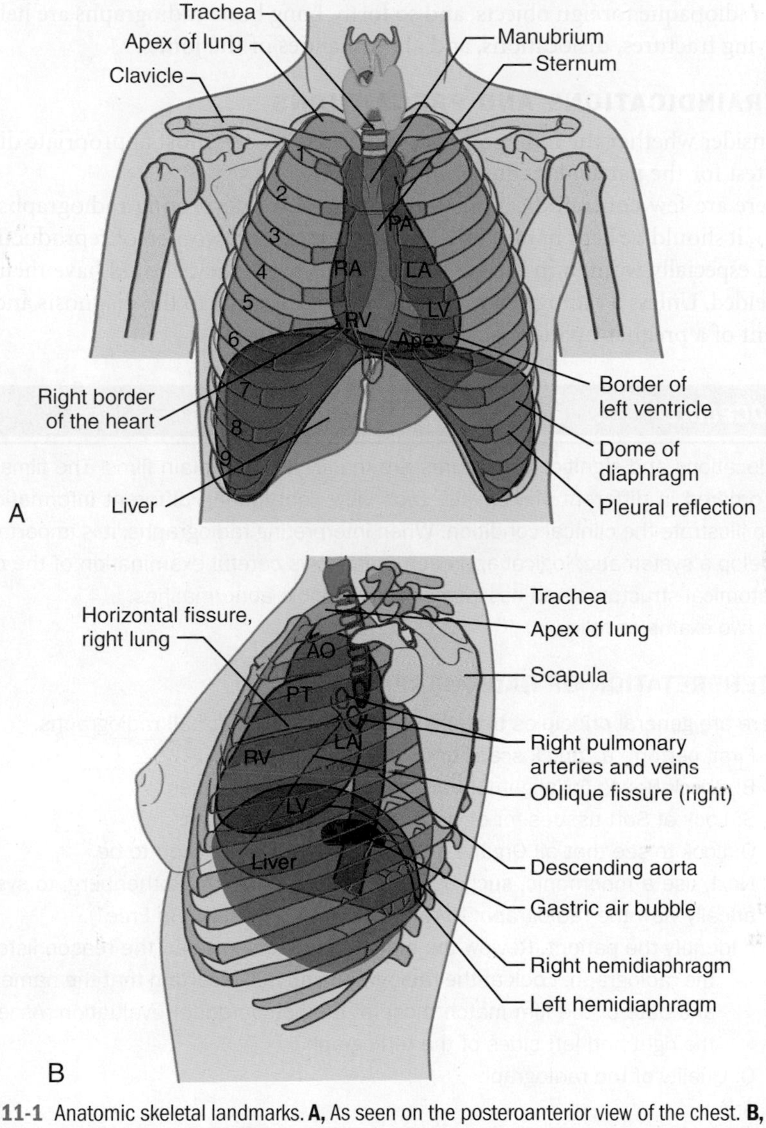

FIGURE 11-1 Anatomic skeletal landmarks. **A,** As seen on the posteroanterior view of the chest. **B,** As seen on the lateral view of the chest. *Ao,* Aorta; *LA,* left atria; *LV,* left ventricle; *PA,* pulmonary artery; *RA,* right atria; *RV,* right ventricle. (Adapted from Patrick J. Lynch, illustrator; C. Carl Jaffe, MD, cardiologist, Yale University Center for Advanced Instructional Media Medical Illustrations by Patrick Lynch, generated for multimedia teaching projects by the Yale University School of Medicine, Center for Advanced Instructional Media, 1987-2000. Patrick J. Lynch, http://patricklynch.net. Creative Commons Attribution 2.5 License 2006.)

INDICATIONS

Basic radiography is often performed before other diagnostic imaging because it is cost effective and noninvasive. Radiographic evaluation of the chest may help identify possible rib fractures, infiltrate patterns suggestive of parenchymal disease, increased pulmonary vasculature suggestive of pulmonary edema, cardiac enlargement, among others.

Basic abdominal radiographs are helpful in identifying bowel air-fluid levels and obstruction, free air associated with possible bowel perforation, kidney and bladder stones, radiopaque foreign objects, and so forth. Long bone radiographs are helpful in identifying fractures, dislocations, and abnormalities of the joints.

CONTRAINDICATIONS AND PRECAUTIONS

- Consider whether the radiographs (plain films) are the most appropriate diagnostic test for the particular clinical situation.
- There are few contraindications to ordering and interpreting radiographs; however, it should be kept in mind that children, men, and women of reproductive age, and especially women in the first trimester of pregnancy, should have their pelvis shielded. Unless a radiographic examination is essential to the diagnosis and treatment of a pregnant patient, it should be deferred.

Procedure

Dislocations and significant fractures are readily seen on plain films. The films may be ordered in different views, with each view contributing different information to help illustrate the clinical condition. When interpreting radiographs, it is important to develop a systematic, logical approach that allows careful examination of the chest anatomical structures and assessment for possible abnormalities.

Two examples follow.

INTERPRETATION OF RADIOGRAPHS

There are general principles that are important to follow for all radiographs.

1. First, perform a "quick scan" or BSO.

   B: Check Bones for alignment or for obvious abnormalities.

   S: Look at Soft tissues for obvious abnormal shadowings.

   O: Look to see that all Organs are where they are supposed to be.

2. Next, use a mnemonic, such as one coined by Mikel A. Rothenberg, to systematically view the radiograph: IQAWBF ("I Quit And Wanna Be Free").

   I: Identify the patient. Review the material on the chart and the reason listed for the radiograph. Look at the radiograph and make certain that the name, sex, and date of the film match those of the person under evaluation. Ascertain the right and left sides of the radiograph.

   Q: Quality of the radiograph

   A: Air

   W: Water (fluid densities)

   B: Bone

   F: "Funny-looking things" (abnormal calcifications, growths, foreign bodies, tubes, pacemakers, and so on)

Clinicians commonly need to evaluate the chest, abdomen, and extremities when viewing radiograph films. The following are some of the specific things that should be considered in viewing films from these areas.

Chest Radiographs: Develop a System and Stick with It!

1. Determine whether the radiograph is technically adequate.
   a. Positioning: Is it the correct film?
      (1) *Posteroanterior (PA):* Posterior to anterior (reduces magnification and enhances sharpness)
      (2) *Anteroposterior (AP):* Anterior to posterior; most portable films are AP

(3) *Lateral:* Left or right chest against film cassette
(4) *Oblique:* Helps radiologists localize lesions
(5) *Lordotic-AP:* Patient leans back 30 degrees; projects apices of lung, right middle lobe, and lingula

Try to position the problem area of the patient as close to the cassette as possible to decrease magnification and distortion.

b. Adequate inspiration
(1) Is there adequate inspiration that allows for optimal visualization of the structures?
(2) Count ribs to the diaphragm. Should be able to count 5 to 6 anterior ribs or 8 to 10 posterior ribs.

c. Rotation
(1) Is the patient facing forward or slightly turned?
(2) The medial ends of the clavicles should be an equal distance from the spinous process. Lung fields should appear uniform.

d. Adequate x-ray penetration
(1) Should be able to barely see the vertebral bodies through the cardiac silhouette.
(2) Radiographs distinguish objects based on relative densities. Air appears black; fat, soft tissues, and fluids appear gray; and bone appears white.

2. Evaluate the diaphragm.

Note its level and shape (curved, elevated, flattened). Is there evidence of air in the subdiaphragmatic space? It should be dome-shaped with distinct margins, with the right hemidiaphragm 1 to 3 cm higher than the left hemidiaphragm because of the anatomic location of the liver; the costophrenic angle should be symmetric and sharply defined.

3. Evaluate the subdiaphragmatic area.

Are the margins clearly visible? Does fluid appear to be present?

4. Heart

Examine the size, shape, and location of the heart. Measure the *cardiothoracic width* (the widest width of the heart divided by the widest width of the chest). When the widest part of the heart is greater than half the widest width of the chest, the *cardiac silhouette* is increased.

5. Evaluate the trachea. Look at the position and upper paravertebral shadows. The column of radiolucency is readily visible above the clavicles and extends inferiorly to the bifurcation at the carina. Its position should be midline; its width should be fairly even.

6. Evaluate the hila.

The hila normally have a butterfly-like appearance. Evaluate the central pulmonary arteries and veins; the left hilum is slightly higher than the right hilum.

7. Evaluate the mediastinum.

Examine the blood vessels (a normal width ratio with the remainder of the chest cavity width no more than 1:3). Look for the presence of air. The size will vary with age and sex.

8. Evaluate the lung fields.

These form the largest and most radiolucent area of the chest. They should be equally lucent without opacities, cysts, or air-fluid levels. Bronchi are NOT normally distinctly visible. Peripheral lung fields should be easily seen. Visceral and parietal pleura appear as a thin hairline along the apices and lateral chest wall. Look for the prominence of vessels and abnormal opacities.

9. Evaluate the skeletal system.

a. Skeletal structures

Look for rotation of vertebrae (normally, posterior spinous processes will line up in the same plane). Trace each rib contour out to the lateral edges; some fractures can be quite subtle. Note the size, shape, and symmetry of the right and left hemithoraces and the individual bones. Note the width of the spaces and the angles of the intercostal spaces between the ribs. Calcifications may be seen in chondral cartilages (usually multiple, in line with the ribs, and within the inner third of each lung field).

10. Evaluate the shadows.

Define the position of the breasts and nipples in women and the position of the nipples in men. Look for vertebral borders of scapulae. Overlying neck muscles may cloud the apices of both lungs. Subcutaneous fat may make interpretation more problematic.

11. Miscellaneous evaluations

a. Silhouette sign

There are five densities that are seen on radiographs: air, fat, soft tissue, bone, and metal. When two substances of the same density are side by side, they cannot be differentiated from each other with radiography; therefore, if a lesion of water density (i.e., pneumonia) is in anatomic contact with an area of increased soft tissue density, there will be loss of the normal silhouette. Thus compare films on a side-to-side and top-to-bottom basis.

Use the silhouette sign to recognize some of these anatomic relationships.

(1) Uppermost part of cardiac border and ascending aorta in contact with right upper lobe; if you cannot see heart border: right mid lobe infiltrate pneumonia

(2) Obliteration of left heart border: lingular infiltrate

(3) Right heart border: against right mid lobe

(4) Upper part of left heart border: against left upper lobe

(5) Ascending aorta: against right upper lobe

(6) Upper right cardiac border: against right upper lobe

(7) Aortic knob: against left upper lobe

b. Air bronchogram sign

(1) Bronchi are not normally seen on radiographs; the branching markings are vessels.

(2) In the normal chest, bronchi are surrounded by air in the alveoli, but if the bronchi contain air and the alveoli contain fluid, their respective densities change. This allows visualization of the bronchi *air bronchogram sign,* which demonstrates a pulmonary lesion (pneumonia, pulmonary edema, or infarct).

(3) Pleural, mediastinal, and chest wall diseases cannot cause an air bronchogram because they do not contain bronchi.

c. Atelectasis
   (1) *Atelectasis* refers to a lobe or segment whose volume has been diminished.
   (2) Possible signs of significant atelectasis include displacement of fissures, increased radiopacity, and vascular or bronchial crowding.
   (3) Indirect signs suggestive of atelectasis, lung collapse, and partial lung collapse include hilar displacement, elevation of diaphragm, shift of mediastinal structures, or compensatory hyperaeration.

Skeletal Radiographs

Using the BSO format, look at the bones first.

1. *Overall size and shape of bone:* Look for extra calcification and/or abnormal contour.
2. *Local size and shape of bone:* Keep the patient's age in mind. Is there appropriate skeletal maturity? Are epiphyseal growth plates open or closed?
3. *Cortex:* Look at thickness, contour, and integrity. Normal adult cortex thins with age. At any age, a lytic lesion that involves more than 50% of the cortex is an indication for surgery, prophylactic fixation, or both.
4. *Trabecular pattern:* This is more easily seen in larger bones (iliac crest, greater trochanter, femoral neck). Look for unusual density, lucency, or tumor.
5. *Bone density:* The density of the entire bone should, in general, be consistent. Before changes in density become apparent, 30% to 35% of bone mass must be lost. With local density changes, look for evidence of fracture (new or healed), tumor, or sclerosis.
6. *Margins of local lesions:* Are there calcifications in the surrounding tissue? Do lesions invade the medullary canal or in the surrounding soft tissue? *Chronic osteomyelitis* may show bone and soft tissue inflammation.
7. *Bone continuity:* Look for fracture lines or displacement of fracture fragments. Look at the symmetry of the joint lines; for example, no more than 2 mm of difference between the joint spaces should be present in an intact ankle mortise.
8. *Periosteal change:* Periosteal thickening may be the only objective initial evidence of a stress fracture or an acute inflammatory process. Chronic osteomyelitis will show changes in soft tissues overlying infected bone. Continuing the BSO format, look at the soft tissue next for foreign bodies and gas. Then look for changes in organ position and for breaks in the skin. To obtain good radiographs, immobilize injured extremities before the radiographic examination. Remove all clothing and jewelry to prepare for the examination so that metallic snaps, zippers, pins, rings, and other metal objects do not occlude findings on film. Usually request that the joint nearest to a suspected fracture is included in the radiograph; sometimes include the joint proximal or distal to the area of interest.

Abdominal Radiographs

1. Flat plate and upright radiographic views are usually ordered. A left lateral decubitus and chest PA views are ordered if there is a suspicion of free air.
2. Inspect for the presence of any foreign bodies in the abdominal cavity.
3. Bone: Systematically inspect the skeletal system in the abdominal area.
   a. Identify all major anatomic landmarks and look for any abnormalities.
   b. Look for evidence of demineralization.

c. Look for lack of continuity or symmetry of skeletal structures that may represent fractures, metastases, or dislocations.
d. Look for calcifications of the lumbosacral spine, iliosacral region, pelvis, acetabulum, and femur, and look particularly for the presence of any pathologic calcifications.

4. Systematically examine soft tissues.
5. Organs
   a. General appearance of bowel loops (e.g., air/fluid levels; distention).
   b. Examine diaphragm for air and/or fluid pattern.
   c. Examine major organ structures.
      (1) *Liver:* Look for uniform density of hepatic shadow and sharp visualization of hepatic edge.
      (2) *Spleen:* Splenic flexure of the colon not usually visible unless splenomegaly is present. Splenic shadow is generally hidden by a gastric air bubble.
      (3) *Kidneys:* Are often visible on radiographs. They lie at T12 to L3 and the left kidney is usually slightly higher than the right kidney.
      (4) *Bladder:* Appears as round, homogeneous mass, if filled.
      (5) *Pancreas:* Renal shadow and uterus are generally not clearly visible.
      (6) *Stomach:* Gastric bubble is generally located at the midline to the left upper quadrant.
      (7) *Intestines:* There is a random and nonspecific air shadow pattern throughout the abdominal cavity. It is difficult to determine normal from abnormal presentations.

      The small intestine has circular folds (valvulae conniventes) that are noted around the entire circumference of the small bowel, which resembles a "coiled spring" in appearance. The small intestine lies centrally in the abdomen. The large intestine has small pouches caused by sacculation. These pouches are called haustra and give the large intestine a segmented appearance. The large intestine lies peripherally in the abdomen and may have feces present.
         (a) Bowel *displacement* may be suggested when there is an abnormal concentration of abdominal gas in one location and/or a unilateral appearance of the air gas pattern on one side with the absence of any air on the opposite side.
         (b) *Paralytic ileus* may be suggested when there is a dilated bowel proximally and decreased air shadows distally.
         (c) Bowel *obstruction* may be suggested when there is dilated bowel with or without air and/or fluid levels proximal to the obstruction and the absence of air shadows distal to the obstruction.
      (8) Peritoneum
         (a) Free *air* in the peritoneal cavity may be caused by disruption of the abdominal wall. Viewed as dark air shadows in the diaphragm and against the inferior hepatic margin.
         (b) Look for intraperitoneal *fluid* that may obscure the hepatic edge or displace the normal abdominal gas pattern.
6. Vascular system: Look for the presence of widening or tortuosity of the aorta or renal arteries or for any calcifications of the vascular structures.

RADIOLOGY INTERPRETATION OF RESULTS

Abnormalities should be reviewed by a qualified physician to differentiate pathology from normal variants.

Chest Radiographs

- The most common pattern of *diffuse lung disease* is pulmonary edema in patients who have congestive heart failure. Diffuse disease involves both lungs. Both interstitial and alveolar edema may be present. Alveolar filling produces poorly defined, but homogeneous opacities. Denseness and radiopacity spread as more alveoli fill up with fluid and less air density is seen. Normal structures become less visible. The loss of the visible margin between the black air-density lung and the adjacent gray soft tissue-density organ is called the *silhouette sign.*
- Air bronchograms indicate *diffuse alveolar filling.* An air bronchogram is the black radiolucency of airways that become visible as a result of the contrast provided by adjacent alveoli that are no longer filled with air (see "Air bronchogram sign").
- *Interstitial lung disease* is illustrated by indistinct vessels with small, well-defined reticular, nodular, or reticulonodular opacities in the central hilar areas and in the lung periphery. The fluid in the lung tissue and periphery collects in characteristic *Kerly B* or *septal lines,* which are fine horizontal lines seen in the periphery of the lung along the chest wall. These fluid-containing lines are septae between anatomic lung lobules.
- In *congestive heart failure,* there is cephalization or vascular redistribution of blood flow to the upper lobes due to reflex vasoconstriction of the lower lobe vessels.
- Localized alveolar infiltrates are most often caused by *infection* and are usually *bacterial.* Pneumonia is a commonly seen localized alveolar opacity. It may appear as lobar, segmental, or nonsegmental consolidation. There is loss of the visible margin of the right heart border due to the replacement of air by fluid in the alveoli of the lung adjacent to the margin of the fluid-density heart (silhouette sign). Other characteristics of focal alveolar (air-space) consolidation include (1) focal densities that are homogeneous and have irregular "fluffy margins" and (2) visible air bronchograms. Alveolar diseases that are acute may change relatively rapidly. Some alveolar diseases, such as pneumonia, tuberculosis, coccidioidomycosis, and malignancy, may form cavitations.
- Also look for symptoms of pleural effusions, pneumothorax, and hyperlucency.

PATIENT EDUCATION POSTPROCEDURE

- Instruct the patient that radiographic examinations may have to be repeated after a reasonable length of appropriate treatment.
- Pulmonary infections may require follow up in 1 to 2 weeks to document resolution of infiltrates.
- Fractures should be reevaluated once immobilization has been discontinued.

■ CPT BILLING

71010—Radiologic examination, chest; single view, frontal ■ **71020**—Radiologic examination, chest; 2 views, frontal and lateral ■ **73000 – 73140**—Radiologic examinations of the upper extremities

11

■ **73500 – 73660**—Radiologic examinations of the lower extremities ■ **74000**—Radiologic examination, abdomen; single anteroposterior view

REFERENCES AND RELATED RESOURCES

Connolly MA: Black, white, and shades of gray: common abnormalities in chest radiographs, *AACN Clin Issues* 12:259, 2001.

Dehn RW, Asprey DP: *Essential clinical procedures*, ed 3, Philadelphia, 2013, Elsevier.

Herring W: *Learning radiology: recognizing the basics*, ed 2, Philadelphia, 2012, Elsevier Mosby.

Pezzotti W: Chest x-ray interpretation: not just black and white, *Nursing* 44:41, 2014.

Radiology Masterclass. http://www.radiologymasterclass.co.uk website. (n.d.). http://www.radiologymasterclass.co.uk. Accessed June 22, 2015.

Smith W, Farrell T: *Radiology 101: basics and fundamentals of imaging*, ed 4, Philadelphia, 2014, Lippincott Williams & Wilkins.

Watters J: A systematic approach to basic chest radiograph interpretation: a cardiovascular focus, *Can J Cardiovasc Nurs* 24:4, 2014.

Sample Checklist for Certification

____

[Procedure]

____

[Name and Credentials of Health Care Professional]

[Date]

Procedure process reviewed	________
Reading relevant to procedure completed	________
Procedure observed	________
Completes procedure under direct supervision	________
Had equipment ready	________
Followed correct order of steps	________
Gave adequate preprocedure instruction	________
Gave follow-up instruction	________
Verbalized contraindications	________
Verbalized how to assess for complications	________
Completes procedure with backup available	________
Supervision and certification given by qualified expert	________

____

[Signature certifying individual/date]

Comments:

Sample Consent Form for Procedure

[On company letterhead]

Consent Form for Procedure

I authorize (Dr/NP/PA) ____________________ to perform ____________________, which is necessary because ____

____.

This procedure was explained to me in detail and all of my questions were fully answered. I understand this procedure has certain risks, including ____.

The alternatives, which include ____, were also explained to me, along with their relative risks and benefits.

I wish to proceed with this procedure.

Patient ____

(Parent or guardian if a minor)

Witness ______________________________________

Date ___________________________

Index

Page numbers followed by *b* indicate boxes; *f*, figures; *t*, tables.

B

E

F

H

I

R

S

U

Z